# Fetal Growth Re...
# Diagnosis and Treatment

Editors

**Asim Kurjak, M.D., Ph.D.**
Professor and Chairman
Ultrasonic Institute
World Health Organization Collaborating
Center for Diagnostic Ultrasound
Zagreb, Yugoslavia

**John M. Beazley, M.D., Ph.D.**
Dean of the Faculty of Medicine
University of Liverpool
Liverpool, England

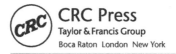

**CRC Press**
Taylor & Francis Group
Boca Raton  London  New York

CRC Press is an imprint of the
Taylor & Francis Group, an **informa** business

CRC Press
Taylor & Francis Group
6000 Broken Sound Parkway NW, Suite 300
Boca Raton, FL 33487-2742

© 1989 by Taylor & Francis Group, LLC
CRC Press is an imprint of Taylor & Francis Group, an Informa business

First issued in paperback 2019

No claim to original U.S. Government works

ISBN 13: 978-0-367-45105-9 (pbk)
ISBN 13: 978-0-8493-4765-8 (hbk)

**Visit the Taylor & Francis Web site at**
**http://www.taylorandfrancis.com**

**and the CRC Press Web site at**
**http://www.crcpress.com**

Library of Congress Card Number 88-26296

**Library of Congress Cataloging-in-Publication Data**

Fetal growth retardation : diagnosis and treatment / editors, Asim
  Kurjak, John M. Beazley.
      p.    cm.
  Includes bibliographies and index.
  ISBN 0-8493-4765-3
  1. Fetus--Growth retardation.      I. Kurjak, Asim.   II. Beazley,
John M.
  [DNLM: 1. Fetal Growth Retardation--diagnosis.   2. Fetal Growth
Retardation--therapy.     WQ 211 F4198]
RG629.G76F48 1989
  618.3'2--dc19
  DNLM/DLC
  for Library of Congress                                              88-26296
                                                                            CIP

# FOREWORD

Fetal growth retardation remains an important problem in obstetrics and neonatology, and interest in this subject has grown considerably in recent years. The primary aim of the Editors and Publisher has been to offer comprehensive reviews and authoritative comments on the progress being made in this rapidly growing field, and we should like to thank the contributors for their enthusiasm and willingness to collaborate in the production of this book. It is our hope that the book will prove to be useful to obstetricians, pediatricians, pathologists, geneticists, and hospital and scientific personnel who may be confronted with this difficult problem.

# EDITORS

**Asim Kurjak, M.D., Ph.D.,** is chairman of the department and professor of Obstetrics and Gynecology at the University of Zagreb, Yugoslavia. He is also head of the Ultrasonic Institute of Zagreb which is the World Health Organization Collaborative Center for Diagnostic Ultrasound.

Dr. Kurjak obtained his training at the University of Zagreb, receiving his M.D. degree in 1966 and his Ph.D. degree in 1977. He served as an assistant professor at the Department of Obstetrics and Gynecology, University of Zagreb from 1968 to 1980. In 1971, as a British scholar, he was research assistant for 1 year at the Institute of Obstetrics and Gynecology, University of London. From 1983 to 1985 he was external examiner at the University of Liverpool. It was in 1983 that he assumed his present position.

Dr. Kurjak is a member and past president of the Yugoslav Society of University Professors Academy of Croatia. He is member of the advisory board of four international scientific journals. He served as vice president of the European federation for ultrasound in medicine and biology. He has been the recipient of many research grants from the Scientific Council from Yugoslavia and is currently the WHO coordinator for the use of ultrasound in developing countries. Among other awards, he is an honorary member of Ultrasonic Society of Obstetrics and Gynecology of Italy, Poland, and Hungary.

Dr. Kurjak has presented over 70 invited lectures at major international meetings and approximately 100 guest lectures at universities and institutes. He has published more than 200 research papers and 14 books in the English language. His current major research interests include ultrasound diagnosis, and fetal and Doppler studies of fetoplacental and maternal blood flow.

**Reverend John M. Beazley, M.D., F.R.C.O.G.** is Dean of the Faculty of Medicine, University of Liverpool, and Chairman of the Department and Professor of Obstetrics and Gynecology at the University of Liverpool.

He obtained his training at the University of Manchester, receiving the M.B., Ch.B. degree in 1957 and the M.D. degree in 1964. He obtained the M.R.C.O.G. qualification in 1962, and the F.R.C.O.G. in 1973. He held medical posts at Manchester, Liverpool, and Sheffield before being appointed Senior Lecturer at Queen Charlotte's Maternity Hospital, London. It was in October 1972 that he assumed his position as Chairman and Professor at Liverpool.

Reverend Beazley is a member of several medical learned societies in the U.K., in the U.S., and in Yugoslavia, including the British Medical Association, the Royal Society of Medicine, the American Association of Obstetrics and Gynecology (Honorary), the Central Travel Club of America, the Yugoslav Association of Societies for Ultrasound in Medicine and Biology (Honorary), and the Yugoslav Association of Obstetricians and Gynaecologists. He has served on several special committees; from 1983 to 1985 he served on the Council of the Royal College of Obstetricians and Gynaecologists as a Fellows representative for England and Wales. In 1981 he was privileged to receive the Order of the Yugoslav Flag with Golden Wreath from the Yugoslav Ambassador for his contribution to the promotion of friendly relationships between Yugoslavia and the U.K. In 1983, to foster subspecialization in the discipline, he established the first University Mastership Degree in Obstetrics and Gynecology at Liverpool.

He is author of more than 100 medical publications in the field of Obstetrics and Gynecology. His current major research interests relate to pediatric gynecology, systems of diagnostic gynecology, and fetomaternal surveillance.

A. Kurjak
J. M. Beazley

# CONTRIBUTORS

**Žarko Alfirević, M.Sc.**
Medical Doctor
Department of Obstetrics and Gynecology
Ultrasonic Institute
University of Zagreb
Zagreb, Yugoslavia

**Domenico Arduini, M.D.**
Specialist and Assistant
Department of Obstetrics and Gynecology
Catholic University of the Sacred Heart
Rome, Italy

**Pall Agustsson**
Department of Obstetrics and Gynecology
Ninewells Hospital
Dundee, Scotland

**R. J. Bradley, M.R.G.O.C.**
Lecturer
Department of Obstetrics and Gynecology
King's College Hospital
London, England

**G. V. P. Chamberlain, M.D.**
Professor and Chairman
Department of Obstetrics and Gynecology
St. George's Hospital Medical School
University of London
London, England

**Peter M. Dunn, M.D.**
Professor of Perinatal Medicine and
  Child Health
University of Bristol
Southmead Hospital
Bristol, U.K.

**Anne S. Garden, M.R.C.O.G.**
Senior Lecturer
Department of Obstetrics and Gynecology
University of Liverpool
Liverpool, England

**Lászlo Kovács, M.D., Ph.D.**
Professor
Department of Obstetrics and Gynecology
Albert Szent-Györgyi Medical University
Szeged, Hungary

**A. Kravka, Engr.**
Computer Laboratory
Research Institute for the Care of Mother
  and Child
Prague, Czechoslovakia

**Višnja Latin, Ph.D.**
Professor
Department of Obstetrics and Gynecology
Medical Faculty
University of Zagreb
Zagreb, Yugoslavia

**F. Mandys, Engr., Ph.D.**
Computer Laboratory
Research Institute for the Care of Mother
  and Child
Prague, Czechoslovakia

**Iain R. McFadyen, F.R.C.O.G.**
Senior Lecturer
Department of Obstetrics and Gynecology
University of Liverpool
Liverpool, England

**K. H. Nicolaides, M.R.C.O.G.**
Deputy Director
Harris Birthright Research Center for
  Fetal Medicine
King's College Hospital
London, England

**Naren Patel**
Department of Obstetrics and Gynecology
Ninewells Hospital
Dundee, Scotland

**Jadranka Pavletić, M.Sc.**
Doctor
Department of Obstetrics and Gynecology
Ultrasound Institute
University of Zagreb
Zagreb, Yugoslavia

**Hana Přibylová, M.D., Ph.D.**
1st Pediatric Department
Research Institute for the Care of Mother
  and Child
Prague, Czechoslovakia

**Joseph G. Schenker**
Professor and Chairman
Department of Obstetrics and Gynecology
Hadassah University Hospital
Jerusalem, Israel

**Giuseppe Rizzo, M.D.**
Specialist and Assistant
Department of Obstetrics and Gynecology
Catholic University of the Sacred Heart
Rome, Italy

**Zdenek Štembera, M.D., D.Sc.,**
Obstetrical Department
Research Institute for the Care of Mother
 and Child
Prague, Czechoslovakia

**Vladimír Šabata, M.D., Ph.D.**
1st Obstetric Department
Research Institute for the Care of Mother
 and Child
Prague, Czechoslovakia

**Danniel Weinstein, Ph.D.**
Associate Professor
Department of Obstetrics and Gynecology
Hadassah University Hospital
Jerusalem, Israel

# TABLE OF CONTENTS

Chapter 1

# THE EPIDEMIOLOGY AND ETIOLOGY OF INTRAUTERINE GROWTH RETARDATION

**Geoffrey Chamberlain**

## TABLE OF CONTENTS

# I. INTRODUCTION

Intrauterine growth retardation (IUGR) is one of the major factors in perinatal death and morbidity. It causes much of the work generated for the obstetricians and neonatal pediatricians in the Western World and probably is the major factor to be tackled next in the more affluent societies which wish to see further reduction in perinatal mortality.

# II. DATA SOURCES

## A. Neonatal Data

Intrauterine growth retardation used to be diagnosed at birth. It was considered to be present when a baby was below the tenth centile on a birthweight gestation distribution for a given population. In some areas, the fifth centile or even the second standard deviation below the mean of a distribution curve of birthweight were taken as the cutoff point. These are now used less often as indices in the Western World for both are too restrictive; further, the second, which would include about 2.5% of the population, should apply only if the distribution of birthweight was a truly Gaussian one.

One of the problems of this definition is that it was generated from, and should strictly be applied to, certain populations living in specific communities. Inside that community, there are a variety of types of women who make up the mix who constitute the total. Later in this chapter, we will be discussing many of the associations of IUGR; different communities have different mixes of women with these various components. In consequence, some epidemiologists have endeavored to derive subsets of women who would have good nutrition, live at sea level, are nonsmoking, and do not drink alcohol. In addition, these women would in retrospect have been shown to have had no pathological conditions in pregnancy and to have produced a singleton normal baby. This would be called *a normal subset*. However, even to constitute this group, the epidemiologists can choose only those factors of which they have some knowledge to set the limits of their subset. There must be other factors of which we are still ignorant. The definition of the population chosen is arbitrary; however, the usefulness of any definition of intrauterine growth retardation depends upon its ability to be used clinically to act as a flag, warning obstetricians and pediatricians of impending problems and to give a prompt for some variation in management. This means it is most useful if it is capable of being applied to the total population looked after by groups of obstetricians and pediatricians.

It is important to derive data generated from the population served by the individual group of obstetricians to consider birthweight for any given gestation. Too often, the original data derived from one center have been unthinkingly applied elsewhere. A good example has been the international use of the Denver data published in the early 1960s by Lubchenco et al[1]. This town is about a mile above sea level with a population containing many underprivileged people of mixed racial origin who have their own background of nutritional and disease problems. In the U.K., there has been a similar indiscriminate use of the data published at various times from Aberdeen where there is a particularly good statistical input into their obstetrics. Aberdeen is a granite fishing port in the northeast of Scotland with a very tight population. Data derived there would not apply to the southerners of the U.K. and particularly not to the recent immigrants such as those who come from Pakistan and live in Birmingham.

There are many difficulties in deriving birthweight-gestational data but recent help has come from Carr-Hill and Pritchard.[2] These statisticians, working in the Aberdeen maternity and neonatal data bank, have derived a series of standardizations that can be applied to many populations. Their book is essential to anyone wishing to construct their own birthweight-gestation charts allowing for the numerous factors referred to later in this chapter.

## B. Fetal Data

More recently, the term intrauterine growth retardation has been applied before birth to fetuses who are still *in utero*. The fetal measurements provided by ultrasound scanning allow the growth of the infant to be checked. This is dealt with in detail in Chapter 7 but it is important to follow the background philosophy of these measurements to realize the difference in their application from those used by pediatricians.

Most women of Great Britain have an ultrasound estimation performed before the 20th week of pregnancy. The biparietal diameter of the fetal head is measured early and this allows the fetus to be placed correctly on a distribution chart of ultrasound measurements by week of gestation derived from a population of women previously attending that particular unit. Subsequent biparietal diameter measurements in the last trimester of pregnancy could then confirm or refute that growth is proceeding inside the normal range of the population. If it does not, the fetus may show growth retardation occurring in a symmetrical or asymmetrical fashion. Probably measurement of the fetal abdominal area is a more valid ultrasound estimation in later pregnancy and this too is considered in Chapter 7. However, it must be noted that ultrasonographers use as their normal range the population within two standard deviations of the mean. Thus, about 2.5% of fetuses would be considered in the zone of intrauterine retardation compared with the 10% enclosed in the less rigorous birth weight definition used by pediatricians.

Whichever method is used, ultrasound has now brought IUGR into the prospective and predictive obstetrical field. As well as conferring benefit, it has brought some new dilemmas in management.

## C. Incidence

If we define IUGR as being those below the tenth centile of birthweight, then by definition, the incidence at birth should be 10%; if below the second standard deviation below the mean, then 2 to 3% of babies are so designated. Minor variations of this proportion obviously will occur but the incidence is laid down by the basic mathematics of the definitions. It does not add to the clarity of the subject, particularly for those for whom English is not the mother tongue, when one reads of large units in Britain reducing their intrauterine growth retardation rates from X to X/2%, an impossibility if the definitions are set as a fixed proportion of the population delivering either, i.e., 10% if the tenth centile is used or 2 to 3% when considering ultrasound diagnoses.

The term small-for-dates is commonly used as a synonym for IUGR; it refers to one point in time when the baby is being measured rather than the general condition of lack of growth. This reflects the cross-sectional aspect of the use of birthweight definitions and is less useful when the dynamic longitudinal definitions of fetal growth are considered.

Placental insufficiency is another phrase commonly used in association with poor growth of the fetus. This begs the question, for more commonly in the Western World, IUGR is associated with a placental bed problem and it is not of necessity the placenta that is insufficient. Unfortunately the obstetrical profession had got into a habit of measuring placental function through the estimation of various aspects of its metabolism, such as the oestriol production or human placental lactogen manufacture. These may have had some relationship to the transfer of nutrients or oxygen but these associations were loose and varying ones; the use of these estimates have mostly been abandoned. Further, all functions of transfer may not go at the same pace. The same baby for whom amino acids and calories have been reduced by poor transfer during pregnancy does not have to suffer from hypoxia in labor due to poor transfer of oxygen. Placental insufficiency as a phrase is therefore probably best avoided in this context for it is too loose a concept and it probably draws attention to the wrong place.

## III. SIGNIFICANCE OF IUGR

Dobson et al.[3] from Melbourne examined mortality and morbidity among babies after IUGR and in a separate publication in 1982,[4] the same workers assessed the antenatal pregnancy complications of this problem. They examined 500 consecutive pregnancies complicated by IUGR and compared them with selected controls where babies were of normal weight for gestation. The perinatal mortality was significantly increased (52 per thousand compared with 12 per thousand total births). Examining the same population for antenatal complications, they found that the early onset of pre-eclampsia before 37 weeks, the incidence of both diabetes mellitus and of abruptio placenta were more common, at a significance level of $p < 0.05$, among women with such a complication.

Many have followed up babies born after IUGR and this is detailed in Chapter 13. In general, they seem not to catch up in height and weight over the next 10 years and are differentiated from the low birthweight babies that are born correct for gestational age. A good example of such a study was published by Van den Berg.[5]

There is also an increased chance of IUGR recurring in a subsequent pregnancy. This was well shown by Fedrick and Adelstein[6] examining the British Births 1970 Survey population. Bakketeigh et al.[7] showed that mothers who had previously produced a baby with IUGR had a three times increased risk of producing a second child with the same problem.

When looking for predisposing factors to disease, physicians often tend to be causal. Going back to the beginning of this century, the cause of all diseases was thought to be understood. Bacteria caused infections and trauma caused bone fractures; therefore why should not every disease have such a simple associated cause. It was only in the 1930s that it was realized that many etiological factors were statistically associated with specific diseases by more than chance. They did not cause the disease but may have made the onset of disease more likely. The teleologic minded tried to rationalize these by labeling them as prodromal factors. In fact, they are only associations and should not be taken for more than that.

In the case of IUGR, the actual cause is either a genetic problem so that the parents are coded to produce a small baby or alternatively there is some deficiency in nutrients arriving at the fetus. In the Western World, the latter is most commonly due to a diminution in transfer of nutrients because of poor placental bed blood flow (Chapter 9). Behind these simple causes, however, lie a large number of associated factors, often interlinked. In order to consider them, we will analyze them independently although in real life these factors are often found grouped together to make clusters of biological, social, or environmental features as recognizable to the epidemiologist as are clinical syndromes (Table 1).

## IV. MATERNAL BACKGROUND FACTORS

**A. Age**

It has always been considered that younger women are at a greater risk to produce a fetus with IUGR. Figure 1 shows the mean birthweight by various age groups. At all lengths of gestation, the proportions of small-for-dates babies among mothers in the median age group (25 to 29 years) and the group above 35 years are similar, but at all stages of gestation the mothers aged 14 to 19 had lighter babies.

These data, from the British Births 1970 Survey, do not stand percentile breakdown but others have done this and showed that there was a younger age association (Selvin and Janerich[8]). However, many others have not found this to be so, i.e., Scott and Usher.[9]

Carr-Hill and Pritchard,[2] in their analysis of the factors affecting birthweight, show that materal age in gestation/sex/parity groups, after adjusting for the effects of maternal height, are only significantly associated in one small subgroup (for boys from parity 1 +, born at 34 weeks of gestation). They conclude therefore that the use of maternal age in any estimate

**Table 1**

**SOME DOCUMENTED ETIOLOGICAL FACTORS OF INTRAUTERINE
GROWTH RETARDATION**

| Maternal factors | | | | |
|---|---|---|---|---|
| **Biological background** | **External environment** | **Milieu interieur** | **Diseases** | **Fetal factors** |
| Age | Work | Nutrition | Congenital abnormalities of the uterus | Sex |
| Parity | Altitude | Smoking | | Multiple pregnancy |
| Social class | | Alcohol | Pre-eclampsia | Genetic abnormalities |
| Race | | Drugs | Hypertension | |
| Past obstetric performance | | | Infections | |

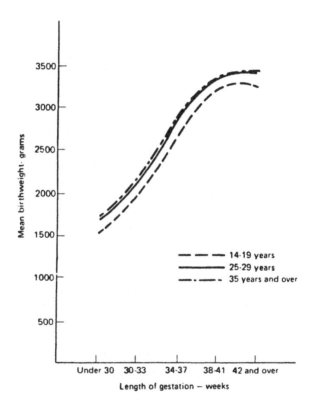

FIGURE 1.   Mean birthweight and length of gestation by certain maternal age groups. (From British Births Survey 1970.)

involving gestation/sex/parity can be discarded for it does not significantly affect the calculations. They stress that this is not the same thing as saying that maternal age has no effect on birthweight but that it does not affect the relationship between the statistical model they present and the observation that the model describes. This is a very careful statement and epitomises the paradoxes which are found through the whole of the consideration of the etiological data of birthweight/gestation, that we are perhaps not asking the right questions and therefore are not getting the correct answers.

## B. Parity

There is an association between increase in birthweight and increase in parity. Primi-

**Table 2**

**MEAN BIRTHWEIGHT AND SD BY WEEK OF
GESTATION ACCORDING TO PARITY —
SINGLETONS, L.N.M.P. CERTAIN**

| | Length of gestation — weeks[a] | | | | |
| --- | --- | --- | --- | --- | --- |
| | <30 | 30—33 | 34—37 | 38—41 | 42 and over |
| All firstborn | | | | | |
| N | 30 | 58 | 384 | 4010 | 575 |
| Mean (g) | 1267 | 1932 | 2664 | 3287 | 3381 |
| SD (g) | 792 | 846 | 572 | 469 | 494 |
| All laterborn | | | | | |
| N | 50 | 92 | 623 | 6889 | 867 |
| Mean (g) | 1486 | 2039 | 2930 | 3417 | 3480 |
| SD (g) | 985 | 703 | 560 | 480 | 514 |

[a]   Where both birthweight and length of gestation are known.

From Chamberlain, R., Chamberlain, G., Howlett, B., and Claireaux, A.,
*British Births 1970*, Vol. 1, William Heinemann Medical Books, London,
1975, 75. With permission.

gravidae are likely to give birth to more babies small for gestational age than multipara. In
the British Births Survey 1970 study,[10] firstborn babies were lighter than later born, especially
in the under 37 weeks gestation, as is shown in Table 2.

This analysis, like many others, extends only to the difference between primigravidae
and multigravidae. Billewicz and Thomson[11] have shown an increase in birthweight over
the woman's whole reproductive life. Carr-Hill and Pritchard[2] come to the conclusion that
the birthweight changes associated with parity relate more to maternal weight before pregnancy than to the position of the child in the family.

## C. Social Class

Socio-economic class is a flag for a large number of other, less easily measured variables.
It relates to the woman's past pattern of nutrition, education, and disease when she was a
child and in her teenage life. In this country, the social class is usually coded from the
husband's occupation using the Classification of Occupations of the Registrar General. Social
Class I is the professional class and the grades descend to Social Class V, the untrained
classes. Women who are divorced, widowed, or separated and single women are not classified
in this group; neither theoretically are those married to the unemployed but so many are
now in this group that observers often use the last occupation when employed. This system
therefore has many deficiencies but data from it constantly parallel trends derived from
independent features such as perinatal mortality or congenital abnormalities. Practically, it
is the most commonly used classification and so it will be used in this chapter.

In Figure 2, women from Social Class I and II are compared with those in Social Classes
IV and V. Intrauterine growth retardation (below the ten percentile) does not seem to be
associated with social class until after 36 weeks of gestation when the effect becomes more
dramatic in Social Class IV and V. These features have been documented by many others.

Much of the effect of social class on the fetus is probably brought about by maternal
height and smoking. Figure 3 from the National Birthday Trust's British Births 1970 Survey
shows the similar increase in babies born under the tenth percentile of weight from about
36 weeks of gestation among women under 62 inches (157.5 cm). Carr-Hill and Pritchard[2]
came to a similar conclusion for they showed that much of social class gradient in the mean
corrected standardized birthweight scoring can be accounted for by factors of maternal size
and smoking.

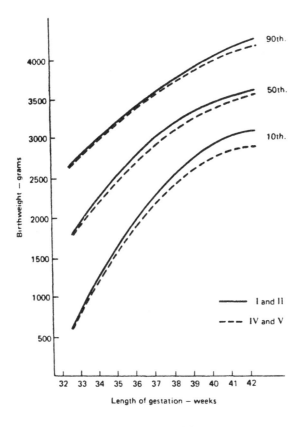

FIGURE 2. Mean birthweight and tenth percentile by week of gestation in Social Classes I and II and IV and V. (From British Births Survey 1970).

## D. Race

People from different racial backgrounds produce different sized babies. This relates to the genetics of any given race as well as to nutrition in early life and behavior in pregnancy. This lack of worldwide applicability was one of the problems that existed when a low birthweight baby was defined as one below 5 ½ lb or 2500 g. The cutoff point had been agreed upon in the Scandinavian countries in the early 1920s and was adopted by the League of Nations and then the World Health Organization after the second World War. It did not allow for the difference between low birthweight due to delivery at too short a period of gestation and that due to low birthweight from poor intrauterine growth, and it also made no allowance for the different races of the world. Using such a definition in the U.K., about 7% of babies are born with low birthweight; this figure does not vary from one year to another. In Sweden, the proportion of babies born with weight below 2500g is 4% while in Delhi it is 40%. Boldman and Read[12] have published a large table showing the percentage of low birthweight babies by countries in various decades since the second World War and the table ranges from 4.7 (Finland) to 45% (Kanpur, India).

IUGR obviously plays some part in this but much is due to the different genetics of women whose chromosomes are programmed to produce smaller babies. In addition, certain diseases exist more commonly in some parts of the world and this can be found as a variable with geographical locations; for example Tuck et al.[13] found IUGR among 42% of women with a hemoglobin SS compared with only 18% of those women with hemoglobin SC. Such changes relate strongly to geography and therefore might be cross-related with race.

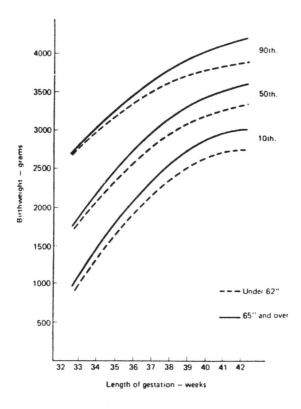

FIGURE 3.  Mean birthweight and tenth percentile by week of gestation in women below 62 in. and those above 65 in. (From British Birth Survey 1970).

**Table 3**

**INCIDENCE OF INTRAUTERINE GROWTH RETARDATION AMONG SECOND BABIES IN RELATION TO BIRTHWEIGHT OF FIRST BABY[7]**

| Weight of first baby | n | % | Relative risk of second baby being below 10th percentile |
|---|---|---|---|
| >90th percentile | 8,470 | 1.6 | 0.2 |
| 10th—90th percentile | 57,602 | 6.7 | 1.2 |
| <10th percentile | 10,457 | 23.0 | 3.4 |

From Bakketeigh, L. S., Hoffman, H., and Harley, E., *Am. J. Obstet. Gynecol.*, 135, 1086, 1979. With permission.

## E. Past Obstetrical Performance

One of the strongest indicators of a multiparous woman's performance in labor is her previous obstetrical performance. The work of Bakketeigh et al.[7] has already been referred to. Table 3 shows the data of their study in more detail.

It is of interest to note that the authors also show no evidence of recurrence of the medical complications which are commonly attributed as causes of low birthweight such as pre-eclampsia. It is probable that this increased risk of producing recurrent IUGR exists because of the background of the woman rather than an assigned medical reason.

# V. ENVIRONMENTAL FACTORS

## A. Work

More women are now working in pregnancy and they are working to a later stage of gestation. In a recent review of the subject, Chamberlain[14] showed that in the U.K. roughly 50% of women were working into pregnancy and three-quarters of them were working into the last trimester.

It is difficult to sort out the multiple effects of work. It may be that work itself, with the concomitant stress of travel to and from the place of work, is a feature. Certainly exercise can reduce uterine bed blood flow both absolutely and relatively (Hytten[15]). Further, male observers should remember that all women work at home as well as some accepting paid work outside the home.

Some of the best research on the effect of work in general in pregnancy comes from very detailed studies performed by the Institute National de la Sarté et la Recherche Médicale in France.[16,17] In the 1972 study, they showed that women who are working to be of greater risk for producing babies with a birthweight below the fifth percentile, a stricter criterion than usually used for IUGR. Of the employed, 6.1% compared with 3.9% for the nonemployed had babies below this birthweight distribution. It is of interest that in the 1976 study from the same source, the employed to nonemployed were 5.0 and 5.8%, implying that there had been a change.

It is data like these that confound the whole issue of the general effect of work in pregnancy. It may well be that this factor is like socio-economic class and may be acting as a warning sign without being a specific entity. Maybe it is not the work itself or even the fatigue that work generates, but the other aspects of life which affect the growth of the fetus. Perhaps those who go to regular work are more likely to be able to get to regular antenatal care. They may lead a more orderly life; they may earn more money and thus be able to pay for their food more readily. The tangled skein of the general effects of work are well laid out by Joffe[18] in his review on this subject.

As well as the general effects of work, certain occupations may carry specific hazards because of their environmental or chemical involvement. Here, the hazard of IUGR relates strongly to the presence of congenital abnormalities. Much work has been done in this area on lead, mercury, anaesthetic agents, and copper; the epidemiological associations are complex. The reader is referred to Murray[19] for a review of the problem of specific congenital abnormalities related to teratogens found at work.

The proof of growth retardation being caused by physical work is yet to come. It is possible that the women who work are an entirely different population from those who do not; the other variables referred to in this chapter are possibly more important and they are being reflected in the woman's work pattern.

## B. Altitude

With increasing distance from sea level, the atmospheric pressure is reduced and therefore the partial pressure of oxygen is less. It is noticed by those who usually live at lower altitudes and climb mountains. Those who live in such high altitudes adapt through their hemoglobin systems so that a relative polycythaemia occurs. Sabrevilla et al.[20] showed a marked reduction in birthweight in those born in extremely high altitudes but the number in the study is not very great. McCullough et al.[21] found a greater population of babies with IUGR among those born at high locations in the Rockies than those born at Denver (a town itself about 5000 feet above sea level). Gibson[22] took the argument a stage further when he showed an inverse relationship in the mean birthweight to hemoglobin levels in pregnancy. These high hemoglobin levels can be associated with a proportionately low increase in plasma volume;[23] thus this might be the real reason for any association of fetal growth and altitude.

## VI. MATERNAL MILIEU INTERIEUR

### A. Nutrition

One of the great folk myths is that a woman eats in pregnancy to feed her unborn child. If she eats too little, the child will suffer. More recently, the myth has stretched to eating the right foods. Associations between IUGR and maternal nutrition before and in pregnancy have been shown at the extremes of poor nutrition. Some studies, detailed in this section, indicate that intervention by feeding women can improve fetal growth but this is an area where one cannot go further to cross-correlate perinatal mortality with low birthweight. It cannot be assumed that by improving birthweight, one would of necessity improve perinatal mortality any more than by raising birthweight the expected perinatal mortality level will alter to that of the new birthweight group. This was well shown by Rush et al.[24] assessing the impact of the Women, Infants and Children Programme (WIC Programme), used in America to provide food supplements and nutrition education to the poorer women of that country through the aegis of the U.K. Department of Agriculture.

Many of the studies on nutrition that have been performed in an observational or an interventional nature are flawed for they were either not controlled correctly or data were collected in a patchy fashion. Many do not control tightly, with no allowance for social class, parity, or age; other use as controls the previous years of population. Rush et al.[25] examined a randomized controlled trial on nutrititional supplements among the black poorer population in New York City and found that a balanced protein and calorie complement was associated with a significantly lower proportion of low birthweight babies (<2500 g) and a slightly longer duration of gestation. This would imply that IUGR was reduced. Undoubtedly dietary restriction can be associated with a lower birthweight but the intervention by giving extra protein or low caloried supplements do not always help the ultimate outcome. It is probable that diet is not the major means through which social deprivation has its effect on IUGR.

### B. Cigarette Smoking

Some of the best data on the influence of external events on IUGR are probably in the field of cigarette smoking. In 1958, Butler and Bonham[26] showed an association of babies with a reduced birthweight among women who smoked during pregnancy. They also showed that women who gave up smoking before the 16th week of pregnancy reverted to the birthweight pattern of nonsmokers.

Chamberlain et al.[10] examined this phenomenon in the 1970 British Births Survey showing a difference of 170 g between those who smoked and those who were not smoking at the time of birth (see Figure 4). There is undoubtedly a dose-related effect here for the more cigarettes a woman smokes each day, the greater is the affect on the baby and so the greater the incidence of IUGR. Multivariant analyses have been performed on smoking mothers in which allowance has been made for age, parity, and social class. Smoking has been shown repeatedly to be independently related to the incidence of IUGR. A good review of this is given by Sexton.[27]

### C. Alcohol

This tissue poison has attracted attention because it is used so much in Western society. Prospective studies have shown an increase in intrauterine growth deficiency in a dose-related fashion with the consumption of alcohol. A good example of this is given by Hanson et al.[28] who examined the data from the pregnant women attending two Seattle hospitals in the mid-1970s. The fetal growth effect is found usually at a much lower level of alcohol consumption than the required to produce true fetal alcohol syndrome which is more usual in heavy drinkers. Moderate drinkers do have an effect on their fetal birthweight.

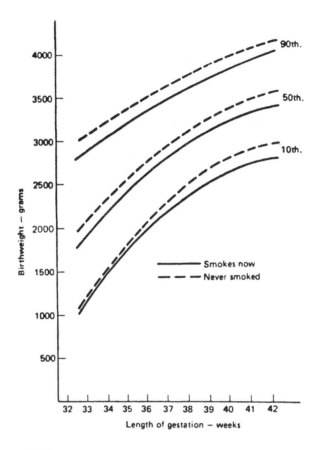

FIGURE 4. Mean birthweight and tenth percentile by week of gestation according to smoking habits. (From British Births Survey 1970).

## D. Other Addictive Drugs

Addictive drugs other than alcohol and tobacco affect fetal development but they are, so far, abused less in the Western World than are the two major toxic agents of society. There is a fivefold increased relative risk of fetal growth retardation among opiate addicts.[29] The effect of opiates alone is hard to apportion for many other social, medical, and biological co-variables exist alongside the actual taking of an addictive drug.

## VII. MATERNAL DISEASES

### A. Congential Abnormalities of the Uterus

The blood supply to the uterus comes from the uterine arteries arriving bilaterally in the base of the broad ligament. Thence they pass upwards from the level of the cervix to provide branches which pass through the myometrium into the endometrium. When the common wall between the two embryonic tubes fails to break down, this produces a series of uterine abnormalities varying from a true uterus didelphys to a slightly dimpled subseptus uterus. The extra median wall of the malformed uterus, which will have a poorer blood supply than do the normal lateral walls for the septum, is at the far end of vessels which travel across the fundus then down into the septum. Should a pregnancy implant on the median wall of an abnormal uterus, it too will have reduced blood supply and it might be expected that the developing fetus would suffer from intrauterine malnutrition.

## B. Hypertensive Diseases

Probably the best identified cause of IUGR among babies born to women in the Western World are hypertensive diseases, either preexisting pregnancy or coming on during the pregnancy itself. Some workers estimate that both sets of hypertensive conditions are responsible for up to a third of all fetal growth retardation.

Pregnancy-induced hypertension, particularly if it is associated with proteinuria has a greater risk of association with IUGR (Moore and Redmond[29]). If pregnancy-induced hypertension with proteinuria is superimposed on preexisting hypertension, the risk worsens even more. Further, the degree of effect increases among those women in whom the condition is found earlier in pregnancy and those who have a longer duration of hypertension. All this relates to the state of the placental bed arterioles and the degree of trophoblast invasion of their walls as first described by Brossens et al.[31] and considered in more detail in Chapter 3.

A similar pattern of fetal retardation occurs in women who have essential hypertension when they become pregnant. If the condition is mild, the weight of the baby does not seem to be affected but if it is severe then growth retardation is increased (Dunlop[32]).

## C. Infections

Acute infections may affect the fetus temporarily because of maternal pyrexia. Chronic infections act mostly on the fetus by passing across the placenta and actually altering the growth of the cells. A few however attack the utero-placental transfer mechanisms, so the fetal growth retardation is a consequence on the depressed supply of nutrients.

Malaria is probably the most common infection in the world and IUGR is common in this condition. This may be a mixed problem with nutrition for there is an infiltration of the placenta by parasites in up to 20% of women with malaria (McGregor et al.[33]). Extensive villus damage occurs and birthweight is reduced.

Cytomegalovirus is commonly associated with congential abnormalities of the fetus. Approximately 40% of infants born with the condition have IUGR noted at birth (Stagno et al.[34]). The earliest common infection in which IUGR was noted was rubella. Cooper et al.[35] found up to 60% of infants with congenital rubella to be below the tenth percentile of birthweight for gestation. The mechanism here is both of limitation of cell multiplication in the fetus and an infection of the vascular endothelium of the villus capillaries, thus impeding circulation.

Virus infections such as herpes and hepatitis have been occasionally reported as associated with IUGR. Readers are referred to a good review of this by Waterson[36], who outlines the problems of dealing with data in this field while similar information on bacterial infections may be found in a review by Hurley.[37]

## VIII. FETAL FACTORS

## A. Sex

In all studies, male babies are found to be heavier than female babies at any given gestational age. Chamberlain et al.[10] in the British Births 1970 Study, found among 17,000 babies that the average male birthweight was 3367 g and the female 3249 g, 118 g different. This is consistent with many other studies. What was different about the British Births Survey, however, was they found that this birthweight difference went back to less than 30 weeks of gestation. Thomson et al.[38] did not show any difference before the 32nd week of gestation while Milner and Richards[39] showed the effect of birthweight by the 28th week of gestation.

Chamberlain et al.[10] further analyzed their data by sex and parity combined (Figures 5 and 6). They showed that the IUGR against length of gestation is not quite the same in the

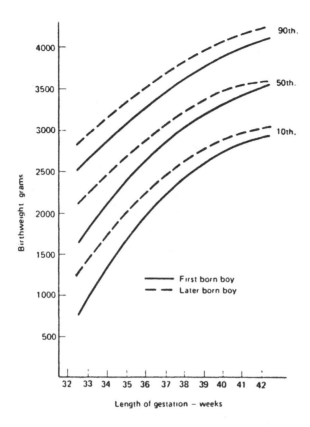

FIGURE 5. Mean birthweight and tenth percentile of boys by week of gestation according to order of birth. (From British Births Survey 1970).

two sexes; the difference associated with parity in the boys was more emphasized in lower gestational ages than it was in the girls. They caution that there may have been a small group of larger immature girls born this particular survey week, which would thus bias the information, but this trend is seen in both the centile charts of the boys.

It must be emphasized this statistical difference does not imply that the female genetic makeup in any way retards the girl but more girls would appear below a tenth percentile line birthweight gestation chart if the distribution curve was made up of both sexes. It is therefore wise always to have charts made up for each sex as well as for primiparous and multiparous mothers.

## B. Abnormalities

Certain abnoralities are associated with IUGR, i.e., anencephaly (Usher and Maclean[40]) and renal malformations (Keirse and Meerman[41]). The growth retardation is probably due to changes in fetal function but in some instances chromosomal abnormalities are constantly linked with the malfunction so there might well be a genetic component as well. Turner's Syndrome and Down's Syndrome are well documented as being associated with poor fetal growth (Wright[42]).

## C. Multiple Pregnancy

About a third of multiple pregnancies finish preterm. In addition to this, however, these babies show IUGR compared with singleton babies. This might be expected with the sharing of the same placental bed. When judging standards of growth of babies, twin babies cannot

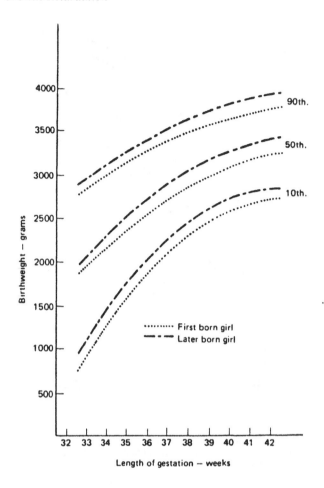

FIGURE 6.    Mean birthweight and tenth percentile of girls by
week of gestation according to order of birth. (From British Births
Survey 1970).

be assessed in the same distribution charts as singleton babies. So much is this the point
that most studies ignore twins for they are too difficult to assess, yet here is a perfect example
of a shared intrauterine environment which may affect the different individuals in different
ways. Monozygotic twins tend to have more growth retardation that dizygotic twins (Bulmer[43]).
There is a similar higher incidence of growth retardation in the birthweight of mono-amniotic
twins (Wharton et al.[44]) and this would fit with the zygosity association.

## IX. CONCLUSIONS

The epidemiology of IUGR is a tangled skein. There are many external associations that
are known and can be spotted in the antenatal period. The common etiological factor for
many of these is probably in the flow of blood through the placental bed. If this is diminished,
then the fetus will be deprived of nutrients and will be small for gestational stage. Having
been born, such a fetus may well catch up when he receives extrauterine nutrition. The
future pathways of sorting out the epidemiological conditions lie in the identification of
those women with poor flow in the placental bed early in pregnancy. Thus, a population at
higher risk could be identified and associations could be better worked out to provide more
precise quantification of identifying factors which may be seen in the antenatal clinic.

# REFERENCES

1. **Lubchenco, L., Hansman, C., Dresslor, M., and Boyd, E.,** Inrauterine growth as estimated from live born birthweight data, *Paediatrics,* 32, 793, 1963.
2. **Carr-Hill, R. and Pritchard, C.,** *The Development & Exploitation of Empirical Birthweight Standards,* 1st ed., Stockton Press, New York, 1985.
3. **Dobson, P., Abell, A., and Beischer, N.,** Mortality and morbidity of fetal growth retardation, *Aust. N.Z. J. Obstet. Gynaecol.,* 21, 69, 1981.
4. **Dobson, P., Abell, A., and Beischer, N.,** Antenatal pregnancy complications and fetal growth complications, *Aust. N.Z. J. Obstet. Gynaecol.,* 22, 203, 1982.
5. **Van den Berg, B. J.,** Epidemiological observations in prematurity, in *Epidemiology of Prematurity,* Reed, D. M. and Stanley, F., Eds., Urban & Schwarzenberg, Baltimore, 1977, 159.
6. **Fedrick, J. and Adelstein, P.,** Factors associated with low birthweight infants delivered at term, *Br. J. Obstet. Gynaecol.,* 85, 1, 1978.
7. **Bakketeigh, L. S., Hoffman, H., and Harley, E.,** The tendency to repeat gestational age and birth weight in successive births, *Am. J. Obstet. Gynecol.,* 135, 1086, 1979.
8. **Selvin, S. and Janerich, D.,** Factors influencing birthweight, *Br. J. Prev. Soc. Med.,* 25, 12, 1971.
9. **Scott, K. and Usher, R.,** Fetal malnutrition, *Am. J. Obstet. Gynecol.* 94, 951, 1966.
10. **Chamberlain, R., Chamberlain, G., Howlett, B., and Claireaux, A.,** *British Births 1970,* Vol. 1, William Heinemann, London, 1975, 75.
11. **Billewicz, W. and Thomson, A.,** Birthweights in consecutive pregnancies, *J. Obstet. Gynaecol. Br. Commonw.,* 80, 491, 1973.
12. **Boldman, R. and Reed, D.,** Worldwide variations in low birthweight, in *Epidemiology of Prematurity,* Reed, D. and Stanley, F. Eds., Urban & Schwarzenberg, Baltimore, 1977, 41.
13. **Tuck, S., Studd, J., and White, J.,** Pregnancy in sickle cell disease in the U.K., *Br. J. Obstet. Gynaecol.,* 90, 112, 1983.
14. **Chamberlain, G.,** Women at work in pregnancy, in *Pregnant Women at Work,* Chamberlain, G., Ed., Macmillan, London, 1984, 1.
15. **Hytten, F.,** The effect of work on placental function, in *Pregnant Women at Work,* Chamberlain, G., Ed., Macmillan, London, 1984, 15.
16. **Saurel Cubizothes, M., Kaminski, M., and Rumean Rocquette, C.,** Activite professionnelle des femmes enceintes, *J. Gynecol. Obstet. Biol. Reprod.,* 11, 959, 1982.
17. **Mammelle, N., Lauman, B., and Lazar, P.,** Prematurity and occupational activity during pregnancy, *Am. J. Epidemiol.,* 119, 309, 1984.
18. **Joffe, M.,** Women's work and pregnancy, in *Prepregnancy Care,* Chamberlain, G. and Lumley, J., Eds., John Wiley & Sons, Chichester, 1986, 245.
19. **Murray, R.,** Hazards of work in pregnancy, in *Pregnant Women at Work,* Chamberlain, G., Ed., Macmillan, London, 1984, 31.
20. **Sabrevilla, L. et al.,** Low oestrogen excretion during pregnancy at high altitude, *Am. J. Obstet. Gynecol.,* 102, 823, 1968.
21. **McCullough, R., Reeves, J., and Liljegren, R.,** Fetal growth retardation at high altitudes, *Arch. Environ. Health,* 32, 26, 1977.
22. **Gibson, H.,** Plasma volume in pregnancy, *J. Obstet. Gynaecol. Br. Commonw.,* 80, 1067, 1973.
23. **Pirani, B., Campbell, D., and MacGillivray, I.,** Plasma volume in normal first pregnancy, *J. Obstet. Gynaecol. Br. Common.,* 80, 884, 1973.
24. **Rush, D., Alvir, J., and Lessfor, J.,** Histological Study of the Special Food Programme for Women, Infancts, & Children to Pregnancy Outcome, Food & Nutrition Service, Department of Agriculture, Washington, D.C., 1985.
25. **Rush, D., Stein, Z., and Susser, M.,** A randomized controlled trial of prenatal nutritional supplements in New York City, *Pediatrics,* 65, 683, 1980.
26. **Butler, N. and Bonham, D.,** *Perinatal Mortality,* Livingstone, Edinburgh, 1963.
27. **Sexton, M.,** Smoking, in *Prepregnancy Care,* Chamberlain, G. and Lumley, J., Eds., Wright, Chichester, 1986, 141.
28. **Hanson, J., Streissgoth, A., and Smith, D.,** The effects of moderate alcohol consumption on fetal growth, *J. Pediatr.,* 92, 457, 1978.
29. **Ostrea, E. and Chaver, C.,** Perinatal problems in maternal drug addiction, *J. Pediatr.,* 94, 292, 1979.
30. **Moore, M. and Redman, L.,** Case controlled study of severe pre-eclampsia at early onset, *Br. Med. J.,* 287, 580, 1983.
31. **Brosens, I., Robertson, W. B., and Dixon, H. G.,** *Obstetrics and Gynecology Annual,* Wynn, R. M., Ed., Appleton-Century-Crofts, New York, 1972, 177.
32. **Dunlop, J.,** Chronic hypertension and perinatal mortality, *Proc. R. Soc. Med.,* 59, 838, 1966.

33. **McGregor, I., Wilson, M., and Billewicz, W.,** Malarial infection of the placenta, *Trans. R. Soc. Trop. Med. Hyg.,* 77, 232, 1983.
34. **Stagno, S., Poss, R., Dworsky, M., and Alford, C.,** Congential and perinatal cytomegalovirus infections, *Semin. Perinatology,* 7, 31, 1983.
35. **Cooper, L. et al.,** Neonatal thrombocytopaenic puerpera and other manifestations of rubella contracted in utero, *Am. J. Dis. Child.,* 110, 416, 1965.
36. **Waterson, A.,** Virus infections during pregnancy, *Br. Med. J.,* ii, 564, 1979.
37. **Hurley, R.,** Serious infections of the newborn, *Clin. Obstet. Gynecol.,* 10, 65, 1983.
38. **Thomson, F., Billewicz, W., and Hytten, F.,** The assessment of fetal growth, *J. Obstet. Gynaecol. Br. Commonw.,* 75, 903, 1968.
39. **Milner, R. and Richards, B.,** Analysis by birthweight of infants born in England and Wales, 1967—1971, *J. Obstet. Gynaecol. Br. Commonw.,* 81, 956, 1974.
40. **Usher, R. and Maclean, F.,** Normal fetal growth and the significance of fetal growth retardation, in *Scientific Foundation of Paediatrics,* Davis, J. and Dobbing, J., Ed., William Heineman, London, 1974, 69.
41. **Keirse, M. and Meerman, R.,** Antenatal diagnosis of potter's syndrome, *Obstet. Gynecol.,* 52, 645, 1978.
42. **Wright, E.,** Chromosomes and human fetal development, in *The Biology of Human Fetal Growth,* Roberts, D. and Thomson, A. Ed., Taylor & Francis, London, 1976, 237.
43. **Bulmer, M.,** *The Biology of Twinning in Man,* Oxford University Press, Oxford, 1970.
44. **Wharton, B., Edwards, J., and Cameron, A.,** Monoamniotic twins, *J. Obstet. Gynaecol. Br. Commonw.,* 75, 158, 1968.

Chapter 2

# EPIDEMIOLOGY OF FETAL GROWTH RETARDATION IN DEVELOPED COUNTRIES

## Z. Štembera, A. Kravka, and F. Mandys

## TABLE OF CONTENTS

# I. INTRODUCTION

Epidemiology is a new, developing branch, the aim of which is to study (1) the distribution and dynamics of diseases in population subgroups delimited locally, temporally, and materially (e.g., by age, sex, environment, etc.), (2) the causes of diseases and the conditions of their origin, course, duration, and consequences, and (3) to propose practical measures for prevention of the diseases and for maintenance and improvement of health of the society.

# II. BASIC PROBLEMS OF IUGR EPIDEMIOLOGY

If the general epidemiologic principles are applied to a special obstetric and neonatologic problem concerning intrauterine growth retardation (IUGR), then the results should provide a basis to answer the following fundamental questions:

1.  Does IUGR still belong among the serious problems of perinatal medicine in those countries with high quality obstetrical and neonatal care, i.e., characterized by perinatal mortality rate of, say, less than 15/1000?
    If yes, then:
2.  What are the main etiologic causes of IUGR, or, by what criteria is it possible to identify the "at risk" group of women endangered by occurence of IUGR?
3.  In given conditions, what is the optimal intervention strategy that could lead to either a decrease of the incidence of IUGR in the population, or, to a limitation of the adverse effect of IUGR upon further development of these infants?

As the results of each epidemiologic study are based on analysis of data collected in a certain region, they are influenced by different regional conditions (e.g., social, cultural, health condition of the inhabitants, and by the system of health care). Therefore, the general validity of the answers is always, in a certain sense, limited by the quoted different local conditions.

# III. DEFINITION OF IUGR AND METHODS OF DATA COLLECTION

From the methodologic point of view, an exact definition of IUGR must be the first step when beginning such a study. If IUGR is, at present, conventionally defined as a birthweight below a certain average for gestational age, then knowledge of these lower variables is necessary. Thus, although birthweight is readily and objectively obtained, different criteria are used to determine the lower borderline of birthweight for gestational age, e.g., 2 SD below the mean,[1] or, below the third percentile,[2] below the tenth percentile,[3] or below the fifth percentile. Also, these different criteria are based on different mean birthweights for a given gestational age, depending on geographic and ethnic differences, also on the sex of the newborn, and on the parity of the mother (Table 1).

We have chosen for our study, the tables with the fifth percentile calculated by Poláček,[4] whose data, concerning the average birthweight, correspond best to the conditions in central Europe (Table 2). (To standardize this calculation for international comparison, it will be suitable, in the future, to use a unified mode of the average growth curve plus the relevant deviation for each different population, as recommended, by the International Federation of Gynecology and Obstetrics or FIGO[7]).

In our previous study[8] we have drawn attention to the inaccuracy of using a subjective statement of the last menstrual period to calculate gestational age. By means of ultrasound anthropometry at the 16th week of pregnancy (i.e., when different influences have not significantly affected fetal growth), deviations greater than 2 weeks were found in gestational age, (2.8% older, 2.0% younger). Therefore, in the present study, ultrasound screening of all pregnant women was employed in the 16th week of pregnancy.

## Table 1
### MEAN BIRTHWEIGHT AND DIFFERENT CALCULATIONS OF THE LOWER LIMIT FOR THE 40TH GESTATIONAL WEEK, BY SEX AND PARITY, IN FOUR DEVELOPED COUNTRIES

| Country | Parity | Mean | Male SFD Limit | Male SFD Calculation | Mean | Female SFD Limit | Female SFD Calculation | Ref. |
|---------|--------|------|-------|-------------|------|-------|-------------|------|
| Sweden | Total | 3650 | 2850 | −2 SD | 3510 | 2740 | −2 SD | 5 |
| Iceland | First | 3580 | 3080 | <10% | 3460 | 2950 | <10% | 6 |
| | Subsequent | 3745 | 3155 | <10% | 3600 | 3060 | <10% | |
| Japan | First | 3170 | 2560 | −1.5 SD | 3110 | 2560 | −1.5 SD | 1 |
| | Subsequent | 3330 | 2720 | −1.5 SD | 3220 | 2690 | −1.5 SD | |
| ČSSR | Total | 3425 | 2738 | <5% | 3149 | 2370 | <5% | 4 |
| | | | 2890 | <10% | | 2542 | <10% | |

## Table 2
### MEAN BIRTHWEIGHT—FIFTH AND TENTH PERCENTILE

| Weeks of pregnancy | Male 5% | Male 10% | Male Mean | Female 5% | Female 10% | Female Mean |
|---------|-----|------|------|-----|------|------|
| 24 | 639 | 709 | 954 | 628 | 676 | 844 |
| 25 | 739 | 804 | 1034 | 680 | 728 | 897 |
| 26 | 846 | 903 | 1105 | 793 | 843 | 1017 |
| 27 | 991 | 1041 | 1218 | 912 | 965 | 1155 |
| 28 | 1097 | 1147 | 1324 | 1003 | 1059 | 1258 |
| 29 | 1222 | 1275 | 1463 | 1112 | 1169 | 1369 |
| 30 | 1331 | 1394 | 1616 | 1277 | 1339 | 1560 |
| 31 | 1524 | 1595 | 1846 | 1392 | 1471 | 1748 |
| 32 | 1656 | 1735 | 2012 | 1559 | 1645 | 1947 |
| 33 | 1791 | 1875 | 2171 | 1672 | 1771 | 2122 |
| 34 | 1928 | 2027 | 2377 | 1841 | 1946 | 2318 |
| 35 | 2048 | 2165 | 2578 | 1979 | 2095 | 2503 |
| 36 | 2183 | 2313 | 2773 | 2112 | 2241 | 2699 |
| 37 | 2386 | 2524 | 3013 | 2246 | 2394 | 2918 |
| 38 | 2568 | 2711 | 3214 | 2273 | 2444 | 3045 |
| 39 | 2677 | 2829 | 3368 | 2326 | 2500 | 3115 |
| 40 | 2738 | 2890 | 3426 | 2371 | 2543 | 3149 |
| 41 | 2813 | 2968 | 3516 | 2502 | 2663 | 3230 |

Data from Polacek, K., *High Risk Pregnancy,* Stembera, Z., Polacek, K., and Vlach, V., Eds., Avicenum, Prague, 1979, 217.

The study sample comprises 2005 newborns representing a population sample from one of the Prague districts, who were born in the years 1981 and 1982 in our institute, and whose complete data, (pre-, intra-, and postnatal, plus data concerning their mothers), are a part of the database in our Hewlett-Packard computer (Figure 1). Cases of IUGR caused by nonviable malformations (four cases out of six), and by multiple pregnancies (no case of IUGR and no case of perinatal death out of 16 newborns) were analyzed separately due to dissimilarity in etiology.

The remaining 1983 newborns were divided into three main groups: 53 corresponded to the criteria for small-for-date (SFD) newborns; 38 of them had a birthweight lower than

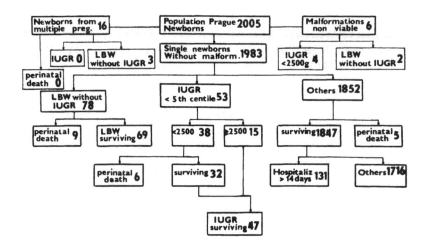

FIGURE 1. IUGR Newborns, LBW newborns without IUGR, and other newborns in the population sample of Prague.

2500 g, out of whom 6 died perinatally. Among the 15 newborns with a birthweight of 2500 g and more, there was no perinatal death. Consequently, altogether, 47 SFD survived. The second group consists of 78 low birthweight newborns (LBW) without malformations. Out of them 9 died perinatally and 69 survived. In the last group there are the remaining 1852 newborns, with only five perinatal deaths. One hundred and thirty-one mothers from the group of 1847 surviving newborns had a "high-risk" pregnancy, requiring antenatal hospitalization longer than 2 weeks. The remaining 1716 pregnancies were considered "non-risk" or "lowrisk".

## IV. PERINATAL MORTALITY IN IUGR

The population sample is large enough to analyze the perinatal mortality rate (PMR) and provide a basis to answer the first question quoted in the introduction.

Out of a total of 26 perinatal deaths; 10 (38.5%) babies are growth retarded, i.e., 12.9% of the total PMR. Hepburn and Rosenberg[9] also found, among randomly selected newborns from Glasgow, a three times greater PMR amongst the growth-retarded group (i.e., 23.3%), when compared with the incidence in the hospital population as a whole (i.e., 7.6%). Low and Galbraith[10] have shown that the perinatal mortality rate in IUGR, (50%), is more than three times greater than that in the total studied population, (i.e., 15.6%). These results indicate that IUGR remains an important problem to correct, in order to further decrease the PMR, even in developed countries.

In the present study all deaths among the IUGR newborns occurred in babies with a birthweight lower than 2500 g. Table 3 shows that the mortality of newborns in the group, LBW *with* IUGR (15.8%) exceeded the group LBW *without* IUGR (10.7%). (Similar results were recorded by Eggermont et al.[11] who analyzed a group two times larger and found a difference of 12 and 10%, respectively). Even more striking is the difference found in the subgroup with a birthweight lower than 1500 g, where the PMR is 60% *with* IUGR, and 28.6% *without* IUGR.

Amongst the subgroups of very low birthweight (VLBW) infants *with* or *without* IUGR the specific PMR is 43 and 20%, respectively (birthweight 1000 to 1499 g), and in the group of extremely low birthweight infants (ELBW = <1000 g) it is 100 and 50%, respectively.

Although the number of infants is small, the difference noted is important, because the

## Table 3
## LBW NEWBORNS WITH AND WITHOUT IUGR: NUMBER OF SURVIVORS, PERINATAL DEATHS, AND THE SPECIFIC PERINATAL MORTALITY RATE

| Birthweight (g) | LBW with IUGR | | LBW without IUGR | | Specific perinatal mortality rate | | |
|---|---|---|---|---|---|---|---|
| | Survived | Perinatal death | Survived | Perinatal death | LBW with IUGR | LBW without IUGR | Total |
| <1000 | 0 | 3 | 2 | 2 | 100 | 50 | 71.4 |
| 1000—1499 | 4 | 3 | 8 | 2 | 43 | 20 | 29.2 |
| 1500—2499 | 28 | 0 | 65 | 5 | 0 | 7.1 | 5.1 |
| Total | 32 | 6 | 75 | 9 | 15.8 | 10.7 | 12.3 |

## Table 4
## ALL IUGR NEWBORNS, WITH AND WITHOUT NONVIABLE MALFORMATIONS: NUMBER OF SURVIVORS AND PERINATAL DEATHS

| Week of pregnancy/ birthweight (g) | Survived (without nonviable malformations) | Perinatal death | | Total | | |
|---|---|---|---|---|---|---|
| | | Without nonviable malformations | With nonviable malformations | Survived | Perinatal death | Total |
| <28/<800 | 0 | 2 | 0 | 0 | 2 | 2 |
| 28—33/800—1499 | 4 | 4 | 3 | 4 | 7 | 11 |
| >33/1500—2499 | 28 | 0 | 1 | 28 | 1 | 29 |
| >37/2500—2800 | 15 | 0 | 0 | 15 | 0 | 15 |
| Total | 47 | 6 | 4 | 47 | 10 | 57 |

IUGR fetuses have a greater gestational age at the same birthweight. Eggermont[11] found that, even when the gestational age is the same — (32 to 34 weeks) — the mortality of LBW newborns *with* IUGR is twice that the LBW infants *without* IUGR, (16 against 7%), but this difference was no longer present at a gestational age of 35 to 36 weeks.

Table 4 shows that when the group LBW *with* IUGR is further differentiated into three subgroups, according to birthweight and gestational age, all perinatal deaths (with the exception of one newborn with a nonviable malformation occurred before the 34th week of gestation, and that the birthweight did not exceed 1500 g.

These results indicate that, in growth-retarded fetuses, the PMR risk is increased if infants are born before the 35th week of gestation with a birthweight less than 1500 g. Also, their PMR is substantially greater than in LBW newborns without IUGR.

## V. IUGR AND LBW INFANTS

An important international study by Vilar and Belizán[12] compared the results from 11 regions in the developed world and from 25 developing areas. In this vast group, involving several millions of deliveries, a straight correlation was observed, in developing countries, between the total LBW incidence (10 to 43%) and that of IUGR-LBW. In the large majority of cases the incidence of IUGR amounted to 70 to 90% of all LBW infants. By contrast, data from the developed populations, where the LBW incidence was 4 to 7%, showed opposite results. From these results it was concluded that when the incidence of LBW is greater than 10%, it is almost exclusively due to the increase of IUGR-LBW infants. Prematurity remains almost unchanged. When the LBW incidence is less than 10%, preterm infants represent the major component of LBW.

The results of the present study correspond with the above finding. The IUGR newborns

**Table 5**
**IUGR NEWBORNS, WITH AND WITHOUT**
**NONVIABLE MALFORMATIONS, BY**
**BIRTHWEIGHT AND GESTATIONAL AGE**

| Weeks | Birthweight (g) | Without nonviable malformations | | With nonviable malformations | |
|---|---|---|---|---|---|
| | | n | % | n | % |
| ≥37 | <2500 | 26 | 49.1 | 26 | 45.6 |
| ≥37 | ≥2500 | 15 | 28.3 | 15 | 26.3 |
| <37 | <2500 | 12 | 22.6 | 16 | 28.1 |
| Total | | 53 | 100 | 57 | 100 |

with a birthweight <2500 g, and a gestational age of >37 weeks, amount to only 31% of all LBW infants. This group is the most numerous in the developing countries but, in our series, as in other developed countries,[13] is less than half of all the IUGR newborns (Table 5). In the remainder, the newborns with a gestational age more than 37 weeks and birthweight 2500 to 2700 g, (predominantly males), equal the newborns with a gestational age <37 weeks and birthweight <2500 g.

The observed differences in IUGR, between developing and developed countries, closely corresponds with the differences in the two basic causes of IUGR. Thus, whereas in the developing countries, IUGR is predominantly induced by nutritional risk factors, (i.e., the main component of environmental conditions), in developed countries, the prevalence of these conditions is less, and biomedically related, nonnutritional risk factors, are of greater importance.

## VI. RISK FACTORS CONNECTED WITH IUGR

Several authors have identified different partial risk factors[14-19] for each of the two basic causes of IUGR. From the database of our series (Figure 1), 24 risk factors were chosen which are most frequently quoted in the literature in connection with the onset of IUGR (Table 6). In addition, each case was characterized by a further 14 items, out of which three concerned intervention during pregnancy and labor, and 11 related to different outcomes of the fetus and newborn. Each of the 38 items was further subdivided into two to nine variables.

Analysis of the importance of the 24 risk factors in IUGR was performed by calculation of a relative risk factor, (RR). For this purpose the IUGR group and the "nonrisk" plus "low-risk" group was used, and a comparison was made between the incidence of IUGR in the population *with* risk factors and the incidence of IUGR in the population *without* risk factors (Table 7).

The results show that only six risk factors had a RR of 1.4 and greater. If a RR of 2 and more is taken as the borderline of significance, then only three risk factors are significant, i.e., a small average weekly increase in maternal weight from the 13th to the 40th week of pregnancy, high and low age of the mother, and high and low maternal blood pressure.

As these risk factors are of a continual character, it was necessary to find a "cutoff" point at which the risk factor attains the highest RR. Surprisingly, this revealed that an initial maternal weight of ≤55 kg, and not of ≤50 kg, had a greater RR. The two other risk factors have two borderlines: a maternal age of 34 years and more, or of 18 years and less; and a systolic blood pressure 145 mm Hg and more, or of 105 mm Hg and less.

Whereas all the mentioned risk factors have a positive correlation with the occurrence of SFD, in women whose height is 170 cm and more IUGR occurs significantly less frequently, and the same results were observed also by Ounsted et al.[15]

## Table 6
## IDENTIFICATION OF RISK FACTORS RELATED TO
## IUGR

A. Maternal risk factors
  1. General history
    Age
    Parity
    Weight (preconceptional)
    Height
  2. Social
    Status
    Education
    Occupation
    Smoking
  3. Previous pregnancy
    Artificial abortion
    Spontaneous abortion
    Newborn <2500 g
  4. Diseases before pregnancy
    Diabetes mellitus
    Hypertension
    Menstrual cycle disorders
  5. Present pregnancy
    Time elapsed from the last
     pregnancy
    Weight gain
    Twins
    Breech presentation
    Placenta previa
    Premature separation of
     placenta
    1st trimester bleeding
    Anemia <10 g%
    Urinary tract infection
    EPH gestosis

B. Fetus-newborn-infant outcome
  Prepathological CTG
  Meconium in the amniotic fluid
  Birthweight
  Length
  Gestational age
  Apgar Score
    1 min
    5 min
    10 min
  NICU admission (d)
  Nonviable malformations
  Perinatal death
C. Antenatal actions
  Admission (more than 14 d)
  Labor induction
  Caesarean section

## Table 7
## RISK FACTORS AND A RELATIVE RISK (RR) GREATER THAN
## 1.4 IN IUGR BY SURVIVAL AND PERINATAL DEATH

| | | RR | | Incidence | |
|---|---|---|---|---|---|
| Risk factors | Cutoff points | + | − | Surviving n = 47 | Perin. death n = 6 |
| Parity | Primipara | 1.4 | — | 32 | 5 |
| Weight | ≤50 kg | 1.4 | — | 11 | 1 |
| (before pregnancy) | ≤55 kg | 1.6 | — | 25 | 5 |
| Weight gain 13—40 weeks | <0.25 kg/week | 2.3 | — | 5 | 2 |
| Age | ≥34 | 2.7 | — | 3 | 1 |
| | ≤18 | 3.0 | — | 4 | — |
| Blood Pressure | ≥145 90 mm Hg | 12.8 | — | 3 | 1 |
| | ≤105 | 1.6 | — | 22 | 2 |
| Height | ≥170 cm | — | 1.9 | — | — |

**Table 8**
**SENSITIVITY, SPECIFICITY, AND YOUDEN**
**INDEX FOR SOME OF THE RISK FACTORS**
**WITH A GREATER RR VALUE**

| Risk factors | Sensitivity (%) | Specificity (%) | Youden index |
|---|---|---|---|
| Primipara | 69.8 | 53.2 | 0.23 |
| Weight ≤55 kg | 56.6 | 67.9 | 0.25 |
| Blood pressure ≥145/90 | 7.6 | 99.5 | 0.07 |
| Weight gain | 14.1 | 95.1 | 0.09 |

To evaluate the importance of RR in the problem of SFD infants, it is important to know the incidence of RR factors in the general population. We have quoted this separately for surviving newborns, and those who died perinatally. Because of the small number of cases only the absolute values were shown.

The risk factors with a low RR have a relatively high incidence in the population. By contrast, the risk factors with a high RR have a relatively low incidence. Since only the risk factors with a high incidence and a relatively high RR are suitable for effective screening purposes, these results show that none of the mentioned risk factors can be used in this way.

This finding is even more objectively documented by the calculation of sensitivity and specificity for the mentioned risk factors, and their mutual correlation as expressed by the Youden index (Table 8). A risk factor suitable for screening must have a high sensitivity and specificity, and the Youden index a value of at least 0.50. The first two risk factors have a balanced but only average sensitivity and specificity, so that the Youden index attains only a half of the necessary value, corresponding to the lower borderline. Increased blood pressure, and small weight gain, have a high specificity, which means that when they occur the probability of IUGR is high. However, their incidence in the SFD group is very small. Therefore, these signs have a low sensitivity, and the value of the Youden index is also very low. Even in developed countries Ounsted et al.[15] comment, "The relative risks associated with pre-eclampsia were high, but because these pathological factors are fairly uncommon, their contribution for the SFD population as a whole is very small".

## VII. SCREENING OF IUGR

Since there is a possibility of a synergistic effect of some of the analyzed risk factors in the etiology of IUGR,[20,21] we tried to identify the "at risk" pregnant women by looking at combinations of risk factors in a multifactorial sequentional discriminant analysis. Unfortunately, this did not increase the value of the method when compared to the simple scoring system already described. In the developing countries, however, where some risk factors attain both a high RR and a high incidence in the population, it is possible to work out an effective scoring system for screening of IUGR. Risk factors related to nutritional defects provide a good example.

As risk factors do not provide an effective means of screening for IUGR even in developed countries, it seems that greater attention must be paid to new procedures which evaluate individual fetal parameters. Ultrasound is a simple, noninvasive method that does not inconvenience the woman, and is easily performed.

Only a few years ago, the detection of IUGR by means of ultrasound examination had a detection rate of about 50%.[22,23] By measurement of the trunk at liver level, which is a more efficient method of detecting IUGR,[24-27] ultrasound detection increased, so that it met the demands made on mass screening tests.[28,29] By using two-stage ultrasound examination

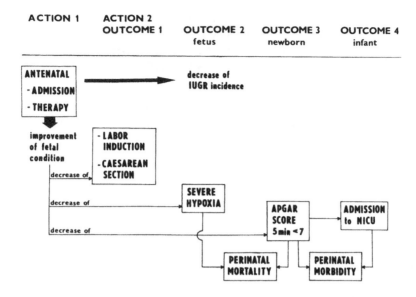

FIGURE 2.   Relationship between antenatal action (admission, labor induction, Caesarean section) and fetus-newborn-infant adverse outcome.

during early pregnancy, followed by measurement of fetal length from crown to rump, and estimation of the area of the fetal trunk during the third trimester, the sensitivity of the test increased to 94% with a specificity of 90%[30] (see Chapters 7 and 8).

## VIII. ANTENATAL ADMISSION OF IUGR

Without early detection of IUGR, timely and effective intervention, to promote improvement in the outcome of these cases, is not possible. If, however, we wish to search for an optimal intervention strategy, then precise data are needed concerning the different methods of antenatal treatment. (Such action is here defined as an antenatal admission for further fetal monitoring, and, as required, appropriate therapy, or elective delivery before the 40th gestational week). The correlation between antenatal action and fetal outcome is schematically shown in Figure 2.

Inability to diagnose IUGR has been one of the main reasons in the past for the infrequent use of antenatal action. More recently, retrospective studies of different types of antenatal actions, in postnatally verified IUGR cases, have been performed. The number of actions reported, however, varies between 6%[9] (i.e., 8 out of 129 cases) and 14%[23] (i.e., 31 out of 226 cases).

In the present study an analysis was performed separately for antenatal admission, induction of labor, and delivery by Caesarean section.

The effect of antenatal admission was studied only in patients hospitalized for 2 weeks or longer. According to the indication for hospitalization, three groups of surviving newborns were assessed: IUGR, imminent premature labor (without IUGR) and those hospitalized for other reasons. Each of these groups was further divided according to gestational age (Table 9).

The result of the analysis of these groups reveals that antenatal admission to hospitals occurs in 40% of subjects with IUGR and LBW without IUGR. This is nearly six times more often than occurs in the other group of newborns. However, whereas in the LBW without IUGR, hospitalization occurs prior to the 30th week of pregnancy in more than half, in the IUGR group, hospitalization occurs most frequently after the 36th week. When

**Table 9**
**ANTENATAL ADMISSION LONGER THAN 14 D IN 3
DIFFERENT SUBGROUPS, ACCORDING TO
GESTATIONAL AGE**

| n | Group of surviving newborns | | Weeks of gestation | | | |
| --- | --- | --- | --- | --- | --- | --- |
| | | | <28 | 28—36 | >37 | Total |
| 47 | IUGR | n% | 0 | 9 | 12 | 19 |
| | | | 0.0 | 19.1 | 25.6 | 40.4 |
| 69 | LBW without IUGR | n% | 17 | 11 | — | 28 |
| | | | 24.6 | 15.9 | — | 40.5 |
| 1847 | Others | n% | 70 | 47 | 13 | 131 |
| | | | 3.8 | 2.6 | 0.7 | 7.1 |

compared with the group of other newborns, hospitalization in the IUGR group is seven times more common between the 30th and 36th week of gestation and 36 times more frequent after the 37th week.

The high frequency of longer hospitalization for IUGR includes two different subgroups. In one of these, the indication for admission was chiefly preventive. This may explain, for example, why the incidence of the risk factor, "increased blood pressure", was smaller in the group of women with IUGR than in other studies. Also a lower incidence of hypertension may reflect the preventive effect of hospitalization, or, possibly, early delivery prior to the onset of the related signs.

## IX. ANTENATAL ACTION AND FETAL-NEWBORN-INFANT OUTCOME

The second, substantially greater of antenatal admissions, results from the early detection of IUGR. This group was examined in relation to different forms of prenatal treatment. The favorable result of antenatal admission, possibly related to therapy, can manifest itself in two ways: either by a decreased incidence of IUGR in the population, because of increased fetal growth, or, if the fetal weight remains within the limits for IUGR, by an improvement of the infant's intrauterine condition (e.g., metabolic, circulatory, etc.), cf. Figure 2.

Evidence of the beneficial effects of therapy upon the weight of growth retarded fetuses can be obtained in two ways: (1) by comparing the incidence of IUGR in treated and untreated groups, (preferably with a randomized study) and (2) by comparing the IUGR incidence in different studies using different types of antenatal action. This type of evaluation is influenced by numerous variables (e.g., defining IUGR, selecting patients, etc.).

In our study, most antenatal admissions for IUGR resulted in some form of therapy,[31] and a comparison of the treated and untreated group reveals a decrease in the incidence of IUGR by 1%.[32]

Neilson et al.[30] reported a study similar to ours. They used the fifth percentile to classify IUGR and a two-stage ultrasound examination to screen for IUGR. This resulted in a 25% antenatal admission of women with IUGR fetuses, (which is the biggest percentage in any of the studies we have examined). It is striking that between the incidence of IUGR (2.84%) in our series, (i.e., with long-term hospitalization and prenatal therapy) and IUGR incidence (3.76%) in Neilson's cases, (i.e., with a short-lasting hospitalization without any further therapy) there is again a difference of 1%. This is the same decrease we found when evaluating our antenatal action.

When antenatal action does not "cure" IUGR, other favorable effects may be reflected in an improvement of the IUGR outcome. The first indicator of a favorable effect is delivery prior to term by either induction of labor or, by Caesarean section. These actions usually

### Table 10
### PERINATAL MORBIDITY OF
### IUGR FETUSES AND THEIR
### RELATIVE RISK (RR) AND
### INCIDENCE

|  | | RR | Incidence (%) |
|---|---|---|---|
| 1. Intrapartal | | | |
| CTG Prepathology | | 6.0 | 20.9 |
| Pathology | | 4.7 | 27.9 |
| 2. Postpartal | | | |
| APGAR 5' | 1—5 | 8.7 | 4.3 |
|  | 6—7 | 2.7 | 19.1 |
| APGAR 10' | 1—6 | 12.8 | 6.4 |
|  | 7—8 | 6.3 | 17.0 |
| 3. Early neonatal | | | |
| Disorders of adaptation | | | |
| 2—3 d | | 29.8 | 14.9 |
| >3 d | | 17.0 | 8.5 |

result from deterioration of the intrauterine fetal condition. In our series the increased RR for labor induction (1.8) and in Caesarean section (7.3) in IUGR cases, favors the more frequent use of this antenatal action. If, however, we compare the incidence of both these antenatal actions in our series (21.4 and 23.4%) with those in the Neilson series (33 and 42%, respectively), then it is evident that the incidence of these actions is less in our series.

Turning now to the intrapartum, postpartum, and early neonatal outcome of the fetus with IUGR, cf. Figure 2, we observed a large RR and a large incidence of intrauterine hypoxia in IUGR, as based upon pathological or prepathological CTG tracings (Table 10). We were unable to find comparable data in other publications, which confirm only that in IUGR, intrauterine hypoxia occurs more frequently, as evidenced by a decreased Apgar score.[14] Neilson reports that a low value (i.e., less than 7 after 5 min) occurs three times more frequently (i.e., in 18% of all IUGR newborns) than in our series (6.4%). He also reports the incidence of Caesarean section is 30 to 42%. In our series it is 23%. We take these figures to bear witness to a better capability of the IUGR fetuses, in our series, to cope with the stress of uterine activity, and of the favorable effect of our intensive antenatal action.

On the basis of the analyses performed in the last part of this paper, it is possible to formulate the following intervention strategy, when IUGR is effectively detected antenatally:

1. Ensure long-term hospitalization, and employ the known effective therapeutic, and admit in the first half of the third trimester, or even at the end of the second trimester.
2. If possible, avoid delivery before the 34th week of gestation, thereby preventing the undesirable combination of IUGR and prematurity.
3. If necessary, deliver when fetal monitoring reveals deterioration, thus preventing the undesirable combination of intrauterine hypoxia and IUGR.

## REFERENCES

1. **Nishida, H., Sakamoto, S., and Sakanoue, M.,** New fetal growth curves for Japan, *Acta Paediatr. Scand.*, Suppl. 319, 62, 1985.
2. **Ounsted, M. and Ounsted, C.,** On fetal growth rate, in *Clinics in Developmental Medicine*, No. 46, Heinemann, London, 1973.

3. **Lubchenko, L. O. et al.,** Intrauterine growth as estimated from liveborn birth-weight data at 24 to 42 weeks of gestation, *Pediatrics,* 32, 793, 1963.

4. **Poláček, K.,** The small for dates neonate, in *High Risk Pregnancy* (in Czech), Štembera, Z., Poláček, K., and Vlach, V., Eds., Avicenum, Prague, 1979, 217.

5. **Karlberg, P., Niklasson, A., Ericson, A., Fryer, J. G., Hunt, R. G., Lawrence, C. J., and Munford, A. G.,** A metodology for evaluating size at birth, *Acta Paediatr. Scand.,* Suppl. 319, 26, 1985.

6. **Biering, G., Snaedal, G., Sigvaldason, H., Ragnarsson, J., and Geirsson, R. T.,** Size at birth in Iceland, *Acta Paediatr. Scand.,* Suppl. 319, 68, 1985.

7. Report of the FIGO Sub-Committee on Perinatal Epidemiology and Health Statistics, International Federation of Gynecology and Obstetrics (FIGO) Secretariat, London, 1986.

8. **Štembera, Z., Kovařik, J., and Jungmannová, Č.,** Frequency of fetal growth deviations diagnosed by ultrasonic measurement and analysis of their causes, *Acta Paediatr. Scand.,* Suppl. 319, 48, 1985.

9. **Hepburn, M. and Rosenberg, K.,** An audit on the detection and management of small-for-gestational age babies, *Br. J. Obstet. Gynaecol.,* 93, 212, 1986.

10. **Low, J. A. and Galbraith, R. S.,** Pregnancy characteristics of intrauterine growth retardation, *Obstet. Gynecol.,* 44, 122, 1974.

11. **Eggermont, E., Devlieger, H., Standaert, L., Dalasre-Van Hee, A. M., Snoel, L., Bhavani, S., and Jaeken, J.,** The neonate who is small for gestation age, in *Fetal Growth Retardation,* Van Assche, F. A., Robertson, B., and Liningstone, Ch., Eds., Edinburg, London, 1981, 90.

12. **Vilar, J. and Belizán, J. M.,** The relative contribution of prematurity and fetal growth retardation to low birth weight in developing and developed societies, *Am. J. Obstet. Gynecol.,* 98, 793, 1982.

13. **Metcoff, J.,** Maternal nutrition and fetal development, *Early Hum. Dev.,* 4, 99, 1980.

14. **Hedberg, E. and Holmdahl, P. K.,** On relationship between maternal health and intrauterine growth of the fetus, *Acta Obstet. Gynecol. Scand.,* 29, 225, 1970.

15. **Ounsted, M., Moar, V. A., and Scott, A.,** Risk factors associated with small-for-dates and large-for-dates infants, *Br. J. Obstet. Gynaecol.,* 92, 226, 1985.

16. **Rudolph, A. J.,** Failure to thrive in the perinatal period, *Acta Paediatr. Scand.,* Suppl. 319, 55, 1985.

17. **Naeye, R. L. and Tafari, N.,** Biologic bases for international fetal growth curves, *Acta Paediatr. Scand.,* Suppl. 319, 164, 1985.

18. **Peters, T. J., Golding, J., Butler, N. R., Fryer, J. G., Lawrence, C. J., and Chamberlain, G. V. P.,** Plus ca change: predictors of birthweight in two national studies, *Br. J. Obstet. Gynaecol.,* 90, 1040, 1983.

19. **Fedrick, J. and Adelstein, P.,** Factors associated with low birth weight of infants delivered at term, *Br. J. Obstet. Gynaecol.,* 85, 1, 1978.

20. **Butler, N. R. and Alberman, E. D.,** *Perinatal Problems,* Livingstone ES, Edinburg, 1969.

21. **Aickin, D. R., Duff, G. B., Evans, J. J., and Legge, M.,** Antenatal biochemical screening to predict low birthweight infants, *Br. J. Obstet. Gynaecol.,* 90, 129, 1983.

22. **Hal, M. H., Chang, P. K., Mac Gillivray, I.,** Is routine antenatal care worthwhile?, *Lancet,* 11, 78, 1980.

23. **Rosenberg, K., Grant, J. M., and Hepburn, M.,** Antenatal detection of growth retardation: actual practice in a large maternity hospital, *Br. J. Obstet. Gynaecol.,* 80, 12, 1982.

24. **Campbell, S. and Wilkin, D.,** Ultrasonic measurement of fetal abdomen circumference in the estimation of fetal weight, *Br. J. Obstet. Gynaecol.,* 82, 689, 1975.

25. **Wladimiroff, J. W., Bloemsa, C. A., and Wallenburg, H. C. S.,** Ultrasonic assessment of fetal head and body sizes in relation to normal and retarded fetal growth, *Am. J. Obstet. Gynecol.,* 131, 857, 1978.

26. **Warma, T. R., Taylor, H., and Bridges, C.,** Ultrasound assessment of fetal growth, *Br. J. Obstet. Gynaecol.,* 86, 623, 1979.

27. **Kurjak, A., Kirkinen, P., and Latin, V.,** Biometric and dynamic ultrasound assessment of small-for-dates infants: report of 260 cases, *Obstet. Gynecol.,* 56, 281, 1980.

28. **Wittmann, B. K., Robinson, H. P., Aitchison, T., and Fleming, J. E. E.,** The value of diagnostic ultrasound as a screening test for intrauterine growth retardation: comparison of nine parameters, *Am. J. Obstet. Gynecol.,* 134, 30, 1979.

29. **Warsof, S. L., Pearce, J. M., and Campbell, S.,** The present place of rutine ultrasound screening, *Clin. Obstet. Gynaecol,* 10, 445, 1983.

30. **Neilson, J. P., Munjanja, S. P., and Whirfield, C. R.,** Screening for small-for-dates fetuses: a controlled trial, *Br. Med. J.,* 289, 1179, 1984.

31. **Šabata, V.,** Die Therapie der intrauterinen Mangelernährung, *Gynakologe,* 17, 236, 1984.

32. **Šabata, V.,** Prenatal therapy of fetal growth-retardation by long-term glucose infusions. XII. Concluding considerations (in Czech), *Cesk. Gynekol.,* 48, 406, 1983.

Chapter 3

# THE PATHOPHYSIOLOGY OF INTRAUTERINE GROWTH RETARDATION

## I. R. McFadyen

## TABLE OF CONTENTS

## I. DEFINITION OF FETAL GROWTH RETARDATION

Fetal growth retardation describes the consequences of a complex pathology. The complexity lies not only in the processes involved but also in the different reasons for the disturbed growth. Some fetuses grow abnormally because their cells are deprived of nutrients, and some because they have a reduced number of cells. Inaccurate gestational age accounts for some being labeled "light-for-dates" when they are truly premature and in others the significance of physiological factors affecting birthweight have been ignored. Such differences have to be recognized before the underlying physiopathology can be reviewed. There is also another group of fetuses which is difficult to classify: those whose birthweight is within the normal range but whose growth has slowed insufficiently or too late for it to reduce the mass of fetal tissues by a clinically apparent amount. They may be recognized by abnormally rapid weight gain after delivery or other postnatal parameters, by ultrasound during pregnancy, or by abnormalities of cord blood constituents. The clinical significance of such occult growth retardation is not known. The consequences of the severe quantifiable variety are well established: stillbirth or fetal distress in labor, severe neonatal problems, and deficits in later development. The severely growth retarded are at risk for many types of physical or mental handicap.

Definition of growth-retarded fetuses as those whose birthweight is 2 standard deviations (2 SD) or more below the mean includes the lightest 2.3% of births. This is similar to the 2 to 3% incidence of severe growth retardation (runting) which occurs spontaneously in animals.[1,2] Many studies of human growth retardation include all with birthweights on or below the fifth centile. These babies are similar to those included in the 2 SD definition, but those between the fifth and tenth centiles are not. The group less than the fifth centile are significantly different from the remainder of the population, whereas the fifth to tenth centile resemble the general population. "Significance" here has both statistical and clinical meaning. Birthweight has a bimodal distribution with the lightest 2 to 5% being apparently different from the general population,[2,4] and they are different clinically. They are more likely than heavier babies to be delivered by mothers whose circulatory adjustments to pregnancy have been unphysiological,[5,6] to have severe abnormalities of umbilical artery flow,[7] to have low levels of blood glucose a few hours after delivery,[8] and to develop cerebral palsy or other problems.[9,10] Their increased hazard is not in doubt.

## II. GENERAL FACTORS AFFECTING FETAL GROWTH

Even if birthweight is accurately measured and recorded it cannot be given a centile value until it has been adjusted for gestational age and the other physiological factors which affect it: maternal size and parity, and the sex of the fetus. Tall and heavy mothers have heavier babies than do small and light women; first babies are lighter than subsequent ones; boys are 5% heavier than girls.[11] The ideal reference range has such adjustments available and has been constructed from the population into which the baby is born. Few populations have reference ranges of their own, and calculated adjustments for maternal height and the other variables are rare. The range constructed from data on 52,004 normal singleton pregnancies in Aberdeen women is, however, appropriate for most white European populations delivered between 32 and 41 weeks, and it comes complete with appropriate adjustments.[11] Other ranges are available for earlier delivery but they do not have adjustments. In deciding which range to use it is necessary to know the populations used for their construction. Mean birthweight falls by 100 g for each 1000 m[12] increase in altitude so data derived from births at 2000 m are not appropriate for use at sea level. Ethnicity also has a real effect: negro birthweights are greater than white at 34 to 35 weeks, but are lighter at term.[13] Hindu Indian mean birthweight at term is 150 g lighter than white or Muslim Indians even when allowance

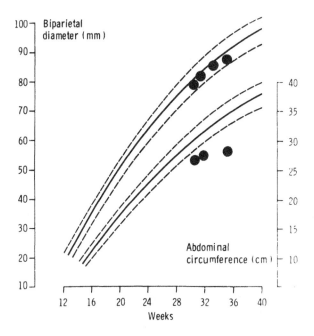

FIGURE 1.    This fetus shows asymmetric growth retardation in the ultrasound scan at 30 weeks. During the next 6 weeks the asymmetry becomes increasingly obvious due to the small increase in abdominal circumference while the biparietal diameter remains within the normal range. Delivered the day after the last scan at 36 weeks he weighed 1.68 kg.[22]

is made for the differences in maternal size.[14] Inbreeding, migration, and other variables affect birthweight and have to be taken into account for the most accurate assessment of weight at delivery, but even the roughest estimate is not possible without an accurate gestational age, preferably confirmed by an ultrasound examination early in pregnancy.

That fetal growth is retarded may be recognized in the second trimester.[15] Then and later it may be suspected because the uterus is small and the volume of liquor is reduced, or because the mother develops hypertension or some other abnormality of pregnancy associated with the fetus being born light for dates. This suspicion can be investigated with ultrasound. Measurement of the biparietal diameter, limb length, and abdominal circumference is the best available assessment of fetal growth, particularly if sequential observations are possible. It also permits separation of these fetuses into those with symmetrical or with asymmetrical retardation. Symmetrical retardation describes a small but correctly proportioned fetus, as is found in those with rubella, chromosome anomalies, or those with congenital heart disease.[16] Asymmetric growth occurs in natural runting,[17,18] animal models of fetal nutritional deprivation,[19] the undergrown fetuses of hypertensive mothers, and stillbirths with no obvious cause.[20,31] It occurs because growth of the brain, heart, and long bones continues normally for weeks after the liver, thymus, and other viscera have become measurably smaller than normal.[22,23] (Figure 1) The smaller the abdominal circumference relative to the biparietal diameter the more growth retarded is the fetus.

Many associations of disease with fetal growth retardation have been described. In some of these, such as the rubella-affected fetus, the underlying mechanism is known. In others, such as maternal hypertension or leprosy, the underlying pathology has been described in detail but the stimulus for this maldevelopment is not understood. There are, however, many fetuses whose growth is impaired without an obvious cause. Among all fetuses the variance in birthweight has been calculated to be 38% hereditary (18% fetal and 20% maternal), 6%

maternal health during pregnancy, and the remainder environmental or unknown.[24] The physiopathology of fetal growth retardation similarly involves the fetus, the placenta, the mother, or a combination of all of these.

## III. THE FETUS

Fetal growth rate is determined by several weeks. The cells have an intrinsic growth potential. The genes controlling this are different from those which determine final size and may operate differently in different ethnic groups.[25] Whether or not this potential is fully realized is determined by the health of the cell, by the supply of nutrients, and the use to which these are put. The nutrient supply is dependent on the fetal circulation as well as on placental transfer. The quality of the nutrients depends on the maternal diet, absorption, metabolism, and transfer. Competition by a sibling sharing the uterus and possibly the same circulation, also may affect growth.

### A. Cell Size, Number and Replication

Both the number and size of the cells may be reduced. This combination is not invariable. Cell number is smaller than normal in chromosomally abnormal fetuses, in some of these affect by viruses, and in some with congenital heart lesions, but the size of these cells may be normal or increased.[26] In mild fetal malnutrition cell size and number are little affected, but in severe malnutrition both are reduced.[27] While some of these differences are related to a restricted nutrient supply, others are due to disorders of cell replication.

Abnormalities of both autosomes and sex chromosomes affect cell division. In trisomies 18 and 21, the rate of replication is reduced.[28] Additional X chromosomes have the same effect, birthweight being reduced by 300 g for each additional X chromosome in the nucleus.[29] Any similar effect of the Y chromosome is not so well established, but XO cells divide more rapidly than normal.[30] This suggests that birthweight in Turner's syndrome might be increased but in fact it is reduced, probably because excessively rapid cell division disorganizes the patterns of fetal growth leading to a high rate of spontaneous abortion as well as to low birthweight among the survivors. Intrinsic hormonal deficiency is unlikely to be the cause of the growth deficit in these fetuses because they experience a growth spurt at puberty.[31]

The chromosomally abnormal are symmetrically growth-retarded fetuses.[32] The placenta, however, may be of normal weight despite having the same basic cellular structure as the light fetus.[33] This is in accord with the pregnanediol excretion in the maternal urine being normal even when oestrogen excretion is reduced.

Some viral infections affect cell replication. Chronic infection with the rubella virus slows cellular growth and the organs of these fetuses have reduced numbers of cells.[34] Not all viruses have such pronounced effects but cytomegalovirus may be more severe with cell death and an increased inflammatory response by the fetus.[35]

Chromosome breakage may occur in severe malnutrition,[36] in some inherited metabolic diseases, and in fetuses born to mothers addicted to heroin.[37] This also produces disordered replication and reduced fetal size.[38] The reduction in birthweight associated with inbreeding is probably also due in part to abnormalities of chromosomal function but these have not yet been identified.

### B. Nutrient Supply

The supply of oxygen to the fetus is maintained at an adequate level by adjustments in both maternal and fetal blood flow to the placenta even when there are wide variations in maternal blood concentration.[39] The uses the oxygen is put to are in general similar to that in adult but there are subtle differences.[40-42] It is used to metabolize fatty acids, ketone bodies, and lactic acid as well as glucose which is the principal fuel for the fetus. Although it is a less efficient way of releasing energy, the fetus metabolizes glucose to lactate rather than to $CO_2$. The lactate may be used in the hepatic synthesis of glycogen and fatty acids.

The fetus stores calories in the form of glycogen and fatty acids, particularly in the third trimester. These are synthesized from glucose, lactate, alanine, and other gluconeogenic amino acids in the liver, muscles, and elsewhere. The brain stores only glycogen but it can use effectively circulating ketone bodies as sources of energy. By term the largest stores are in the body fat. All of these sources of energy are required by the neonate because the enzymes required for gluconeogenesis are less active in the fetal than in the child's liver and do not mature until some time after delivery, which limits gluconeogenesis from amino acids. The advantage of this to the fetus is that amino acids are required for protein construction, and are best used for this. The fetus requires all of the amino acids which are essential for the adult, but also tyrosine and histidine, which must be provided by placental transfer because there is not an active cystathionase in the fetal metabolic system.

Other nutrients which the fetus requires are trace elements and vitamins. Anabolic activity is increased insulin, glucocorticoids, human placental lactogen, and other hormones. Drugs such as the β mimetics may also have some anabolic effects.[43]

The asymmetrically growth retarded fetus has not only reduced cell numbers but cellular activity is lower than normal.[44] Glycogen and fat stores are reduced. These effects are not equally severe in all organs: brain metabolism is preserved unless growth retardation is very severe. Slowing fetal growth slows the rate at which organs mature: they may catch up after delivery, but this is less likely if growth retardation starts before 26 weeks.[45] The fetal organs (particularly myocardium and brain) have a greater capacity to compensate for hypoxia than the adult: the younger the fetus the greater is the ability.[46] In severe hypoxia, hypoxanthine is released into the blood stream from breakdown of ATP and this can be used in the central nervous system to generate ATP.[47] Fetal blood levels of hypoxanthine and other products of ATP breakdown can be used to assess the severity of hypoxia which had existed before delivery.[48] The normal weight fetus may outgrow its energy supply before term[49] or in postmaturity.[50] Small fetuses also appear to be able to slow their growth rate, but they have little or no margin of safety. Even the normal healthy fetus may clamp down its metabolism to survive. The fetal temperature is about 1°C above the maternal yet it is "irreducible" ATP consumption is lower: possibly the effect of shunting thyroid hormone to an inactive form and the sedative effects of progesterone.[51,52] The energy charge in the fetal liver and brain are lower than in the placenta, so failure at this metabolic level will tend to occur earlier in the fetus than in the placenta.[50]

## C. Growth Factors

Growth hormone is not necessary for fetal growth. Anencephalic fetuses achieve a birthweight close to the mean even though their proportions are abnormal.[53] Insulin, however, is essential for normal growth.[54] It encourages transfer of amino acids into cells, and thus protein production, and it increases Krebs cycle activity which leads to fat deposition. Fetal insulin levels are raised in poorly controlled maternal diabetes because of the transfer of excessive quantities of glucose from mother to fetus which develops increased numbers of large cells leading to organomegaly as well as excessive quantities of adipose tissue. In growth retardation the islets of Langerhans are reduced in size[55] and the occasional fetus which totally lacks insulin is very markedly underweight.[56]

Human placental lactogen, prolactin, erythropoetin, and other hormones also are necessary for growth.

Somatomedin and other growth factors also are involved in fetal development. Somatomedin is the best characterized of these but epidermal growth factor and other generally or locally acting factors are relevant. The fetal liver, lungs, and other tissues synthesize somatomedin: it does not cross the placenta. Cord blood levels are directly related to birthweight, being low in the growth retarded.[57]

## D. Fetal Circulation

This shows both qualitative and quantitative differences between the normally grown and the growth retarded. In the former there is progressive reduction in peripheral vascular resistance as the placental villi develop and the fetus matures, slowing during the third trimester.[58,59] Near term about 55% of fetal aortic flow passes through the umbilical arteries while the remainder supplies the viscera and lower part of the body.[60] Umbilical venous flow is 60% to the liver with the remainder passing through the ductus venosus:[61] this is 75% of the blood flow to the liver, but 20% is from the portal vein and 5% via the hepatic artery.

In growth-retarded fetuses the peripheral resistance remains higher than normal. This is the result of raised vascular tone in the fetus, obliteration of placental tertiary stem villi,[62] and reduction in the feto-placental circulating volume, although the total body water in the fetus is not reduced.[63] Obvious consequences of these changes are the desquamating skin of the severely growth retarded and the thin umbilical cord from which it is difficult to obtain blood after delivery. Other results are a fall in umbilical flow and increased shunting of umbilical venous flow through the ductus venosus.[61] Although this reduces oxygen delivery to the liver and other organs they compensate by increasing oxygen extraction.[64] As the condition becomes more severe there is a linear fall in umbilical flow with decreasing oxygen tension.[65] There is also a marked reduction in umbilical and aortic flow due partly to changes in these vessels themselves and also the more marked alterations in the vessels downstream.[66-68] While most organs have (like the liver) reduced flow there is vasodilatation with increased flow in the brain, myocardium, and adrenals.[59,69] Surprisingly, the changes in aortic and umbilical flow are the same in chromosomally abnormal and in normal fetuses whose growth is reduced for other reasons.[70] They are, however, most marked in those fetuses who have the greatest problems in recovery after delivery.[71]

Circulating volume decreases, producing increases in total blood viscosity.[72] This does not affect fetal aortic flow, nor does viscosity at low shear rates (which reflects red cell aggregation and rouleaux formation). Viscosity at high shear rates (which is related to red cell rigidity) is, however, significantly associated with reduced flow in the umbilical artery.[73]

The fetal heart rate falls in normal but not in hypertensive pregnancy, which frequently is complicated by growth retardation.[74] In conditions of stress there are considerable differences in the cardiovascular reactions of the normal and of the undergrown, the principal being an even greater proportion of the combined ventricular output being directed to brain, heart, and adrenals with reduction in the umbilical flow: this possibly being a consequence of reduced catecholamine production by the stressed and decompensating fetus.[75]

The marked growth retardation and anaemia of one twin with a heavy plethoric sibling is associated with unbalanced flow to each.[76] Arteries rising from the umbilical arteries of the smaller communicate with veins running to the larger.[77] Not only does this lead to differences in weight and blood volume, but to differences in visceral weight and development. In extreme cases both fetuses may develop heart failure, but in other cases the smaller twin may die and the other have a normal haematocrit.

## E. Individual Organs

The altered circulation and nutrient supply lead to differences in weight and health of many organs.[78,79] Liver weight is reduced early and considerably: the greater the asymmetric growth retardation the relatively lighter the liver. Hepatic glycogen stores are reduced and development of enzymes may be reduced or delayed.[80] An even greater relative reduction in weight occurs in the thymus although this may be due as much to immunological exhaustion as to nutritional deprivation. Both the thymus and the kidney are histologically appropriate for gestational age but not for their weight. Renal weight also is reduced, as is urine formation, which reduces the fetal contribution to the amniotic fluid and leads to oligohydraminios.[81]

The myocardial weight is proportionately reduced only in the most severely affected cases, but there is reduction in its glycogen content which frequently is associated with marked fatty infiltration.[82,83] It is not surprising that growth retarded fetuses have increased intra-ventricular conduction time[84] and reduced heart rate variability.[85]

The myocardial fat deposition is a degenerative change, but subcutaneous fat shows the opposite trend. In those growth retarded from nutritional deprivation fat deposits are reduced in proportion to the severity of their condition, while those who have chromosomal or similar problems have normal amounts of subcutaneous fat.[86] The less the subcutaneous fat the lower is the neonatal blood glucose 4 h after delivery.

The last and least affected organ is the brain. Neuronal numbers and myelination are decreased if the organ is affected. Animal experiments suggest also that metabolism and function may be affected: these brains may be less able to utilize ketone bodies as sources of energy,[87] and neurotransmitter synthesis may be reduced.[88] There is not a uniform effect. The cerebrum has the least reduction in weight and the cerebellum the most. While myelination may catch up after delivery cell numbers cannot;[89] their deficit is permanent.

**F. Milieu Interieur**

The abnormalities of development and of function which are associated with asymmetric growth retardation alter the balance of the constituents of the blood and other extracellular fluids. The more severely the fetus is affected by nutritional deprivation the more deviated from the normal are these constituents. The hematocrit is raised but other changes are not directly related to this; all of them are due to effects of the underlying fetal ill health. Glycogen stores are low but the plasma levels of gluconeogenic aminoacids are raised because of the reduced capacity of the liver to use them.[90] The pH and $PO_2$ are low, and $PCO_2$ and lactate are high.[91] The reduction in variability of the fetal heart rate is partly due to this acidosis[85] which may be aggravated by labor so that clinically significant changes in the pattern of the fetal heart rate are more likely in the growth retarded.[92,93] Raised levels of the products of purine metabolism and other metabolic changes reflect the sickness of the individual,[94] and some affect his functions.

## IV. AMNIOTIC FLUID

The volume of amniotic fluid in the third trimester is directly related to fetal size.[95] In asymmetric IUGR it is, however, reduced to a greater extent than is the fetus. This is due partly to reduced formation of urine by the fetal kidneys; but there may be also reduced formation of fluid by the membranes or cord[96] which are likely themselves to be as unhealthy as the fetus since they are derived from the same tissues. The volume of fluid is reduced also in the growth retardation associated with renal agenesis or obstruction to the bladder outlet. Only if urine could escape through the urachus would fetal urine contribute to the amniotic fluid volume in urinary tract obstruction. Even in the absence of such a leak amniotic fluid is sometimes present so there must be other sources of its formation. These, however, appear to be as reduced as renal function since 83 to 89% of fetuses with oligo-hydramnios on ultrasound are below the tenth centile of birthweight.[97,98] The oligohydramnios has been blamed for "cord compression" patterns in antenatal cardiotocography associated with IUGR[99] but while this may contribute to the abnormal trace, the many fetal disturbances present are likely to be more significant.

## V. THE PLACENTA

The normally grown fetus is four times as heavy as its placenta at 32 weeks but 5 times as heavy at term.[100] The growth-retarded fetus has the same relationship by weight to its placenta.[101,102] If, however, the blood-free weight is measured,[103] or how close the fetus came to achieving its growth potential is assessed by measuring the size of its head or the length of its femur,[104] then many placentas are found to be lighter than would be expected from the fetal birthweight. Some placentas are heavier than expected: Down's fetuses have relatively heavy placentas.[33]

### A. Macroscopic Features

Two other macroscopic features of the placenta are relevant to retarded fetal growth: the presence of infarcts[105] and circumvallate formation.[106,107] In the latter the basal plate (from which the villi arise) is smaller than normal but this reduction is not by itself sufficient to account for its association with growth retardation; possibly there is defective development of the placental bed, but this has not been documented. Infarcts of the placenta also are associated with IUGR if they involve more than 10% of the placenta. Since the placenta has a functional reserve of 50% this relatively small reduction in its tissue would not be expected to affect the fetus unless the remainder of the placenta was also abnormal. Microscopic examination shows this to be true, although there may be areas of healthy tissue in some cases. The infarcts are a consequence of thrombosis probably in maternal spiral arteries which have not undergone physiological changes. This deficient adaptation is not confined to a part of the placental bed but is generalized so there are effects involving the whole placenta.

### B. Microscopic Description

Microscopic examination confirms that there are a number of differences between the placentas of normally grown fetuses and those of the growth retarded. In the normal placenta 78% of the tissue is active parenchyma, and the remainder is supporting stroma.[63,108] The placenta of the growth-retarded fetus, however, is only 67% parenchyma with a corresponding increase in stroma. This is accompanied by a reduction in both stem and villous capillaries with the greater reduction in the peripheral vessels. This may be due to obliteration of tertiary villi which are formed from 30 weeks,[70] but their deficiency may be determined earlier in pregnancy with a reduction in the formation of tertiary villi and their vasculature.[109-111] More subtle differences are revealed by electron microscopy. In a normal placenta each villus is covered with a multitude of microvilli. By the third trimester these increase the absorptive surface available 7 to 10 times.[112] This is maximal around 36 weeks and then decreases to term. In IUGR however, the number of microvilli is considerably reduced with a corresponding decrease in the transfer capabilities of the organ.[113,114] Other changes in the villi are due to reduction of blood flowing in the fetal capillaries and in the maternal spaces between them.[105,114] Clumps of syncitial villi protrude into the intervillous space (syncitial knots); the stroma of the villi and the stem arteries fibrose; areas of syncitial necrosis appear and these villi adhere to each other; fibrin is deposited in the intervillous space. These pathological changes are more marked if the IUGR is complicated by maternal hypertension. Fetal growth is, however, not affected unless more than 30% of villi are obliterated by fibrin, or more than 50% of villi are avascular.

The placental villi may be infiltrated by lymphocytes and histiocytes even if the membranes are intact. This "villitis" may be a consequence of infection with the rubella virus or other organisms but usually there is no reason to suspect such an aetiology. Such cases of idiopathic villitis are associated with symmetrical growth retardation.[115,116] The infiltration of the villi may reflect an immune reaction to maternal tissue,[117] but whatever the mechanism there is a direct relationship between lymphohystiocytic infiltration and IUGR.[118]

The number of cells in the placenta of a growth retarded fetus is less than in a normal organ but is appropriate for the reduced fetal weight unless the growth retardation is associated with severe congenital anomalies: these placentas have normal cell numbers.[119] The size of the cells is, however, normal in all IUGR placentas which suggests that cellular proliferation is arrested early but growth is not. Cell metabolism and chromosome content may also be different in IUGR. Although the fetus and placenta are formed from the same tissue the greater part forms the placenta so there is more chance of chromosome abnormality in it which could affect its growth than in the placenta of a normal fetus.[120] Metabolic changes are complex.

Placental metabolism involves both cell growth and metabolic function. Each of these requires oxygen, carbohydrate, and other nutrients but growth may account for up to 15% of the amino acids which it transfers.[121] In IUGR the synthetic capacity of individual cells may not be decreased,[119,122] but the whole organ's enzyme content[123] and oxygen consumption[124] are reduced. The production of most hormones and proteins is reduced, although this is partly due to reductions in fetal metabolism and some maternal functions. Pregnanediol, human placental lactogen, and some placental proteins do, however, reflect placental function. They are low in cases of intrauterine growth retardation.[125,126]

The many changes which occur in the placenta during pregnancy produce progressive alteration in its ultrasonic appearance.[127] This maturation advances more rapidly in IUGR. It is used to screen groups at risk and to identify those with or developing the problem.

## VI. THE MOTHER

Mother and conceptus meet in the intervillous space. There maternal blood is in direct contact with the placenta. The effect of this blood supply on fetal nutrition and growth depends not only on the feto-placental factors which have been discussed but on the volume of maternal blood perfusing the villi and on the content of that blood. These are related to how well the mother adapts to the pregnancy, to her general health, and to her environment. Multigravid women tend to adapt to pregnancy better than those in their first pregnancy but intercurrent illness, smoking, and age may modify adaptation at all parities as may immunological interaction between mother and fetus. If a multigravid woman has changed partners this may be the first pregnancy by the child's father so in some way she may respond like a primigravida.[128] There are also a few mothers who recurrently produce light-for-dates babies,[129,130] but others produce one in an otherwise normal sequence of birthweights. It is the balance of adaptation in all of the maternal systems which determines her contribution to fetal growth.

### A. Maternal Vessels

The blood vessels which undergo the greatest changes in pregnancy are the spiral arteries of the placental bed. In every pregnancy trophoblast invades the decidual portions of these vessels in the first 12 weeks and converts their musculo-elastic wall to a fibrous funnel-shaped structure which is an effective conduit for the increasing flow of maternal blood into the chorio-decidual space. In some pregnancies there is a second wave of trophoblastic invasion which extends down these vessels into their myometrial segments. This destroys the ability of the spiral arteries to respond to vasoactive stimuli and increases their capacity.[131,132] If this second wave of trophoblastic invasion does not occur the mother is more likely to develop pre-eclampsia and the fetus to be growth retarded.[133,134] Whether or not the spiral arterial physiological adaptation is adequate or not is reflected by the maternal serum uric acid: if trophoblastic invasion has been fully physiological the uric acid level remains below 300 mmol/l but if the invasion has been inadequate and does not involve the myometrial segment then the uric acid level is over 300 mmol/l by delivery, and in many cases has been greater than that for much of the pregnancy.[135]

Mothers who develop proteinuric hypertension in pregnancy may also develop acute atherosis in the spiral arteries. This is an accumulation of lipid-containing foam cells in the arterial wall which are the remains of myointimal cells which have been destroyed: fibrin is deposited in the vessel walls, and the vessel is surrounded by round cells. Acute atherosis is found in vessels which have not undergone physiological changes but although the more severe the proteinuric hypertension the more likely is the lesion to be found its presence is not associated with any greater reduction in mean birthweight than that found with a defective physiological response.[134]

The uterine arteries and its tributaries which lead to the spiral arteries also dilate in normal pregnancy: the diameter of the uterine arteries becomes three times the nonpregnant, of the arcuate arteries ten times, and of the spiral arteries thirty times. The ovarian arteries also dilate and provide a significant contribution to the uteroplacental circulation in 70% of pregnancies. Associated with IUGR, however, the increased capacity of the uterine and other arteries is not so great as in normal pregnancy and an increased proportion of aortic flow passes through the external iliac and gluteal arteries with less going to the uterine arteries via the internal iliac.[136]

Gravidity is relevant to uterine blood flow because a uterus which has previously contained a pregnancy is likely to be more profusely vascularized than one which has never been pregnant, with obvious beneficial effects for the conceptus.[137] Age also may affect the response of the vessels to pregnancy since they tend to become less flexible in those of 35 or more.[138] Thus a primigravid woman of 35 or more is less likely to have satisfactory adaptation of her vasculature. At any age anatomical abnormality of the uterine vessels is associated with poor reproductive performance: this is well documented among those who have two uterine arteries on one or both sides.[139]

## B. Circulating Volume

In a pregnancy with a normally grown fetus the maternal plasma volume increases by about 50% with possibly an additional 5% in the multigravid. The amount of this increase and birthweight are directly related.[140] The circulating hemoglobin also rises but not to the same extent so the concentration of hemoglobin falls. In a healthy woman who is not iron deficient the packed cell volume (PCV) falls from 37/38% in the first trimester to 32/34% at 32 weeks, and then rises again to term and may then be close to the early pregnancy value.[141] Among mothers who consume oral iron regularly during pregnancy the fall in PCV is less marked, usually by about 1%.[142]

In fetal growth retardation the increase in plasma volume may be only half that in a normal pregnancy although birthweight is not diminished by this amount.[143] The increase in plasma volume is least in those who have a history of recurrent abortion, unexplained stillbirth, or growth-retarded fetuses. Such "poor reproducers" show another difference from the rest of the population: the increase in plasma volume is not related to the nonpregnant value in the general population but in "poor reproducers" it tends to be.[144] Not unexpectedly then, poor fetal growth is related to a hemoglobin of 12 G% or over. The pattern of PCV change in IUGR also is different from the normal: it may not decrease by the expected amount or having fallen it may rise earlier or to a greater extent than would be expected. There is some evidence that bed rest does not increase the plasma volume but whether or not this happens may be related to how well the mother has adapted to the pregnancy in other ways.[145]

## C. Viscosity

If plasma volume expansion during pregnancy is less than normal but the red cell volume increases normally then plasma viscosity rises. This rise is not linear; the increase is exponential at high haematocrits. It is due not only to the increase in packed cell volume but also to the raised fibrinogen and tendency to rouleaux formation which occur in normal pregnancy and are greater in maternal hypertension.[146] The increased rigidity of the maternal red cell which is found in IUGR also contributes to the altered viscosity.[146,147] The consequence of this is not only reduced capillary flow but an increased tendency to thrombosis. A combination of maternal haemoglobin over 12 G% and a poor physiological response to pregnancy such as low weight gain or hypertension is associated with large placental infarcts and IUGR.[148] This may be a consequence not only of alteration in the circulation of the intervillous space but in the capillaries of the kidney and other organs.

## D. Clotting

Alteration of some hemostatic factors is found with IUGR which also predispose to thrombosis. The platelet count is reduced,[149] there is an increase in fibrin degradation products in some cases, but no change in soluble fibrin.[150,151] Although not directly related to the changes in viscosity the combination of increased viscosity with changes in coagulation increases the possibility of thrombosis in any vessel.

## E. Vasoactive Substances

The uterine and other maternal vessels respond to vasoactive substances produced locally or elsewhere in the body. The role of prostacyclin, thromboxane, the renin-angiotensin system, and of catecholamines is well documented in maternal hypertension which may lead to fetal growth retardation, but few data are available for idiopathic IUGR. Other humoral substances such as the atrial natriuretic peptide and the renal kallikrein system are almost certainly involved in cardiovascular control which may be modified to the detriment of fetal growth, but their roles are not clearly defined.

Prostacyclin is manufactured by the endothelium of the uterus and decidua where it produces local vasodilatation and has an antiaggregatory effect on platelets.[152] It is also produced by the kidney and other organs where it has the same actions. In normal pregnancy these effects on the vessels and coagulation are balanced by those of the vasoconstrictor and aggregatory protaglandin thromboxane. In pregnancy-induced hypertension (PIH), however, prostacyclin production is reduced so that the balance between it and thromboxane is upset which increases the possibility of vasoconstriction and thrombosis in small vessels.[153]

Prostacyclin also antagonizes the vasoconstrictive hormones angiotensin II (AII) and noradrenaline. In normal pregnancy this is effective but mothers who will develop PIH show an increased response to AII by 18 weeks, before their blood pressure rises.[154] The same is probably true of those who will have growth-retarded fetuses. Angiotensin II also has a sodium-retaining effect mediated through alosterone. In normal pregnancy this is balanced by the natriuretic action of progesterone.[155] The vasoconstrictive response to the catecholamines also is reduced in normal pregnancy but in PIH the uteroplacental vessels respond more actively than in the normotensive.[156] In a small number of women the tendency to thrombosis is aggravated by the presence of the lupus anticoagulant. This is an immunoglobulin found in systemic lupus erythematosis but also in ''poor reproducers''. It inhibits prostacyclin production and also predisposes to thrombosis by its action on the prothrombin system.[157]

One simple hypothesis which would integrate these observations is that an unsatisfactory physiological response by the mothers leads to reduced production by the uterine and placental bed of prostacyclin and other vasodilator substances such as $PGE_2$ (Figure 2). This exposes the spiral arteries which are still able to respond to vasoactive substances to these, and this may be aggravated by increased production of renin from the uterus. The effect on the placenta is to reduce the production of progesterone which increases sodium retention and thus aldosterone production further. This increases the tubular reabsorption of uric acid so the maternal serum level rises. Other factors would need to be taken into account for a complete theory but it is likely that the underlying vascular physiopathology has this basis. A comparable situation appears to exist on the other side of the placenta. Fetal prostacyclin levels are low in IUGR which will reduce circulation through the umbilical cord as well as having feto-placental effects.[158]

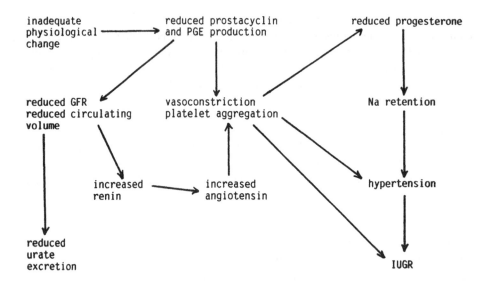

FIGURE 2.    Humoral control of vasomotor tone in normal pregnancy is maintained within the physiological range by the balance of a number of agents. The equilibrium between prostacyclin and thromboxane is a significant part of this mechanism. If prostacyclin production is reduced there is a relative increase in the vasoconstrictive effect of thromboxane, and an increased tendency to platelet aggregation. If the spiral arteries of the placental bed have not undergone a satisfactory physiological change during the pregnancy they are still able to respond to such vaso-active stimuli. That inadequate physiological change in these vessels is directly related to reduced prostacyclin production remains hypothetical.

## F. Blood Flow

Fetal weight is directly related to placental blood flow.[159,160] So is the extent to which the fetus achieves his growth potential: the greater the maternal flow to the placenta the heavier is the fetal liver in relation to the brain.[161] In normal human pregnancy uterine blood flow increases 20- to 30-fold between early pregnancy and term but in IUGR the increase may be only a quarter of this.[162] Both idiopathic growth retardation and maternal hypertension are associated with reduced flow and the effect of hypertension is increased if there is also proteinuria.[163] Flow is increased 10% by rest,[164] but exercise does not necessarily by itself reduce it. A healthy woman accustomed to exercise can maintain her uterine flow during exertion[165] but this may not be true if the fetus is on the border of being compromised.[166] The reduction in birthweight which occurs in women who have to toil during most of their pregnancy is a result of a combination of many factors: intercurrent infection probably being particularly relevant.

While the proportion of the cardiac output which passes through the maternal brain and kidneys falls during pregnancy the actual blood flow to them increases as the cardiac output increases. In normal pregnancy the glomerular filtration rate rises by 50% or more early in pregnancy and falls slowly to term. The increase in GFR is related to birthweight, but not only is the increase less in IUGR but the fall from mid-pregnancy is greater.[143] In a woman with healthy kidneys this is not a cause of growth retardation but is a reflection of her unsatisfactory response to the pregnancy.

## G. Blood Pressure

Birthweight has a variable relationship with maternal blood pressure. In mild pre-eclampsia without proteinuria the distribution of birthweight is the same as in a normotensive population.[167] In severe pre-eclampsia with proteinuria, however, mean birthweight is reduced in those delivered before term but not in those who reach or pass term: possibly because the severely affected start premature labor spontaneously or are delivered electively before term.[15,167-169] When birthweight is reduced the growth retardation tends to be asymmetric with growth of the head and increasing length of the body continuing after other organs have slowed or stopped. Essential hypertension also is associated with increasing birthweight.[170] The mechanism of increased birthweight is, in part, uterine blood flow which increases until a critical level of blood pressure is reached.[171] This level is around 90 mm Hg diastolic[172] but it is variable:[173,174] it depends on the degree of maternal adaptation to the pregnancy. Among those who have an apparently satisfactory adaptation (edema but no proteinuria) birthweight continues to rise until the diastolic blood pressure reaches 100 mm Hg. If proteinuria is present mean birthweight stops rising or falls when the diastolic pressure is above 85 to 90 mm Hg. The threshold is even lower among mothers who do not have edema or proteinuria, but who are thin and have little weight gain during the pregnancy: in them the critical level may be as low as 70 to 75 mm Hg.

Review of maternal blood volume change and the condition of her spiral arteries along with the level of blood pressure emphasizes the importance of physiological adaptation to birthweight. The heaviest babies are born to normotensive mothers with normal expansion of the blood volume whose spiral arteries have undergone physiological change. The most growth retarded are delivered by hypertensive mothers with proteinuria whose blood volume expansion is abnormal and whose spiral arteries have not adapted physiologically or have developed acute atherosis.[141]

Fetal growth may be retarded for some time before hypertension appears and the rise in blood pressure has been interpreted as a compensatory response to maintain placental flow. It could be mediated through the changes in circulating volume and electrolytes which also appear before the hypertension. If the spiral arteries have not, however, undergone physiological changes adequately they may constrict as the blood pressure rises with adverse effects on fetal nutrition.

## H. Nutrient Content of Blood

Acute deprivation of food for the mother reduced birthweight by the weight of the fetal subcutaneous fat: these babies are thin but of normal length.[175] Chronic deprivation of energy sources will reduce birthweight and the number of cells in the fetus and placenta, but only if the calorie intake is very low.[176] In most women, even those in Third World countries, the total supply of energy to the mother does not have a critical effect on birthweight.[177] Fat women have lighter babies than thin mothers of the same height.[178]

Individual constituents of the diet may affect birthweight, either directly or through metabolic consequences of their deficiency. Maternal levels of serine, lysine, and other amino acids are positively related to birthweight as is the level of carotene.[179] Vitamin D deficiency also may be related to IUGR.[180] Carbohydrate metabolism too may be relevant. Mothers who have a reduced rise in blood sugar in one or more values during a glucose tolerance test have a significantly increased probability of delivering a growth retarded fetus.[181] Other constituents of the diet can affect the availability of carbohydrate: bitter gourd (a vegetable used in Indian salads) reduces the rise in blood sugar for a given carbohydrate intake,[182] as do some fiber-rich foods.

The effects of diet on birthweight are complex. Vitamins, trace elements, the season of the year, the frequency of meals, and other factors are relevant to fetal growth. Transfer across the placenta of glucose stimulates increased fetal insulin secretion and thus increased growth. Amino acid transfer likewise stimulates fetal metabolism. Supply and stimulation are both necessary.

## I. Maternal Disease and Behavior

The chronic maternal diseases most likely to reduce fetal growth are the renal disorders. Renal disease without hypertension is associated with retardation of fetal growth, but the

**Table 1**
## MECHANISMS WHEREBY SMOKING MAY AFFECT BIRTHWEIGHT

| | | Ref. |
|---|---|---|
| Fetus | Increased blood carbon monoxide | 193 |
| | Increased blood thiocyanate | 194 |
| | Increased blood viscosity | 195 |
| | Thrombo cytopenia | 196 |
| | Increased heart rate and myocardial contractility | 197 |
| Umbilical cord | Thickening of vessel walls | 198 |
| | Reduced prostacyclin production | 199 |
| Placenta | Increased weight relative to fetus | 200 |
| | Increased fibrosis of villi | |
| | Decreased vascularization of villi | 201 |
| | Decreased microvilli | |
| Mother | Reduced intervillous blood flow | 202 |
| | Reduced expansion of plasma volume | 203 |
| | Increased blood carbon monoxide | |
| | Increased packed cell volume | 204 |
| | Increased viscosity — Buchan | 195 |
| | Increased thio cyanate | 206 |
| | Mean pregnancy length 1.5 d shortened | 205 |

*Note:* Maternal smoking during pregnancy reduces mean birthweight by 10—13 g for each cigarette smoked each day.[14,207] Growth retardation is symmetrical.[208-210] This is not a dietary effect as calorie intake is maintained.[210,211] If the mother stops smoking in the first trimester, birthweight is in the normal range.[212,213] If the father smokes but the mother does not, the reduction in birthweight is 66% of that of maternal smoking.[184] Many of the effects are directly related to the nicotine content of the cigarettes smoked.[214]

risk is increased if the blood pressure is raised.[169,182] The proportion of fetuses who are growth retarded is determined by the nature of the disease affecting the kidney.[169] With nephrosclerosis about 9% will have a birthweight below the tenth centile, but this rises to 39% if pre-eclampsia is superimposed: a combination of pre-eclampsia with glomerulonephritis raises the proportion further to 46%. Many other chronic or acute diseases which do not affect the fetus directly (as rubella and other infections) also retard fetal growth. Malaria and bacturiuria are two of the most frequent.

The maternal behavior which most commonly reduces fetal growth is smoking, not only by the mother but by those in her vicinity.[183,184] Passive smoking reduces birthweight. Since smoking wives frequently are married to smoking husbands, this is likely to be a truly familial risk factor. Some of the mechanisms whereby smoking may affect birthweight are shown in Table 1, but more general attributes of the mother are associated with the habit and may act synergistically with them. Smokers tend to drink more alcohol than others, to exhibit neurotic traits, to change husbands, to have a young menarche, and to have a higher rate of twinning.[183] Behavioral characteristics such as these are also associated with low educational attainment and social class which are themselves linked to fetal growth retardation. Nonattendance for antenatal care is more common which reduces the opportunities for detection of risk or actual IUGR.

## VII. WHY IS FETAL GROWTH RETARDED?

Fetal growth may be retarded by intrinsic cellular anomalies such as the trisomies or viral infection which affect replication. Abnormalities of cell metabolism also are associated with

IUGR. Major structural anomalies may be found in growth retarded fetuses but the mechanism underlying this frequently is not obvious. Nutrient supply is not a common deficiency either in total quantity or individual constituents. Drugs have been implicated but the disease for which they are given is as likely to be the cause of retarded growth. Only very occasionally intrinsic disease of the placenta lead to abnormalities of fetal growth.

Some observations are still unexplained. The IUGR associated with alcoholism and with living at altitude appear to be cause and effect. The former is dose related[188] and the latter is directly associated with the height above sea level.[12] Alcoholism may affect maternal and fetal metabolism, but altitude must have a more complex physiopathology than just reduced atmospheric oxygen. The feto-placental circulation can compensate for wide ranges of oxygen tension. Alterations in the pulmonary circulation, in blood pressure, in hemoglobin, and possibly in the normal adaptation to pregnancy would be possible contributory factors. It does not appear to be an ethnic effect since it occurs in any population at altitude. Ethnicity, however, does affect birthweight even when the possible effects of inbreeding, nutrition, maternal size, and other variables are accounted for.[14] This effect is an intrinsic parental effect, but migration may also alter mean birthweight and this must be an extrinsic environmental effect.[186]

Poor maternal adaptation to pregnancy accounts for many undergrown fetuses. While the mechanisms by which this leads to poor growth in utero have been described, the reason for the less than physiological changes in the mother frequently is obscure. In some it may be due to preexisting essential hypertension or to disease of the kidneys or other organs. Social class also is associated which may be relevant to nutrition and development in childhood as well as to events during the pregnancy. Many women, however, do not adapt to the pregnancy physiologically: this may have its basis in her immune reaction to the fetus.

The fetus and placenta contain paternal antigens and are therefore immunologically foreign to the mother. She develops antibodies to the trophoblast which prevent rejection of the pregnancy. If sufficient of these are not produced the more likely is the pregnancy to abort.[187] Contrary to this, the more active the reaction between mother and conceptus the heavier will the baby be at birth.[129,188] The first pregnancy is the initial challenge to the maternal immune system. Whether it ends in the birth of a live child or in abortion subsequent babies will, in the majority of women, be heavier than those born from a first conception.[189]

Reduction in the maternal immune reaction leads to retardation of fetal growth. Treatment of the mother with immunosuppressive drugs increases the proportion of light-for-dates births,[190] but there are also naturally occurring examples. Leprosy is one of these.[191] It occurs in two varieties: tuberculous in which there is a powerful cell-mediated response and lepromatous in which there is a poor response. Mothers with leprosy tend to have growth-retarded fetuses, but most of these are born to mothers with lepromatous disease. There also is a tendency for leprosy to deteriorate during pregnancy so possibly this is a paradigm for other infections. Bacteriuria and malaria frequently have exacerbations in the pregnant woman and are associated with IUGR which, at least in part, could have an immunological basis.[192]

Histological observations which support the hypothesis are villitis and the maternal placental bed reaction. In villitis failure of the immune response would allow attack of the placenta by maternal lymphocytes,[115-118] this lack of response is reflected in the relatively sparse infiltration of maternal cells around the spiral arteries when fetal growth is retarded.[134]

Maternal cells may enter the fetus spontaneously across the placenta or as an intrauterine transfusion. Most fetuses can cope with this. If, however, the mechanism is defective or if the immunological resemblance between the fetus and mother is so great that the fetus does not recognize her as foreign then severe IUGR is the result.[193]

All of this assumes that the father is the same for each pregnancy. Changing fathers may change the growth pattern. The incidence of another disease which possibly has an immunological basis, pre-eclamptic toxemia, alters if the father is a new challenge to the mother: she reverts to being a virtual primigravida. The situation with IUGR is not identical because there is not the same predominance of first pregnancies. Change of partners might, however, account for some of the growth retarded fetuses which appear in healthy multigravid mothers whose other children had normal birthweights.

Since retarded fetal growth is a description and not a diagnosis a single pathology would be unlikely. These fetuses are a heterogeneous group and reach their birthweight by a variety of routes. Ultrasound has shown that the most common of these are symmetric retardation from early in pregnancy and asymmetric when growth slows after 28 weeks. Bed rest or other factors may modify the pattern of growth but its basic form is established by the particular pathology which affects that pregnancy.

## REFERENCES

1. **Platt, H.,** Growth and maturity in the equine fetus, *J. R. Soc. Med.,* 71, 658, 1978.
2. **Wootton, R., Flecknell, P. A., Royston, J. P., and John, M.,** Intrauterine growth retardation detected in several species by non-normal birthweight distributions, *J. Reprod. Fertil.,* 69, 659, 1983.
3. **Royston, J. P., Flecknell, P. A., and Wootton, R.,** New evidence that the intrauterine growth-retarded piglet is a member of a discrete subpopulation, *Biol. Neonate.,* 42, 100, 1982.
4. **Wilcox, A. J. and Russell, I. T.,** Birthweight and perinatal mortality. I. On the frequency distribution of birthweight, *Int. J. Epidemiol.,* 12, 314, 1983.
5. **Brosens, I., Dixon, H. G., and Robertson, W. B.,** Fetal growth retardation and the arteries of the placental bed, *Br. J. Obstet. Gynaecol.,* 83, 656, 1977.
6. **McFadyen, I. R., Price, A. B., and Geirrson, R. T.,** The relation of birthweight to histological appearances in vessels of the placental bed, *Br. J. Obstet. Gynaecol.,* 93, 476, 1986.
7. **Nicolini, U.,** personal communication, 1987.
8. **Haworth, J. C., Dilling, L., and Younoszai, M. K.,** Relation of blood-glucose to haematocrit, birthweight and other body measurements in normal and growth retarded newborn infants, *Lancet,* 2, 901, 1967.
9. **Usher, R. H. and McLean, F. H.,** Normal fetal growth and the significance of fetal growth retardation, in *Scientific Foundation of Paediatrics,* David, J. A. and Dobbing, J., Eds., Heinemann, London, 1974, 69.
10. **Hagberg, G.,** Children with IQs of 50—70, in *Major Mental Handicap: Methods and Costs of Prevention,* Ciba Foundation Symposium, Elsevier Excerpta Medica, Amsterdam, 1978, 211.
11. **Thompson, A. M., Billewicz, W. Z., and Hytten, F. E.,** The assessment of fetal growth, *Br. J. Obstet. Gynaecol.,* 75, 903, 1968.
12. **McCullough, R. E., Reeves, J. T., and Lilijegren, R. L.,** Fetal growth retardation and increased fetal mortality at high altitude, *Arch. Environ. Health,* 32, 36, 1977.
13. **Fujikura, T. and Froehlich, L. A.,** Birth weight, gestational age, and renal glomerular development as indices of fetal maturity, *Am. J. Obstet. Gynaecol.,* 113, 627, 1972.
14. **McFadyen, I. R., Campbell Brown, M., Abraham, R., North, W. R. S., and Haines, A. P.,** Factors affecting birthweight in Hindus, Moslems and Europeans, *Br. J. Obstet. Gynaecol.,* 91, 968, 1984.
15. **Page, E. W. and Christianson, M. A.,** The impact of mean arterial pressure in the middle trimester upon outcome of pregnancy, *Am. J. Obstet. Gynecol.,* 125, 740, 1976.
16. **Naeye, R. L.,** Anatomic features of growth failure in congenital heart disease, *Paediatrics,* 39, 433, 1967.
17. **Verges, J. B.,** Physiological factors affecting birth weight, *Proc. Nutr. Soc. Yearb.,* Suffolk Sheep Society, Ipswich, quoted by Hammond. J., 1944, 2, 1939, 8.
18. **Widdowson, E. R.,** Intrauterine growth retardation in the pig. I. Organ size and cellular development at birth and after growth to maturity, *Biol. Neonate,* 19, 329, 1971.
19. **Myers, R. E., Hill, D. E., Holt, A. B., Scott, R. E., Mellits, E. D., and Cheek, D. B.,** Fetal growth retardation produced by experimental placental insufficiency in the rhesus monkey, *Biol. Neonate.,* 18, 379, 1971.
20. **Gruenwald, P.,** Chronic fetal distress and placental insufficiency, *Biol. Neonate,* 5, 215, 1963.
21. **Naeye, R. L.,** Abnormalities in infants of mothers with toxemia of pregnancy, *Am. J. Obstet. Gynecol.,* 95, 276, 1966.

22. **Meire, H. B., Farrant, P., and McFadyen, I. R.,** Measurement of fetal growth by ultrasound, *Br. Congr. Obstet. Gynaecol.,* Sheffield, Royal College of Obstetricians, 1977, 197.
23. **Campbell, S. and Thomas, A.,** Ultrasound measurement of the fetal head to abdomen ration in the assessment of growth retardation, *Br. J. Obstet. Gynaecol.,* 84, 165, 1977.
24. **Penrose, L. S.,** Some recent trends in human genetics, *Caryologia,* Suppl. 6, 521, 1954.
25. **Roberts, D. F.,** Genetics of growth, *Br. Med. Bull.,* 37, 239, 1981.
26. **Naeye, R. L.,** Cardiovascular abnormalities in infants malnourished before birth, *Biol. Neonate,* 8, 104, 1965.
27. **Naeye, R. L.,** Infants of prolonged gestation, a necropsy study, *Arch. Pathol.,* 84, 37, 1967.
28. **Paton, G. R., Silver, M. F., and Allison, A. C.,** Comparison of cell cycle time in normal and trisomic cells, *Hum. Genet.,* 23, 173, 1974.
29. **Barlow, P.,** The influence of inactive chromosomes on human development. Anomalous sex chromosome complements and the phenotype, *Hum. Genet.,* 17, 105, 1973.
30. **Barlow, P. W.,** Differential cell division in human x-chromosome mosaics, *Hum. Genet.,* 14, 122, 1972.
31. **Lemli, L. and Smith, D. W.,** The XO syndrome: a study of the differential phenotype in 25 patients, *J. Paediatr.,* 63, 577, 1963.
32. **Smith, A. and McKeown, T.,** Pre-natal growth of mongoloid defectives, *Arch. Dis. Child,* 30, 257, 1955.
33. **Matsunaga, E. and Tonomura, A.,** Parental age and birthweight in translocation Down's syndrome, *Ann. Hum. Genet.,* 36, 209, 1972.
34. **Naeye, R. L. and Blanc, W.,** Pathogenesis of congenital rubella, *J. Am. Med. Assoc.,* 194, 1277, 1965.
35. **Knox, G. E.,** Influence of infection on fetal growth and development, *J. Reprod. Med.,* 21, 352, 1978.
36. **Betancourt, M., de la Roca, J. M., Saenz, M. E., Diaz, R., and Cravioto, J.,** Chromosome aberrations in protein — calorie malnutrition, *Lancet,* 1, 168, 1974.
37. **Abrams, C. and Liao, P. Y.,** Chromosomal aberrations in newborns exposed to heroin *in utero, J. Clin. Invest.,* 51, 10, 1972.
38. **Naeye, R. L., Blanc, W., Leblanc, W., and Khatamee, M. A.,** Fetal complications of maternal heroin addiction. Abnormal growth, infections and episodes of stress, *J. Paediatr.,* 83, 1055, 1973.
39. **Edelstone, D. T., Caine, M. E., and Fumia, F. D.,** Relationship of fetal oxygen consumption and acid-base balance to fetal hematocrit, *Am. J. Obstet. Gynecol.,* 151, 844, 1985.
40. **Hahn, P.,** Nutrition and metabolic development in mammals, in *Human Nutrition.* I Nutrition pre and postnatal development, Winick, M., Ed., Plenum Press, New York, 1979, 1.
41. **Jones, C. T. and Rolph, T. P.,** Metabolic events associated with the preparation of the fetus for independent life, in *The Fetus and Independent Life, CIBA Foundation Symposium '86,* Elliott, K. and Whelan, J., Eds., Pitman Publishing, London, 1981, 214.
42. **Kimura, R. E. and Warshaw, J. B.,** Metabolism during development, in *The Biological Basis of Reproductive and Development Medicine,* Warshaw, J., Ed., Edward Arnold, London, 1983, 337.
43. **Wager, J., Fredholm, B. B., Lunell, N. O., and Pearson, B.,** Development of tolerance to oral salbutamol in the third trimester of pregnany: a study of circulatory and metabolic effects, *Br. J. Clin. Pharmacol.,* 12, 489, 1981.
44. **Schrader, R. E. and Zeman, F. J.,** Effect of maternal protein deprivation on morphological and enzymatic development of neonatal rat tissue, *J. Nutr.,* 99, 401, 1969.
45. **Wladimiroff, J. W., Bloemsma, C. A., and Wallenburg, H. C. S.,** Ultrasonic assessment of fetal head and body sizes in relation to normal and retarded fetal growth, *Am. J. Obstet. Gynecol.,* 131, 857, 1978.
46. **Friedman, W. F. and Kirkpatrick, S. E.,** Fetal cardiovascular adaptation to asphyxia in intrauterine asphyxia and the developing human brain, Gluck, L., Ed., Year Book Medical Publishers, Chicago, 1977, 149.
47. **Wallenburg, H. C. and Van Kreel, B. K.,** Maternal and umbilical plasma concentrations of uric acid and oxypurines at delivery in normal and hypertensive pregnancy, *Arch. Gynecol.,* 229, 7, 1980.
48. **Harkness, R. A., Giersson, R. T., and McFadyen, I. R.,** Concentrations of hypoxanthine, xanthine, uridine and urate in amniotic fluid at Caesarean section and the association of raised levels with prenatal risk factors and fetal distress, *Br. J. Obstet. Gynaecol.,* 90, 815, 1983.
49. **Trudinger, B. J., Giles, W. B., Cook, C. M., Bombardieri, J., and Collins, L.,** Fetal umbilical artery flow velocity waveforms and placental resistance: clinical significance, *Br. J. Obstet. Gynaecol.,* 92, 23, 1985.
50. **Harkness, R. A., Cotes, P. M., Gordon, H., McWhinney, N., and Sarkar, P.,** Prolonged pregnancy and fetal energy supply, amniotic fluid concentrations of erythropoieth hypoxanthine, xanthine and uridine at the induction of labor in prolonged uncomplicated pregnancy, *J. Obstet. Gynecol.,* 8, 235, 1988.
51. **Crenshaw, M. C., Meschia, G., and Barron, D. H.,** Role of progesterone in inhibition of muscle tone and respiratory rhythm in foetal lambs, *Nature (London),* 212, 842, 1966.
52. **Harkness, R. A., Coade, S. B., Simmonds, R. J., and Duffy, S.,** Effect of a failure of energy supply on adenial nucleotide breakdown in placentae and other fetal tissues from rat and guinea pig, *Placenta,* 6, 199, 1985.

53. **Honnebier, W. J. and Swaab, D. F.**, The influence of anencephaly upon intrauterine growth of fetus and placenta and upon gestation length, *Br. J. Obstet. Gynaecol.*, 80, 577, 1973.

54. **Cheek, D. B. and Hill, D. E.**, Changes in somatic growth after ablation of maternal or fetal pancreatic beta cells in fetal and postnatal cellular growth. Check, D. B., Ed., John Wiley & Sons, New York, 1975, 311.

55. **De Prins, F. A. and Van Assche, F. A.**, Intrauterine growth retardation and development of the endocrine pancreas in the experimental rat, *Biol. Neonate*, 41, 16, 1982.

56. **Sherwood, W. C., Chance, G. W., and Hill, D. E.**, A new syndrome of pancreatic agenesis. The role of insulin and glucagon in somatic and cell growth, *Pediatr. Res.*, 8, 360, 1974.

57. **Foley, T. P., De Philip, R., Perricelli, A., and Miller, A.**, Low somatomedin activity in cord serum from infants with intrauterine growth retardation, *J. Pediatr.*, 96, 605, 1980.

58. **Marsal, K., Eik-Nes, S. H., Lindblad, A., and Lingman, G.**, Blood flow in the fetal descending aorta. Intrinsic factors affecting fetal blood flow, *Ultrasound Med. Biol.*, 10, 339, 1984.

59. **Wladimiroff, J. W., Tonge, H. M., and Stewart, P. A.**, Doppler ultrasound assessment of cerebral blood flow in the human fetus, *Br. J. Obstet. Gynaecol.*, 93, 471, 1986.

60. **Wladimiroff, J. W. and McGhie, J.**, Ultrasonic assessment of cardiovascular geometry and function in the human fetus, *Br.J. Obstet. Gynaecol.*, 88, 870, 1981.

61. **Creasy, R. K., de Sweit, M., Kahanpaa, K. V., Young, W. D., and Rudolph, A.**, Pathophysiological changes in the fetal lamb with growth retardation in foetal and neonatal physiology, in *Proc. Sir Joseph Barcroft Centenary Symp.*, Cambridge University Press, Cambridge, 1973, 641.

62. **Giles, W. B., Trudinger, B. J., and Baird, P. J.**, Fetal umbilical artery flow velocity waveforms and placental resistance: pathological correlation, *Br. J. Obstet. Gynaecol.*, 92, 31, 1985.

63. **Cassady, G. and Milstead, R. R.**, Antipyrinc space studies and cell water estimates in infants of low birth weight, *Paediatr. Res.*, 5, 573, 1971.

64. **Edelstone, D. I., Paulone, M. E., and Holzman, I. R.**, Hepatic oxygenation during arterial hypoxemia in neonatal lambs, *Am. J. Obstet. Gynecol.*, 150, 513, 1984.

65. **Soothill, P. W., Nicolaides, K. H., Bilardo, C. M., and Campbell, S.**, Relation of fetal hypoxia in growth retardation to mean blood velocity in the fetal aorta, *Lancet*, 2, 1118, 1986.

66. **Stuart, B., Drumm, J., Fitzgerald, D. E., and Duignan, N. U.**, Fetal blood velocity waveforms in normal pregnancy, *Br. J. Obstet. Gynaecol.*, 87, 780, 1980.

67. **Griffin, D., Bilardo, K., and Masini, L.**, Doppler blood flow waveforms in the descending thoracic aorta of the human fetus, *Br. J. Obstet. Gynaecol.*, 91, 997, 1984.

68. **Joupilla, P. and Kirkinen, P.**, Umbilical vein blood flow in the human fetus in cases of maternal and fetal anaemia and uterine bleeding, *Ultrasound Med. Biol.*, 10, 365, 1984.

69. **Fan, F. C., Chen, R. Y. Z., Schuessler, G. B., and Chien, S.**, Effects of hematocrit variations on regional hemodynamics and oxygen transport in the dog, *Am. J. Physiol.*, 238, H545, 1980.

70. **Trudinger, B. J. and Cook, C. M.**, Flow velocity waveforms in the maternal uteroplacental and fetal umbilical placental circulation, *Am. J. Obstet. Gynecol.*, 152, 155, 1985.

71. **McGowan, L. M., Erskine, L. A., and Ritchie, K.**, Umbilical artery Doppler blood flow studies in the preterm, small for gestational age fetus, *Am. J. Obstet. Gynecol.*, 156, 655, 1987.

72. **Thorburn, J., Drummond, M. M., Whigham, K. A., Lowe, G. D. O., Forbes, C. D., Prentice, C. R. M., and Whitfield, C. R.**, Blood viscosity and haemostatic factors in late pregnancy, pre-eclampsia and fetal growth retardation, *Br. J. Obstet. Gynaecol.*, 89, 117, 1982.

73. **Giles, W. B. and Trudinger, B. J.**, Umbilical cord whole blood viscosity and the umbilical artery flow velocity time waveforms: a correlation, *Br. J. Obstet. Gynaecol.*, 93, 466, 1986.

74. **Dawson, A. J., Dalton, K. J., and Newcombe, R. G.**, Baseline fetal heart rates from 15 to 38 weeks gestation in normotensive and hypertensive pregnancies, *Br. J. Obstet. Gynaecol.*, 92, 60, 1985.

75. **Block, R. S. B., Llanos, A. J., and Creasy, R. K.**, Responses of the growth retarded fetus to acute hypoxemia, *Am. J. Obstet. Gynecol.*, 148, 878, 1984.

76. **Erskine, R. L. A., Ritchie, J. W. K., and Murnaghan, G. A.**, Antenatal diagnosis of placental anastomasis in a twin pregnancy using Doppler ultrasound, *Br. J. Obstet. Gynaecol.*, 93, 955, 1986.

77. **Arts, N. F. and Lohman, A. H. M.**, The vascular anatomy of monochorionic twin placentas and the transfusion syndrome, *Eur. J. Obstet. Gynecol.*, 3, 85, 1971.

78. **Morison, J. E.**, *Multiple Births in Foetal and Neonatal Pathology*, 3rd ed., Butterworths, London, 1970, 184.

79. **Gruenwald, P.**, Chronic fetal distress and placental insufficiency, *Biol. Neonate*, 5, 215, 1963.

80. **Nitzam, M. and Groffman, H.**, Hepatic gluconeogenesis and lipogenesis in experimental intrauterine growth retardation in the rat, *Am. J. Obstet. Gynecol.*, 109, 623, 1971.

81. **Wladimiroff, J. W. and Campbell, S.**, Fetal urine production rates in normal and complicated pregnancy, *Lancet*, 1, 151, 1974.

82. **Scott, J. M.**, Fatty change in the myocardium of the newborn, *Br. Med. J.*, 2, 1746, 1961.

83. **Shelfey, H. J.**, Carbohydrate reserves in the newborn infant, *Br. Med. J.*, 1, 273, 1964.
84. **Brambati, B. and Bonsignore, L.**, Intraventricular conduction time in fetuses born with growth retardation, *Br. J. Obstet. Gynaecol.*, 89, 900, 1985.
85. **Henson, G., Dawes, G. S., and Redman, C. W. G.**, Characterization of the reduced heart rate variation in growth retarded fetuses, *Br. J. Obstet. Gynaecol.*, 91, 751, 1984.
86. **Whitelaw, A.**, Subcutaneous fat measurement an indication of nutrition of the fetus and newborn, in *Nutrition and Metabolism of the Fetus and Infant*, Visser, H. K. A., Ed., Martinus Nyhoff, The Hague, Boston, 1979, 131.
87. **Dahlquist, G.**, Cerebral utilization of glucose ketone bodies, and oxygen in starving infant rats and the effect of intrauterine growth retardation, *Acta Physiol. Scand.*, 98, 237, 1976.
88. **Cohen, E. L. and Wurtman, R. J.**, Nutrition and brain neurotransmitter, in *Nutrition: Pre- and Postnatal Development*, Winick, M., Ed., Plenum Press, New York, 1979, chap. 7.
89. **Brandt, T.**, Brain growth fetal malnutrition and clinical consequences, *J. Perinat. Med.*, 9, 3, 1981.
90. **Mestyan, J., Soltesz, G., Schultz, K., and Horvath, M.**, Hyperaminoacidemia due to the accumulation of gluconeogenic amino acid precursors in hypo-glycemic small-for-gestational age infants, *J. Pediatr.*, 87(3), 409, 1975.
91. **Soothill, P. W., Nicolaides, K. H., and Campbell, S.**, Prenatal asphyxia, hyperlacticaemia, hypoglycaemia, and erythroblastosis in growth retarded fetuses, *Br. Med. J.*, 294, 1051, 1987.
92. **Lin, C. C., Moawad, A. H., Rosenow, P. J., and River, P.**, Acid-base characteristics of fetuses with intrauterine growth retardation during labor and delivery, *Am. J. Obstet. Gynecol.*, 137, 553, 1980.
93. **Low, J. A., Galbraith, R. S., Muir, D., Killen, H., Karchar, J., and Campbell, D.**, Intrauterine growth retardation. A preliminary report of long-term morbidity, *Am. J. Obstet. Gynecol.*, 130, 534, 1978.
94. **Harkness, R. A.**, Clinical biochemistry of the perinatal period: immaturity, hypoxia and metabolic disease, *J. Clin. Pathol.*, 40, 1128, 1987.
95. **Kurjak, A., Kirkinen, P., Latin, V., and Ivankovic, D.**, Ultrasonic assessment of fetal kidney function in normal and complicated pregnancies, *Am. J. Obstet. Gynecol.*, 141, 266, 1981.
96. **Van Otterlo, L. C., Wladimiroff, J. W., and Wallenburg, H. C. S.**, Relationship between fetal urine production and amniotic fluid volume in normal pregnancy and pregnancy complicated by diabetes, *Br. J. Obstet. Gynaecol.*, 84, 205, 1977.
97. **Manning, F. A., Hill, L. M., and Platt, L. D.**, Qualitative amniotic fluid volume determination by ultrasound: antepartum detection of intrauterine growth retardation, *Am. J. Obstet. Gynecol.*, 139, 254, 1981.
98. **Philipson, E. H., Sokol, R. J., and Williams, T.**, Oligohydramnios: clinical associations and predictive value of intrauterine growth retardation, *Am. J. Obstet. Gynecol.*, 146, 271, 1983.
99. **Druzin, M. L., Gratacos, J., Keegan, K. A., and Paul, R. H.**, Antepartum fetal heart rate testing. VII. The significance of bradycardia, *Am. J. Obstet. Gynecol.*, 139, 194, 1981.
100. **Abramovich, D. R.**, The weight of placenta and membranes in early pregnancy, *J. Obstet. Gynaecol. Br. Commonw.*, 76, 523, 1969.
101. **Molteni, R. A., Stys, S. J., and Battaglia, F. C.**, Relationship of fetal and placental weight in human beings. Fetal/placental weight ratios at various gestational ages and birthweight distributions, *J. Reprod. Med.*, 21, 327, 1978.
102. **Teasdale, F.**, Histomorphometry of the human placenta in maternal pre-eclampsia, *Am. J. Obstet. Gynceol.*, 152, 25, 1985.
103. **Garrow, J. S.**, The relationship of fetal growth to size and composition of the placenta, *Proc. R. Soc. Med.*, 63, 498, 1970.
104. **Woods, D. L. and Malan, A. F.**, Placental size of small-for-gestational age infants at term, *Early Hum. Dev.*, 7, 11, 1982.
105. **Fox, H.**, Villous immaturity in the term placenta, *Obstet. Gynaecol.*, 31, 9, 1968.
106. **Fox, H. and Sen, D. K.**, Placenta extrachorialis: a clinico-pathological study, *J. Obstet. Gynaecol. Br Commonw.*, 79, 32, 1972.
107. **Rolschau, J.**, Circumvallate placenta and intrauterine growth retardation, *Acta Obstet. Gynecol. Scand.*, Suppl. 72, 11, 1978.
108. **Aherne, W.**, Morphometry in the placenta and its maternal supply line, P. Gruenwald, Medical and Technical Publishing Co. Ltd., Lancaster, 1975, 80.
109. **Becker, V.**, *Abnormal Maturation of the Villi in the Placenta and its Maternal Supply Line*, Gruenwald Pediatric Medical and Technical Publishing, Lancaster, 1975, 232.
110. **Teasdale, F.**, Idiopathic intrauterine growth retardation: histomorphometry of the human placenta, *Placenta*, 5, 83, 1984.
111. **Lee, M. M. L. and Yeh, M.**, Fetal microcirculation of abnormal human placenta. I. Scanning electron microscopy of placental vascular casts from small-for-gestational age fetus, *Am. J. Obstet. Gynecol.*, 154, 1133, 1986.

112. **Teasdale, F. and Jean-Jacques, G.,** Morphometric evaluation of the microvillous surface enlargement factor in the human placenta from mid-gestation to term, *Placenta*, 6, 375, 1985.

113. **Lister, U. M.,** *Ultrastructure of the Human Placenta in Modern Trends in Obstetrics*, 4, ed., Kellar, R. J., Ed., Butterworths, London, 1969, 26.

114. **Van der Veen, F. and Fox, H.,** The human placenta in idiopathic intrauterine growth retardation: a light and electron microscopic study, *Placenta*, 4, 65, 1983.

115. **Russel, P.,** Inflammatory lesions of the human placenta. III. The histopathology of villitis of unknown origin, *Placenta*, 1, 227, 1980.

116. **Althabe, O. and Laberrere, C.,** Chronic villitis of unknown aetiology and intrauterine growth retarded infants of normal and low ponderal index, *Placenta*, 6, 369, 1985.

117. **Redline, R. W. and Abramowsky, C. R.,** Clinical and pathological aspects of recurrent placental villitis, *Hum. Pathol.*, 16, 727, 1985.

118. **Mortimer, G., MacDonald, D. J., and Smeeth, A.,** A pilot study of the frequency and significance of placental villitis, *Br. J. Obstet. Gynaecol.*, 92, 629, 1985.

119. **Winick, M.,** Cellular growth of human placenta. III. Intrauterine growth failure, *Pediatrics*, 119, 390, 1967.

120. **Kalousek, D. K. and Dill, F. J.,** Chromosomal mosaicism confined to the placenta in human conceptions, *Science*, 221, 665, 1983.

121. **Carroll, M. J. and Young, M.,** Observations on the energy and redox state and protein synthetic rate in animal and human placentas, *J. Perinat. Med.*, 15, 21, 1987.

122. **Metcoff, J., Wikman-Coffelt, J., Yoshida, T., Bernal, A., Rosada, A., Yoshida, P., Urrusti, J., Frenk, S., Madrazo, R., Velasco, L., and Morales, M.,** Energy metabolism and protein synthesis in human leukocytes during pregnancy and in placenta related to fetal growth, *Pediatrics*, 51, 866, 1973.

123. **Velasco, E. G., Rosso, P., Brasel, J., and Winick, M.,** Activity of alkaline in placentas of malnourished women, *Am. J. Obstet. Gynecol.*, 23, 637, 1975.

124. **Mackay, R. B.,** Oxygen consumption of fresh placental tissue, *J. Obstet. Gynaecol. Br. Emp.*, 65, 791, 1958.

125. **Russell, C. S., Dewhurst, C. J., and Blakey, D. H.,** The pregnancediol excretion in suspected placental insufficiency, *J. Obstet. Gynaecol. Br. Emp.*, 67, 1, 1960.

126. **Westergaard, J. G., Teisner, B., Hau, J., Grudzinskas, J. G., and Chard, T.,** Placental function studies in low birth weight infants with and without dysmaturity, *Obstet. Gynecol.*, 65, 316, 1985.

127. **Fisher, G. C., Garrett, W., and Kossof, G.,** Placental ageing monitored by gray scale echography, *Am. J. Obstet. Gynecol.*, 124, 443, 1975.

128. **Ikedife, D.,** Eclampsia in multipara, *Br. Med. J.*, 280, 985, 1980.

129. **Ounsted, M. and Ounsted, C.,** *On Fetal Growth Rate: its Variations and Consequences*, William Heinemann, London, 1973, chap. 5.

130. **Bakketeig, L. S. and Hoffman, H. J.,** The tendency to repeat gestational age and birth weight in successive births, related to perinatal survival, *Acta Obstet. Gynecol. Scand.*, 62, 385, 1983.

131. **Pijenborg, R., Bland, J. M., Robertson, W. B., and Brosens, I.,** Uteroplacental arterial changes related to interstitial trophoblast migration in early human pregnancy, *Placenta*, 4, 397, 1983.

132. **Robertson, W. B., Brosens, I., and Dixon, G.,** Uteroplacental vascular pathology, *Eur. J. Obstet. Gynecol. Reprod. Biol.*, 5, 47, 1975.

133. **Sheppard, B. L. and Bonnar, J.,** An ultrastructural study of uteroplacental spiral arteries in hypertensive and normotensive pregnancy and fetal growth retardation, *Br. J. Obstet. Gynaecol.*, 88, 695, 1981.

134. **McFadyen, I. R., Price, A. B., and Geirsson, R. T.,** The relation of birthweight to histological appearances in vessels of the placental bed, *Br. J. Obstet. Gynaecol.*, 93, 476, 1986.

135. **McFadyen, I. R., Greenhouse, P., Price, A. B., and Geirsson, R. T.,** The relationship between plasma urate and placental bed vascular adaptation to pregnancy, *Br. J. Obstet. Gynaecol.*, 93, 482, 1986.

136. **Bieniarz, J., Yoshida, T., Romera-Salinas, G., Curuchet, E., Caldeyro-Barcia, R., and Crottogini, J. J.,** Aorta caval compression by the uterus in late human pregnancy. IV. Circulation homeostasis by preferential perfusion of the placenta, *Am. J. Obstet. Gynecol.*, 103, 19, 1969.

137. **Becker, J. C.,** Aetiology of eclampsia, *J. Obstet. Gynaecol. Br. Emp.*, 55, 756, 1948.

138. **Roach, M. R. and Burton, A. C.,** The reason for the shape of the distensibility curves of arteries, *Can. J. Biochem. Physiol.*, 35, 681, 1957.

139. **Burchell, R. C., Creed, F., Rasoulpour, M., and Whitcombe, M.,** Vascular anatomy of the human uterus and pregnancy wastage, *Br. J. Obstet. Gynaecol.*, 85, 698, 1978.

140. **Hytten, F. E. and Paintin, D.,** Increase in plasma volume during normal pregnancy, *J. Obstet. Gynaecol. Br. Commonw.*, 70, 402, 1963.

141. **McFadyen, I. R., Duffy, S., De Chazal, R. C. S., Sarkar, P., Geirsson, R. T., and Price, A. B.,** The relationship of birth weight to the adaptation of maternal placental bed vessels to pregnancy changes in packed cell volume, and mean arterial pressure, submitted for publication.

142. **Taylor, D. J. and Lind, T.,** Haematological changes during normal pregnancy: iron induced macrocytosis, *Br. J. Obstet. Gynaecol.,* 83, 760, 1976.

143. **Gibson, H. M.,** Plasma volume and glomerular filtration rate in pregnancy and their relation to differences in fetal growth, *J. Obstet. Gynaecol. Br. Commonw.,* 80, 1067, 1973.

144. **Croall, J., Sherrif, S., and Mathews, J.,** Non-pregnant maternal plasma volume and fetal growth retardation, *Br. J. Obstet. Gynaecol.,* 85, 90, 1978.

145. **Sibai, B. M., Anderson, G. D., Spinnato, J. A., and Shaver, D. C.,** Plasma volume findings in patients with mild pregnancy-induced hypertension, *Am. J. Obstet. Gynecol.,* 147, 16, 1983.

146. **Thorburn, J., Drummond, M. M., Whigham, K. A., Lowe, G. D. O., Forbes, C. D., Prentice, C. R. M., and Whitfield, C. R.,** Blood viscosity and haemostatic factors in late pregnancy, pre-eclampsia and fetal growth retardation, *Br. J. Obstet. Gynaecol.,* 89, 117, 1982.

147. **Cunningham, F. G., Lowe, T., Guss, S., and Mason, R.,** Erythrocyte morphology in women with severe pre-eclampsia and eclampsia, *Am. J. Obstet. Gynecol,* 153, 358, 1985.

148. **Naeye, R. L.,** Placental infarction leading to fetal or neonatal death. A prospective study, *Obstet Gynecol.,* 50, 583, 1977.

149. **Trudinger, B. J.,** Platelets and intrauterine growth retardation in pre-eclampsia, *Br. J. Obstet. Gynaecol.,* 83, 284, 1976.

150. **Howie, P. W., Prentice, C. R., and McNichol, G. O.,** Coagulation, fibrinolysis and platelet function in pre-eclampsia essential hypertension and placental insufficiency, *J. Obstet. Gynaecol. Br. Commonw.,* 78, 992, 1971.

151. **Elder, M. G. and Muatt, L.,** Coagulation and fibrinolysis in pregnancies complicated by fetal growth retardation, *Br. J. Obstet. Gynaecol.,* 83, 355, 1976.

152. **Ylikorkala, O. and Makila, U. M.,** Prostacyclin and thromboxane in gynecology and obstetrics, *Am. J. Obstet. Gynecol.,* 152, 310, 1985.

153. **Koullabis, E. N., Nicolaides, K. H., Collins, W. P., Rodeck, C. H., and Campbell, S.,** Plasma prostanoids in pregnancy-induced hypertension, *Br. J. Obstet. Gynaecol.,* 89, 617, 1982.

154. **Gant, N. F., Daley, G. L., Chand, S., Whalley, P., and MacDonald, P. C.,** A study of angiotensin II pressor response throughout primigravid pregnancy, *J. Clin. Invest.,* 52, 2682, 1973.

155. **Landau, R. L. and Lugibihl, K.,** Inhibition of the sodium-retaining influence of aldosterone by progesterone, *J. Clin. Endocrinol.,* 18, 1237, 1958.

156. **Nisell, H., Hjemdahl, P., and Linde, B.,** Cardiovascular responses to circulating catecholamines in normal pregnancy and in pregnancy-induced hypertension, *Clin. Physiol.,* 5, 479, 1985.

157. **Gerreras, L. O., De Freyn, G., and Machin, S. J.,** Arterial thrombosis intra-uterine death and lupus anticoagulant: detection of immunoglobulin interfering with prostacyclin production, *Lancet,* 1, 244, 1981.

158. **Stuart, M. J., Clark, D. A., Sunderji, S. G., Allen, J. B., Yambo, T., Elrad, H., and Slott, J. H.,** Decreased prostacyclin production: a characteristic of chronic placental insufficiency syndromes, *Lancet,* 1126, May, 1981.

159. **Wootton, R., McFadyen, I. R., and Cooper, J. E.,** Measurement of placental blood flow in the pig and its relation to placental and fetal weight, *Biol. Neonate,* 31, 333, 1977.

160. **Lunell, N. O., Sarby, B., Levander, R., and Uylund, L.,** Comparison of uteroplacental blood flow in normal and intrauterine growth retarded pregnancy. Measurement with Indium — 113 m and a computer-linked gamma camera, *Gynecol. Obstet. Invest.,* 10, 106, 1979.

161. **McFadyen, I. R.,** Maternal blood flow to the uterus, in *Placental Transfer,* Chamberlain, G. V. P. and Wilkinson, A. W., Eds., Pitman Publishing, Marshfield, MA, 1979, 31.

162. **Uylund, L., Lunell, N. O., Levander, R., and Sarby, B.,** Uteroplacental blood flow index intrauterine growth retardation of fetal or maternal origin, *Br. J. Obstet. Gynaecol.,* 90, 16, 1983.

163. **Dixon, H. G., McClure Brown, J. C., and Davey, D. A.,** Choriodecidual and myometrial blood flow, *Lancet,* 2, 369, 1963.

164. **Morris, N., Osborn, S. B., Wright, H. P., and Hart, A.,** Effective uterine blood flow during exercise in normal and pre-eclampsia pregnancies, *Lancet,* 2, 481, 1956.

165. **Collings, C. N. S., Curet, L. B., and Mullin, J. P.,** Maternal and fetal responses to a maternal aerobic exercise program, *Am. J. Obstet. Gynecol.,* 145, 702, 1983.

166. **Pomerance, J. J., Gluck, L., and Lynch, V. A.,** Maternal exercise as a screening test for uteroplacental insufficiency, *Obstet. Gynecol.,* 44, 383, 1974.

167. **De Souza, S. W., John, R. W., and Richards, B.,** Studies on the effect of maternal pre-eclamptit toxaemia on placental weight and on head size and birthweight of the newborn, *Br. J. Obstet. Gynaecol.,* 83, 292, 1976.

168. **Baird, D., Thomson, A. M., and Billewicz, W. Z.,** Birthweight and placental weights in pre-eclampsia, *J. Obstet. Gynaecol. Br. Emp.,* 64, 370, 1957.

169. **Lin, C. C., Lindheimer, M. D., River, P., and Hoawad, A. H.,** Fetal outcome in hypertensive disorders of pregnancy, *Am. J. Obstet, Gynecol.,* 142, 255, 1982.

170. **Walters, W. A. W.,** Effects of sustained maternal hypertension on foetal growth and survival, *Lancet,* 1214, Dec., 1966.

171. **Gant, N. F., Madden, J. S., Chand, S., Worley, R. J., Strong, J. D., and MacDonald, P. C.,** Metabolic clearance rate of dehydroisoandrosterone sulphate. V. Studies of essential hypertension complicating pregnancy, *Obstet. Gynecol.,* 47, 319, 1976.

172. **Tervila, L., Coecke, C., and Timonen, S.,** Estimation of gestosis of pregnancy (Eph-Gestosis), *Acta Obstet. Gynecol Scand.,* 52, 235, 1973.

173. **Naeye, R. L.,** Maternal blood pressure and fetal growth, *Am. J. Obstet. Gynecol.,* 141, 780, 1981.

174. **Gruenwald, P.,** Growth of the human fetus. 1. Normal growth and its variation, *Am. J. Obstet. Gynecol.,* 94, 1112, 1966.

175. **Hytten, F. E.,** *Nutrition in Pregnancy in Perinatal Medicine,* Thalkammer, O., Baumgaften, K., and Pollak, A., Eds., Georg Thieme Verlag, Stuttgart, 1979.

176. **Winick, M.,** Cellular growth in intrauterine malnutrition, *Pediatr. Clin. North. Am.,* 17, 69, 1970.

177. **Prentice, A. M., Whitehead, R. G., Watkinson, M., Lamb, W. H., and Cole, T. J.,** Prenatal dietary supplementation of African women and birthweight, *Lancet,* 1, 489, 1983.

178. **Campbell Brown, M. and McFadyen, I. R.,** Maternal energy reserves and birthweight, *Lancet,* 1, 574, 1985.

179. **Crosby, W. M., Metcoff, J., Costiloe, J. P., Mameesh, M., Sandstead, H. H., Jacob, R. A., McClain, P. E., Jacobson, G., Reid, W., and Burns, G.,** Fetal malnutrition: an appraisal of correlated factors, *Am. J. Obstet. Gynecol.,* 128, 22, 1977.

180. **Brooke, O. G. and Wood, C.,** Growth in British Asians: longitudinal data in the first year, *J. Hum. Nutr.,* 34, 355, 1980.

181. **Khouzami, V. A., Ginsburg, D. S., Daikoku, N. H., and Johnson, J. W. C.,** The glucose tolerance test as a means of identifying intrauterine growth retardation, *Am. J. Obstet. Gynecol.,* 139, 423, 1981.

182. **Jenkins, D. J., Walever, T. M. S., Taylor, R. H., Barker, H. M., and Fielden, H.,** Exceptionally low blood glucose response to dried beans: comparison with other carbohydrate foods, *Br. Med. J.,* 2, 578, 1980.

183. **Yerushalmy, J.,** The relationship of parent's cigarette smoking to outcome of pregnancy-implications as to the problem of inferring causation from observed causes, *Am. J. Epidemiol.,* 93, 443, 1971.

184. **Rubin, D. H., Krasilniroff, P. A., Leventhal, J. M., Weile, B., and Berget, A.,** Effect of passive smoking on birthweight, *Lancet,* 2, 415, 1986.

185. **Ouellette, E. M., Rosett, H. L., Rosman, N. P., and Weiner, L.,** Adverse effects on offspring of maternal alcohol abuse during pregnancy, *N. Engl. J. Med.,* 297, 528, 1977.

186. **Yudkin, P. K., Harlap, S., and Baras, M.,** High birthweight in an ethnic group of low socioeconomic status, *Br. J. Obstet. Gynaecol.,* 90, 291, 1983.

187. **Taylor, C. and Faulk, W. P.,** Prevention of recurrent abortions with leucocyte transfusions, *Lancet,* 2, 68, 1981.

188. **Ounsted, M. and Ounsted, C.,** *On Fetal Growth Rate: its Variations and Consequences,* Heinemann Medical Books Ltd., London, 1973, chap 6.

189. **Alberman, E., Roman, E., Pharoah, P. O. D., and Chamberlain, G.,** Birthweight before and after spontaneous abortion, *Br. J. Obstet. Gynaecol.,* 87, 275, 1980.

190. **Scott, J. R.,** Fetal growth retardation associated with maternal administration of immunosuppressive drugs, *Am. J. Obstet. Gynecol.,* 128, 668, 1977.

191. **Duncan, M. E.,** Babies of mothers with leprosy have small placentae, low birth weights and grow slowly, *Br. J. Obstet. Gynecol.,* 87, 471, 1980.

192. **Cannon, D. S. H.,** Malaria and prematurity in the western region of Nigeria, *Br. Med. J.,* 2, 877, 1958.

193. **Cole, P. V., Hawkins, L. H., and Roberts, D.,** Smoking during pregnancy and its effect on the fetus, *J. Obstet. Gynaecol. Br. Commonw.,* 79, 782, 1972.

194. **Andrews, J.,** Thiocyanate and smoking in pregnancy, *J. Obstet. Gynaecol. Br. Commonw.,* 80, 810, 1973.

195. **Buchan, P. C.,** Cigarette smoking in pregnancy and fetal hyperviscosity, *Br. Med. J.,* 286, 1315, 1983.

196. **Meberg, A., Halvorseu, S., and Orstavik, I.,** Transitory thrombocytopenia in small-for-dates infants, possibly related to maternal smoking, *Lancet,* 2, 303, 1977.

197. **Sindberg Eriksen, P. and Marsal, K.,** Circulatory changes in the fetal aorta after maternal smoking, *Br. J. Obstet. Gynaecol.,* 94, 301, 1987.

198. **Asmussen, I. and Kjeldsen, K.,** Intimal ultrastructure of human umbilical arteries. Observations on arteries from newborn children of smoking and non smoking mothers, *Circ. Res.,* 36, 579, 1975.

199. **Ahlsten, G., Ewald, U., and Tuvemo, T.,** Maternal smoking reduces prostacyclin formation in human umbilical arteries. A study on strictly selected pregnancies, *Acta Obstet. Gynecol. Scand.,* 65, 645, 1986.

200. **Wingerd, J., Christianson, R., Lovitt, W. V., and Schoen, E. J.,** Placental ratio in black and white women: relation to smoking and anemia, *Am. J. Obstet. Gynecol.,* 124, 671, 1976.

201. **Asmussen, I.,** Ultrastructure of the human placenta at term, *Acta Obstet. Gynecol. Scand.,* 56, 119, 1977.

202. **Lehtovirta, P. and Forss, M.,** The acute effect of smoking on intervillous blood flow of the placenta, *Br. J. Obstet. Gynaecol.,* 85, 729, 1978.

203. **Pirani, B. B. K. and MacGillivray, I.,** Smoking during pregnancy. Its effect of maternal metabolism and fetoplacental function, *Obstet. Gynecol.,* 52, 257, 1978.

204. **Davies, J. M., Latto, I. P., Jones, J. G., Veale, A., and Wardrop, C. A. J.,** Effects of stopping smoking for 48 hours on oxygen availability from the blood: a study of pregnant women, *Br. Med. J.,* 2, 355, 1979.

205. **Naeye, R. L.,** Effects of maternal cigarette smoking on the fetus and placenta, *Br. J. Obstet. Gynaecol.,* 85, 732, 1978.

206. **Hauth, J. C., Hauth, J., Drawbaugh, R. B., Gilstrap, L. C., and Pierson, W. P.,** Passive smoking and thiocyanate concentrations in pregnant women and newborns, *Obstet. Gynecol.,* 63, 519, 1984.

207. **Anderson, G. D., Bledner, I. N., McClemont, S., and Sinclair, J. C.,** Determinants of size at birth in a Canadian population, *Am. J. Obstet. Gynecol.,* 150, 236, 1984.

208. **Davies, D. P. and Abernethy, M.,** Cigarette smoking in pregnancy: associations with maternal weight gain and fetal growth, *Lancet,* 1, 385, 1976.

209. **Murphy, J. F., Drumm, J. E., Mulcahy, R., and Daly, L.,** The effect of maternal cigarette smoking on fetal birthweight and on growth of the fetal biparietal diameter, *Br. J. Obstet. Gynaecol.,* 87, 462, 1980.

210. **D'Souza, S. W., Black, P., and Richards, B.,** Smoking in pregnancy: associations with skinfold thickness, maternal weight gain, and fetal size at birth, *Br. Med. J.,* 282, 1661, 1981.

211. **Meyer, M. B.,** How does maternal smoking affect birthweight and maternal weight gain, *Am. J. Obstet. Gynecol.,* 131, 888, 1978.

212. **MacMahon, B., Alpert, M., and Salber, E. J.,** Infant weight and parental smoking habits, *Am. J. Epidemiol.,* 82, 247, 1965.

213. **Butler, N. R., Goldstein, H., and Ross, E. M.,** Cigarette smoking in pregnancy: its influence on birthweight and perinatal mortality, *Br. Med. J.,* 2, 127, 1972.

214. **Vesey, C. J., Saloojee, Y., Cole, P. V., and Russell, M. A. H.,** Blood carboxyhaemoglobin, plasma thiocyanate, and cigarette consumption: implications for epidemiological studies in smokers, *Br. Med. J.,* 284, 1516, 1982.

215. **Fitzgerald, D. J., Entman, S. S., Mulloy, K., and Fitzgerald, G. A.,** Decreased prostacyclin biosynthesis preceding the clinical manifestation of pregnancy-induced hypertension, *Circulation,* 75, 956, 1987.

216. **Baker, V. V., Kort, B., and Cefalo, R. C.,** Effects of plasma on the platelet antiaggregatory action of prostacyclin in pregnancy, *Am. J. Obstet. Gynecol.,* 156, 974, 1987.

217. **Fievet, P., Gregoire, I., Agnes, E., Herve, M. A., Carayoh, A., Mimtam, A., Boulanger, J. E., and Fournier, A.,** Renin-angiotensin-aldosterone system urinary prostaglandins and kallikrein in pregnancy-induced hypertension: evidence for a disregulation of the renin-angiotensin-prostacyclin loop, *J. Hypertension,* 4, 588, 1986.

Chapter 4

# COLLAGEN DISEASES AND INTRAUTERINE GROWTH RETARDATION

**Danniel Weinstein and Joseph G. Schenker**

## TABLE OF CONTENTS

# I. INTRODUCTION

Collagen or connective tissue diseases are a group of clinicopathological conditions which include systemic lupus erythematosus (SLE), scleroderma (systemic sclerosis), rheumatoid arthritis (RA), dermatomyositis, and polyarteritis nodosa. They occur in young women of reproductive age with pregnancy being a frequent occurrence. The conditions are all characterized by a failure of the normal state of immune tolerance and an excessive production of autoantibodies, which may affect almost any organ. The histologic trait is inflammatory damage to connective tissue and blood vessels, seen often in conjunction with deposition of fibroid material.

The possible effects of pregnancy on collagen diseases, and vice versa, have been the subject of controversy, and have been investigated over many years.[1]

Some of these diseases, especially SLE, scleroderma, and dermatomyositis have a profound effect on the outcome of pregnancy.

The present review summarizes the literature about the influence of collagen disease in pregnancy complicated by intrauterine growth retardation (IUGR). Special attention is paid to the placenta as an etiological factor, as well as its immunological background.

# II. SYSTEMIC LUPUS ERYTHEMATOSUS (SLE)

SLE is the major collagen disease associated with pregnancy.

The predilection of SLE to childbearing age makes its coincidence to pregnancy an important clinical problem.[2,3] It is predominantly a disease of women.

Patients with SLE typically develop a multitude of autoimmune phenomena, including anti-cell, anti-cytoplasmic and anti-nuclear antibodies. The most common presenting features are fever, migratory arthralgia, erythematous eruptions on the face and hands, fatigue, malaise, weight loss, and anorexia. The laboratory findings are rapid sedimentation rate, hemolytic anemia, leucopenia, and thrombocytopenia. Fertility is relatively well preserved.[4-9]

In our patients, fertility rate was without significant change before or after the diagnosis of SLE.[10]

Pregnancy occurs during periods of clinical remission. Most series report an increased incidence of abortions, stillbirth, prematurity, and IUGR.[4,6,7,8,11-14] The spontaneous abortion rate varies between 20 and 30%. Smolen claims a spontaneous abortion rate of up to 80% in active SLE.[9]

The systemic vasculitis, especially if the placenta is affected, may well be responsible for the abortions.[15] The prematurity rate ranges between 13 and 36%.[6,7,13,16] Superimposed preeclampsia occurs in about 25% of patients.[17] In our population, SLE with superimposed preeclampsia occurred in 15%.[10]

The medical treatment required depends on the severity of the disorder and type of organ involved. Aspirin is the most useful agent in the treatment of the minor manifestations of SLE in pregnant patients. Aspirin as a prostaglandin synthetase inhibitor may be associated with an increased incidence of postmaturity and prolonged labor.[18,19]

The second stage of treatment is systemic glucocorticoids which are the keystone of therapy whenever systemic manifestations are present.

The third stage of treatment implies the use of immuno-suppressive agents. Azathioprine (Imuran) is used during pregnancy.

Both steroid and imuran can provoke intrauterine growth retardation of the symmetrical type.

## III. RHEUMATOID ARTHRITIS

Rheumatoid arthritis (RA) is a chronic systemic disease of unknown etiology, manifested primarily by inflammation involving peripheral joints. The systemic manifestations include hematological, pulmonary, neurological, and cardiovascular abnormalities. The peak onset is in the fourth decade. Thus, pregnancy associated with RA. is relatively common. No genetic marker associated with this disease has been identified. However, the pathogenesis of RA may be related to an immune complex or action which appears within the synovial space.[20]

The abortion rate is low in patients with RA, and fertility is not impaired.[21] Involvement of the hip joint, severe enough to prevent vaginal delivery, is unusual.

Proper management of RA during pregnancy includes an appropriate balance of rest and exercise, heat, and physical therapy. Aspirin is the drug of choice for analgesic and antiinflammatory therapy. Prolonged pregnancy may be more common in heavy salicylate users due to interference with prostaglandin synthesis. Neonatal bleeding disorders have occasionally been a problem due to decreased platelet aggregation.

## IV. POLYMYOSITIS AND DERMATOMYOSITIS

Polymyositis and dermatomyositis are inflammatory disorders which affect the striated muscle, skin, and various connective tissue of the body. The diseases are characterized by weakness, usually of the proximal muscles, tenderness and atrophy of involved muscles. The injury to muscle cells releases various enzymes which normally reside within skeletal muscles, such as transaminases and creatinine phosphokinase. The diagnosis is established by the detection of a high level of enzymes, by muscle biopsy, and by electromyogram. The skin changes (dermatomyositis) take the form of localized diffuse erythema, and eruption, or exfoliative dermatitis. Females are affected twice as often as males. The age involvement ranges between 30 and 60 years.

The reports in connection with pregnancy are rare.[22] It is generally agreed that there is an increase in perinatal wastage with infants with IUGR. Perinatal mortality rate may reach 50%.[23]

## V. PERIARTERITIS NODOSA

This rare disease affects primarily medium-sized arteries with an intense segmental necrotizing inflammation, which leads to thrombosis within the vessel and infarction of the organ distal to the diseased artery. Some cases are associated with persistance of hepatitis B virus. It is usually a disease of adulthood. It affects three times more men than women. The early complaints include fever, weakness, anorexia, weight loss, myalgia, and arthralgia. Nodules of 5 to 10 mm occur along the course of the arteries as a result of aneurysm formation. Vascular occlusion of such vessels leads to ecchymosis, ulceration, and gangrene of fingers and toes.

There are only nine case reports of periarteritis nodosa associated with pregnancy.[22,25-31] The main reasons for that are that the diagnosis is more common in men and that the onset of the disease occurs during the fifth and sixth decade.

Pregnancy in patients with periarteritis nodosa carries an extremely grave prognosis.

Of the nine cases reported, five died postpartum and two died postabortion. The two surviving patients were the two who were under good clinical control at the time of pregnancy.[27] During pregnancy the disease process may be more rapid.[28]

In all the cases, the fetuses appear to be unaffected by the disease or the treatment which is mainly based on steroid therapy. In several reports simultaneous cutaneous vasculitis in mothers and infants were reported.

## VI. SCLERODERMA

Scleroderma, or progressive systemic sclerosis is the next most common collagen disorder. It is a disorder of connective tissue leading to fibrosis that involves the skin (scleroderma), with or without fixation to underlying structures, and a variety of internal organs. The clinical picture is of tight, firm skin, which may be present several years before visceral involvement becomes apparent. The onset of the disease occurs usually in the third or fifth decade and is found twice as often in women as in men. The increased fibrosis in the various organ system is considered to be due to the over production of collagen. The etiology and pathogenesis are unknown. The onset of the disease is usually insidious. There is vague weakness, weight loss, diffuse stiffness, aching edema, polyarthritis, and Reynaud's phenomenon. The gastrointestinal tract is most often involved, and there is progressive involvement of the esophagus, narrowing of the mouth, dysphagia, and heartburn. Cardiac failure, due to myocardial and pulmonary fibrosis, are common.

The combination of pregnancy and scleroderma is unusual as this rare disease occurs more often during the fourth and fifth decade, and because patients with scleroderma possibly exhibit a secondary relative infertility.[32-34]

Most information comes from case reports and few larger series.[32-38] With generalized sclerosis, the incidence of stillbirth, premature labor, and perinatal mortality is high.[32,33,37,38]

There is no known specific effect of maternal scleroderma on the newborn[39] but there are two reports[33,40] of infants who have been suspected to have scleroderma of the extreme ties.

## VII. INTRAUTERINE GROWTH RETARDATION (IUGR)

IUGR may be classified by ultrasonography into symmetrical and asymmetrical type.[41,42,43,44] In the symmetrical type, the biparietal diameter (BPD) increases in parallel with, but below the normal growth curve, and the head to abdominal circumference ratio is normal. All body organs tend to be reduced in size, and growth impairment affects both the organs and the head in a similar degree. In the asymmetrical type the BPD is normal or flattened and the head to abdomen circumference ratio is above normal. Some of the body organs are affected more than others.[44] Asymmetrical IUGR can be further divided into phases I and II, which depend on whether the BPD is growing or not.

These two types of IUGR are a result of different etiological factors. The symmetrical IUGR is a result of factors such as genetic, constitutional, chromosomal, early malnutrition, smoking, or intrauterine infections.[45] The causes for the asymmetrical type of IUGR are mainly associated with uteroplacental insufficiency, as in cases of hypertension, renal diseases, advanced diabetes, or placental pathology.

In cases of symmetrical growth retardation, ultrasonography and amniocentesis may be done to exclude fetal malformations.

The different maternal conditions that affect pregnancy should be taken into consideration, and delivery should be planned accordingly. In asymmetrical IUGR, the termination of pregnancy should be considered if the BPD does not grow (phase II).

SLE is associated with IUGR.[46-49] It is hardly possible to distinguish between the effect of the disease and the effect of massive doses of glucocorticoides and azathioprine (imuran). Both medications may induce symmetrical IUGR. Asymmetrical IUGR is seen especially in fetuses of patients with renal involvement and hypertension.[17]

SLE patients may also carry a genetic trait that results in abnormalities of the fetus, and therefore symmetrical IUGR.[9]

Patients with active SLE diseases may have fever, negative nitrogen balance and chronic anemia, immune complexes in the placenta, placental insufficiency, and IUGR.

The pathogenesis of IUGR is probably reduced uteroplacental blood flow[16] and the resultant growth retardation is of the asymmetrical type. In patients who receive heavy medication of corticosteroids and/or azathioprine the growth retardation is concordant for head and body producing symmetrical IUGR. This seems to be more in keeping with the effect of steroids on fetal growth observed in animal models. In those animals, cell number in the brain is reduced and myelination, sympatic growth and locomotor ability are improved.[50,51]

Gene Burkett[52] from the University of Miami reviewed the literature about cases of lupus nephritis from 1952 up to 1985. He found that the incidence of IUGR up to 1979 was approximately 5%.[6,53] Perinatal mortality in that period was reported to be 35%. Since 1979 the incidence of IUGR rose to 8.2%, with overall fetal survival of 82%.

Minz et al.[54] in their study of SLE pregnancies found 5 stillbirths between 22 and 34 weeks, 4 of which had IUGR. Of a total of 85 deliveries, 23% showed IUGR. In the SLE premature births, 30% showed IUGR of the total cases of IUGR, in 65% the mother had active SLE, and in 35%, inactive disease. Statistical analysis did not reach significance when compared to the SLE cases without IUGR. IUGR correlated significantly with prematurity. With active maternal disease there were more premature deliveries and more infants with IUGR. In all IUGR infants, perinatal mortality decreased when fetal distress was followed immediately by cesarean section together with intensive care of the newborn.

Inspection of six reports published prior to 1980, in which 314 pregnancies in patients with established SLE were described,[55] indicates that the incidence of live births was 65%.[56] In hypertensive patients the incidence of IUGR was 9%. When hypertension was associated with primary renal disease the rate of IUGR was 35%.[57] The occurrence of IUGR is associated with the occurrence of hypertension and/or renal insufficiency. No study found any increased incidence of congenital anomalies[58-63] among viable pregnancies. Likewise, no increased anomaly rates have been related to steroid or immunosuppressive therapy. Fine et al.[64] found in their study 21% of IUGR in SLE pregnancies.

Duhring[65] is almost the only one who suggested a relationship between rheumatoid arthritis, placental insufficiency, and IUGR. Most reports[66-68] indicated a lack of adverse effects on fetal growth and development.

In Morris's report,[67] out of 34 pregnancies only one patient was delivered by cesarean section at 37 weeks for IUGR, and 4 other infants weighed less than 2500 g at term. These numbers may indicate a tendency for small for gestational-age babies, but it is unwise to generalize from such a small sample.

In polymyositis and dermatomyositis, there is an increase in perinatal wastage with infants of low birth weight and perinatal mortality of 50%.[23]

## VIII. AUTOIMMUNITY, COLLAGEN DISEASES, AND IUGR

SLE is considered to be the prototype of autoimmune disease due to the vast diversity of autoantibodies detected in the sera. Lupus serum may contain a variety of autoantibodies against nucleic acids (notable DNA), nucleoproteins, cell surface antigens, and phospholids. The tissue afflictions include almost any organ.

One of the most perplexing serological findings in SLE is the lupus anticoagulant (LA), and this has been of interest to the obstetricians.[69,70] Its incidence is not exactly known, and varies between 5 and 10%.[71-73]

LA was found to be associated with drug administration, neoplasia, and even in normal subjects.[74,75]

The presence of LA in pregnancy has been associated with recurrent early abortions and intrauterine death. The response to immunosuppressive therapy was a successful outcome of pregnancy.[76,77]

Aspirin, corticosteroids, azathioprine have beneficial effects in diminishing LA levels and thereby promoting a successful pregnancy.[78,79,80]

The antinuclear antibodies participate in the pathogenesis of SLE by forming antigen antibody complexes with their specific antigens. These complexes have been demonstrated in glomerular basement membrane. Complement is consumed and its serum concentration is decreased, and circulating immune complexes can be detected. Fibrinoid deposits are commonly seen in blood vessels, among collagen fibers, and on serosal surfaces. Immune complex like material, has been found in placentas of SLE patients[81] as well as viral complexes.[82] Antilymphocyte antibodies were found in patients with active SLE.[83,84] Some of these antibodies cross react with trophoblastic antigens and may be responsible for early abortions.[85]

Beck and Rowell[86] found a transplacental influx of maternal antibodies such as have been detected in the fetal circulation.

Premature deliveries may be attributed to placental insufficiency induced by vasculitis or derangement in estrogen metabolism.

All these factors may affect pregnancy in the last weeks. It is speculated that immune complexes which cross the placenta may be the causative mechanism of congenital heart block.[87]

Theofilopoulos et al.[88] proposed that in normal pregnancies the mother responds poorly to fetal antigens and therefore the complexes formed have a very large antigen excess and are of scanty pathological significance. By contrast, in the cases where the mother responds strongly, circulatory immune complexes form at slight antigen or antibody excess, persist in the circulation, activate complement, and lead to decidual vessel lesions similar to those described in SLE. Complement-fixing immune complexes in maternal serum containing IgM may be related to the placental vascular lesions observed in SLE, also in preeclamptic pregnancies with IUGR.[89,90]

Bresnihan et al.[91] reported a raised incidence of antitrophoblast cytotoxic antibody in pregnancies complicated by SLE.

In rheumatoid arthritis the serum and fluid of most patients contain heterogeneous antibodies (rheumatoid factor). Unknown etiological factors set into motion the immunological events that lead to the appearance and the continued production of rheumatoid factor in the pathogenesis of RA. Immunological mechanisms play an important role in the development of synovitis. Antinuclear antibodies, DNA, and breakdown products of complement appear in the synovial fluid with activation of the component cascade which releases inflammatory peptides, causing migration of the inflammatory cells. The release of collagenases causes local damage.[92]

The rheumatic factors do not cross the placenta and there is little evidence of fetal or neonatal involvement in maternal RA.

In periarteritis nodosa, there is some evidence that immune complexes of hepatitis B antigen antibody and complement are present in the arterial lesions.

In scleroderma, hypergammaglobulinemia with an elevated level, mainly of IgG, is found in approximately one-half of the patients. Rheumatoid factors in low titer are present in 25%; antinuclear antibodies are reported in 40 to 80% of the patients. Antinuclear antibody fluorescence is commonly patterned in fine or large speckles.

## IX. THE PLACENTA IN COLLAGEN DISEASES COMPLICATED WITH IUGR

In spite of detailed clinical observation reported in hundreds of pregnant patients with collagen diseases (especially with SLE), very little information has been recorded on the placenta in these cases, with or without IUGR. In the two studies[82,93] in which electron microscopy was performed on placentas of 11 normal and 13 SLE patients, it failed to disclose any increased expression of viral activity in the SLE patients over the normal. On the contrary, some investigations have found viral particles in human placentas from SLE patients.[93,94] Grennan et al.[48] performed immunological studies and found granular deposits of immunoglobulins and $C_3$ in trophoblast basement membranes and nuclei, which may play a role in the poor fetal outcome. In complicated pregnancies, particularly with maternal hypertension or preeclampsia, uteroplacental vessels are altered by occlusive lesions, such as fibrinoid necrosis, inflammation, and infiltration of the vascular wall by large cells with lipid-laden foamy cytoplasm for which the term atherosis was coined.[95,96] Although there is a current controversy on the clinical significance of these lesions, it is generally agreed that impairment of uteroplacental blood flow results in variable placental dysfunction, which may culminate in placental infarction, and, as a consequence, in prematurity, IUGR, and death.

Abramowsky[97] did a histological and immunofluorescence study on 11 placentas of SLE patients. No correlation was found between clinical status, duration of the disease, and pregnancy outcome. Their results are in agreement with those shown previously by Grennan[48] concerning trophoblastic nuclear localization of IgG and IgA. Fluorescent deposits were similar to those described in normal placentas by others.[98,99]

Abramowsky also claims[97] that the decidual arterial lesions reasonably explain the poor fetal outcome seen in the patient in whom they were found.

Labarrere et al.[100] studied, by immunoperoxidase staining, lesions of acute atherosis in 23 placentas from three groups of pregnancies complicated by IUGR. Eleven of them were associated with SLE, 12 were associated with primary induced hypertension (PIH), and 10 without hypertension. Massive intramural glandular deposits of IgM, $C_3$, and slight deposits of IgA and IgG were found in vessels with acute atherosis.

The distribution of the different vascular lesions in the studied SLE group revealed, in only one case, 10% acute atherosis in the basal decidua, while in PIH, or pregnancies without hypertension, the acute atherosis in basal decidua reached 50%.

Deposits of immunoproteins (IgM, IgG, IgA, $C_3$, $Cl_q$) without maternal lesions were the same in the three groups studied.

Lesions of acute atherosis have been described, associated with IUGR, with or without SLE[81] or preeclampsia, with normal birthweight.[95,100] Significant deposits of IgM and $C_3$ have been described associated with vascular lesions of acute atherosis in cases of preeclampsia, SLE, and chronic hypertension. It is important to stress that not in all cases of IUGR was this phenomenon demonstrated.

Relatively little has been written in the obstetrics literature concerning IUGR in collagen diseases. The rates of IUGR varied between 8 and 30%. Both types are encountered: the symmetrical and the asymmetrical IUGR. The symmetrical type is found in patients carrying a genetic trait (which may result also in abnormalities of the fetus) and also in patients receiving massive doses of glucocorticoids and Imuran. Asymmetrical IUGR is due to placental dysfunction, necrotizing vasculitis, and atherosis. When there is renal involvement of the disease, the IUGR is much more severe. The classification of IUGR into symmetrical and asymmetrical is clinically important in giving a clue to the etiology of growth retardation in collagen diseases and in directing further clinical management.

# REFERENCES

1. **Merrill, J. A.,** Cortison in disseminated lupus erythomatosus during pregnancy, *Obstet. Gynecol.,* 6, 637, 1955.
2. **Harney, A. M., Shulman, L. E., Tumulty, P. A. et al.,** Systemic lupis erythematosus: review of the literature and clinical analysis of 138 cases, *Medicine (Baltimore),* 33, 291, 1954.
3. **Shearn, M. A. and Pirofsky, B.,** Disseminated lupus erythematosus. Analysis of 34 cases, *Arch. Intern. Med.,* 90, 790, 1952.
4. **Baum, J. and Ziff, M.,** 7S and macroglobulin antinuclear fluorescence factors in systemic lupus erythematosus and rheumatic arthritis, *Arthritis Rheum.,* 5, 407, 1962.

5. **Cox, J. B.,** Disseminated lupus erythematosus in pregnancy, *Obstet. Gynecol.,* 26, 511, 1965.
6. **Donaldson, L. B. and de Alvarez, R. R.,** Further observation on lupus erythematosus with pregnancy, *Am. J. Obstet. Gynecol.,* 83, 1461, 1962.
7. **Friedman, E. A. and Rutherford, J. W.,** Pregnancy and lupus erythematosus, *Obstet. Gynecol.,* 8, 601, 1965.
8. **Garsenstein, M., Pollak, V. E., and Kark, R. M.,** Systemic lupus erythematosus and pregnancy, *N. Engl. J. Med.,* 267, 165, 1962.
9. **Smolen, J. S. and Steinberg, A. D.,** Systemic lupus erythematosus and pregnancy: clinical, immunological and theoretical aspects, *Prog. Clin. Biol. Res.,* 70, 283, 1981.
10. **Mor-Yosef, S., Navot, D., Rabinowitz, R., and Schenker, J. G.,** Collagen diseases in pregnancy, *Obstet. Gynecol. Surv.,* 39, 67, 1984.
11. **Fraga, A., Mintz, G., Orozco, J. H. et al.,** Systemic lupus erythematosus: fertility, fetal wastage and survival rate with treatment, a comparative study, *Arthritis Rheum.,* 16, 541, 1973.
12. **Madsen, J. R. and Anderson, G. V.,** Lupus erythematosis and pregnancy, *Obstet. Gynecol.,* 18, 492, 1961.
13. **McGee, C. and Makowski, E. L.,** Systemic lupus erythematosus in pregnancy, *Am. J. Obstet. Gynecol.,* 107, 1008, 1970.
14. **Turner, S. J., LeVine, L., and Rothman, A.,** Lupus erythematosus and pregnancy, *Am. J. Obstet. Gynecol.,* 70, 10, 1955.
15. **Ardelt, W. and Boehn, N.,** Abort bei lupus erythematodes visceralis, *Geburtshilfe Frauenheilkd.,* 34, 473, 1974.
16. **Fine, L. G., Barnett, E. V., Danowitch, G. M. et al.,** Systemic lupus erythematosus in pregnancy, *Ann. Intern. Med.,* 94, 667, 1981.
17. **White, C. A.,** Collagen diseases in pregnancy, in *Gynecology and Obstetrics,* Vol. 3, Sciarra, J. J., Ed., Harper & Row, Hagerstown, Md., 1930, chap. 20.
18. **Collins, E. and Turner, G.,** Maternal effects of regular salicylate ingestion in pregnancy, *Lancet,* 2, 335, 1975.
19. **Lewis, R. B. and Schulman, J. D.,** Influence of acetylsalicyclic acid, an inhibitor of prostaglandin synthesis on the duration of human gestation and labor, *Lancet,* 2, 1159, 1973.
20. **Zvailfler, N.,** Rheumatoid synovitis. An extra vascular immune complex disease, *Arthritis Rheum.,* 17, 297, 1974.
21. **Trasler, D. G.,** Aspirin-induced cleft lip and other malformation in mice, *Lancet,* 1, 606, 1965.
22. **Tsai, A., Lindheimer, M. D., and Lamber, S. I.,** Dermatomyositis complicating pregnancy, *Obstet. Gynecol.,* 41, 570, 1973.
23. **Kaplan, D. and Diamond, H.,** Dermatomyositis and pregnancy, *Clin. Obstet. Gynecol.,* 8, 304, 1965.
24. **Burkett, G. and Richards, R.,** Periarteritis nodosa and pregnancy, *Obstet. Gynecol.,* 59, 252, 1982.
25. **Chesley, L. C.,** Maternal deaths, *Bull. Hague Matern. Hosp.,* 2, 91, 1949.
26. **DeBeukelaer, M., Travis, L., and Roberts, D.,** Polyarteritis nodosa and pregnancy, *South. Med. J.,* 66, 613, 1973.
27. **Reed, N. R. and Smith, M. T.,** Periarteritis nodosa in pregnancy. Report of a case and review of the literature, *Obstet. Gynecol.,* 55, 381, 1980.
28. **Siegler, A. and Spain, D.,** Polyarteritis nodosa and pregnancy, *Clin. Obstet. Gynecol.,* 8, 322, 1965.
29. **Tait, J. C. V.,** Polyarteritis nodosa: an unusual cause of obscure puerperal pyrexia, *Aust. N.Z. J. Med.,* 54, 58, 1955.
30. **Variabe, P., Fusco, J. M., Acampot, A. et al.,** Polyarteritis nodosa in pregnancy. Report of a case, *Obstet. Gynecol.,* 25, 866, 1965.
31. **Webb, A. C.,** Periarteritis nodosa in pregnancy, *Arch. Pathol.,* 38, 329, 1944.
32. **Slate, W. G. and Graham, A. R.,** Scleroderma and pregnancy, *Am. J. Obstet. Gynecol.,* 101, 335, 1968.
33. **Spellacy, W. N.,** Scleroderma and pregnancy, *Obstet. Gynecol.,* 23, 297, 1964.
34. **Tischler, S., Zarowitz, H., and Daichman, I.,** Scleroderma and pregnancy, *Obstet. Gynecol.,* 10, 457, 1957.
35. **DeCarle, E. W.,** Pregnancy associated with scleroderma. Case report on a patient with three successful pregnancies, *Am. J. Obstet. Gynecol.,* 89, 356, 1964.
36. **Gunther, R. E. and Hare, W. B.,** Systemic scleroderma in pregnancy. Report of a case, *Obstet. Gynecol.,* 24, 98, 1964.
37. **Johnson, T. R., Banner, E. A., and Winkelmann, R. K.,** Scleroderma and pregnancy, *Obstet. Gynecol.,* 23, 467, 1964.
38. **Karlen, J. R. and Cook, W. A.,** Renal scleroderma and pregnancy, *Obstet. Gynecol.,* 44, 349, 1974.
39. **Winkelmann, R. K.,** Scleroderma and pregnancy, *Clin. Obstet. Gynecol.,* 8, 280, 1965.
40. **Quattrochi, C. and Brocchi, D.,** Sclerodermia e gravidanja, *Clin. Obstet. Gynecol.,* 70, 31, 1968.
41. **Gruenwald, P.,** Chronic fetal distress and placental insufficiency, *Biol. Neonate,* 5, 215, 1963.

42. **Naeye, R. L. and Kelly, J. A.,** Judgment of fetal age. III. The pathologist's evaluation, *Pediatr. Clin. N. Am.,* 13, 849, 1966.
43. **Queenan, J. T.,** *Management of High-Risk Pregnancy,* 1st ed., Medical Economics Co., Oradell, 1980, 455.
44. **Rosso, P. and Winick, M.,** Intrauterine growth retardation. A new systemic approach based on the clinical and biochemical characteristics of this condition, *J. Perinat. Med.,* 2, 147, 1974.
45. **Aubry, R. H., Beydoun, S., Cabalum, N. T., and Williams, M. L.,** Fetal growth retardation, in *Perinatal Medicine. Management of the High Risk Fetus and Neonate,* Bologese, R. J. and Schwarz, R. H., Eds., Williams & Wilkins, Baltimore, 1977, 172.
46. **Bulmash, J. M.,** Rheumatoid arthritis and pregnancy, *Obstet. Gynecol. Annu.,* 8, 223, 1979.
47. **Good, S. V. and Kohler, H. G.,** Maternal death from systemic sclerosis. Report of a case of renal scleroderma masquerading a preeclamptic toxemia, *J. Obstet. Gynaecol. Br. Commonw.,* 77, 1109, 1970.
48. **Grennan, D. M., McCormick, J. N., Wojtacha, D. et al.,** Immunological studies of the placenta in systemic lupus erythematosus, *Ann. Rheum. Dis.,* 37, 129, 1978.
49. **Gudson, J. P.,** Immunologic studies of the fetal allograft, *Obstet. Gynecol.,* 37, 129, 1971.
50. **Howard, E.,** Reduction in size and total DNA of cerebrum and cerebellum in adult mice after corticosterone treatment in infancy, *Exp. Neurol.,* 22, 191, 1960.
51. **Shapiro, S.,** Some physiological, biochemical and behavioral consequences of neonatal hormone administration: cortisol and thyroxin, *Gen. Comp. Endocrinol.,* 10, 214, 1868.
52. **Burkett, G.,** Lupus nephropathy and pregnancy, *Clin. Obstet. Gynecol.,* 28, 310, 1985.
53. **Murray, F. A.,** Lupus erythematosus in pregnancy, *J. Obstet. Gynaecol. Br. Emp.,* 65, 401, 1956.
54. **Minz, G., Niz, J., Gutierrez, G. et al.,** Prospective study of pregnancy in systemic lupus erythematosus. Results of a multidisciplinary approach. *J. Rheum.,* 13, 732, 1986.
55. **Hayslett, J. P. and Reece, A. E.,** Systemic lupus erythematosus in pregnancy, *Clin. Perinatol.,* 12, 539, 1985.
56. **Hayslett, J. P.,** Effect of pregnancy in patients with SLE, *Am. J. Kidney Dis.,* 2(Suppl 1), 223, 1982.
57. **Lin, C. C., Lindheimer, M. D., River, P. et al.,** Outcome of pregnancy in hypertensive disorders of pregnancy, *Am. J. Obstet. Gynecol.,* 142, 255, 1982.
58. **Zurier, R. B., Argyros, T. G., Urman, J. D. et al.,** Systemic lupus erythematosus, *Obstet. Gynecol.,* 51, 178, 1978.
59. **Tozman, E. C. S., Urowitz, M. B., and Gladman, D. D.,** Systemic lupus erythematosus in pregnancy, *J. Rheum.,* 7, 624, 1980.
60. **Hahn, B. H.,** Systemic lupus erythematosus, in Clinical Immunology, Vol. 1, Parker, C. W., Ed., W. B. Saunders, Philadelphia, 1980, 614.
61. **Agnello, V., Cambiaso, C., Lambert, P. H., Dixon, F. J., Zubler, R. H. C. et al.,** A WHO collaborative study for the evaluation of 18 methods for detecting immune complexes in serum, *J. Clin. Lab. Immunol.,* 1, 1, 1978.
62. **Inman, R. D., Fong, J. K. K., Pussell, B. A. et al.,** The $Cl_q$ binding assay in systemic lupus erythematosus, *Arthritis Rheum.,* 23, 1282, 1980.
63. **Hubbard, H. C. and Portnoy, B.,** Systemic lupus erythematosus in pregnancy treated with plasmapheresis, *Br. J. Dermatol.,* 101, 87, 1979.
64. **Fine, L. G. et al.,** Systemic lupus erythematosus in pregnancy, *Ann. Intern. Med.,* 94, 667, 1981.
65. **Durhing, J. L.,** Pregnancy rheumatoid arthritis and intrauterine growth retardation, *Am. J. Obstet. Gynecol.,* 108, 325, 1970.
66. **Felbo, M. and Svarrason, E.,** Pregnancy and the place of therapeutic abortion in rheumatoid arthritis, *Acta Obstet. Gynecol. Scand.,* 40, 116, 1961.
67. **Morris, W. I.,** Pregnancy in rheumatoid arthritis and systemic lupus erythematosus, *J. Am. Med. Assoc.,* 183, 917, 1963.
68. **Persellin, E. H.,** The effect of pregnancy on rheumatoid arthritis, *Bull. Rheum. Dis.,* 27, 922, 1977.
69. **Nilsson, I. M., Astedt, B., Hedner, U., and Berezin, D.,** Intrauterine death and circulating anticoagulant ("anti-thromboplastin"), *Acta Med. Scand.,* 197, 153, 1975.
70. **Carreas, L. O., Machim, S. J., Demoan, R. et al.,** Arterial thrombosis, intrauterine death and lupus anticoagulant detection of immunoglobulin interfering with prostaglandin formation, *Lancet,* 1, 244, 1981.
71. **Reagan, M. G., Landner, H., and Karpatkin, S.,** Platelet function and coagulation profile in lupus erythematosus: studies in 50 patients, *Ann. Intern. Med.,* 81, 462, 1974.
72. **Feinstein, D. L. and Rapaport, S.,** Acquired inhibitors of blood coagulation, *Prog. Hemostasis Thromb.,* 1, 75, 1972.
73. **Meacham, G. and Weisburger, A.,** Unusual manifestations of disseminated lupus erythematosus, *Ann. Intern. Med.,* 43, 143, 1951.
74. **Boxer, M., Ellman, L., and Carvallaero, A.,** The lupus anticoagulant, *Arthritis Rheum.,* 19, 1244, 1976.
75. **Muer, J. R., Herbst, K. D., and Rapaport, S. I.,** Thrombosis in patients with the lupus anticoagulant, *Ann. Intern. Med.,* 92, 156, 1980.

76. **Nakao, K., Nishitani, H., Suzuki, M. et al.,** Antiacetylcholine receptor I$_g$G in neonatal myasthenia gravis, *N. Engl. J. Med.,* 297, 169, 1977.
77. **Lubbe, W. F., Butler, W. S., and Palmer, S. J.,** Lupus anticoagulant in pregnancy, *Br. J. Obstet. Gynaecol.,* 91, 357, 1984.
78. **Gleicher, N. and Friberg, J.,** I$_g$M gammopathy and the lupus anticoagulant syndrome in habitual aborters, *JAMA,* 253, 3278, 1985.
79. **Lubbe, W. F., Butler, W. S., Oalmer, S. J., and Liggins, G. C.,** Fetal survival after prednisone suppression of maternal lupus anticoagulant, *Lancet,* 1, 1361, 1983.
80. **Brauch, W. D., Kochenom, N. K., Hershgold, E. J. et al.,** The lupus anticoagulant. A recently discovered and treatable cause of recurrent abortion and fetal death, *Am. J. Reprod. Immunol.,* 5, 100, 1984.
81. **Abramowsky, C. R., Vagas, M. E., Swinehart, G. et al.,** Decidual vasculopathy of the placenta in lupus erythematosus, *N. Engl. J. Med.,* 303, 668, 1980.
82. **Imamura, M., Phillips, P. E., and Mellors, R.,** The occurrence and frequency of type C virus-like particles in placentas from patients with systemic lupus erythematosus and from normal subjects, *Am. J. Pathol.,* 83, 282, 1976.
83. **Raveche, E. S. and Steinberg, A. D.,** Lymphocytes and lymphocyte function in systemic lupus erythematosus, *Semin. Hematol.,* 16, 334, 1979.
84. **Winfield, J. B., Lobo, O. I., and Singer, A.,** Significance of antilymphocytes in systemic lupus erythematosus, *Arthritis Rheum.,* 21, 215, 1978.
85. **Bridge, R. G. and Foley, P. E.,** Placental transmission of the lupus erythematosus factor, *Am. J. Med. Sci.,* 227, 1, 1954.
86. **Beck, J. S. and Rowell, N. R.,** Transplacental passage of antinuclear antibody, *Lancet,* 1, 134, 1963.
87. **McCue, C. M., Mantakes, M. E., Tingelstad, J. E. et al.,** Congenital heart block in newborns of mothers with connective tissue disease, *Circulation,* 56, 82, 1977.
88. **Theofilopoulos, A. N., Gleicher, N., Pereira, A. B., and Dixon, F. J.,** The biology of immune complexes and their possible role in pregnancy, *Am. J. Reprod. Immunol.,* 92, 105, 1981.
89. **Gleicher, N., Adelsberg, B. R., Liu, T. L. et al.,** Immune complexes in pregnancy. III. Immune complexes in immune complex-associated conditions, *Am. J. Obstet. Gynecol.,* 142, 1011, 1982.
90. **Labarrere, C., Manni, J., Salas, P., and Althabe, O.,** Intrauterine growth retardation of unknown etiology. I. Serum complement and circulating immune complexes in mothers and infants, *Am. J. Reprod. Immunol. Microbiol.,* 8, 87, 1985.
91. **Bresnihan, B., Grigor, R. R., Oliver, M. et al.,** Immunological mechanism of spontaneous abortion in systemic lupus erythematosus, *Lancet,* 2, 1205, 1977.
92. **Harris, E. D., Jr. and Krane, S. M.,** Collagenase, *N. Engl. J. Med.,* 291, 652, 1974.
93. **Dirksen, E. R. and Levy, J. A.,** Virus-like particles in placentas from normal individuals and patients with systemic lupus erythematosus, *J. Natl. Cancer Inst.,* 59, 1187, 1977.
94. **Kalter, S. S., Helmke, R. J., Heberling, R. L. et al.,** C-type particles in normal placentas, *J. Natl. Cancer Inst.,* 50, 1081, 1973.
95. **Robertson, W. B.,** Uteroplacental vasculature, *J. Clin. Pathol.,* Suppl. 29, 9, 1976.
96. **Sheppard, B. J. and Bonnar, J.,** Uteroplacental arteries and hypertensive pregnancy, in *Pregnancy Hypertension,* Bonnar, J., McGillivray, I., and Symonds, M., Eds., University Park, Baltimore, 1978, 213.
97. **Abramowsky, C. R.,** Lupus erythematosus, the placenta, and pregnancy. A natural experiment in immunologically mediated reproductive failure, in *Reproductive Immunology,* Alan R. Liss, New York, 1981, 309.
98. **Faulk, W. P. and Johnson, P. M.,** Immunological studies of human placentae: identification and distribution of proteins in mature chorionic villi, *Clin. Exp. Immunol.,* 27, 365, 1977.
99. **Johnson, P. M., Natvig, J. B., Ystehede, U. A. et al.,** Immunological studies of human placentae: the distribution and character of immunoglobulins in chorionic villi, *Clin. Exp. Immunol.,* 31, 145, 1977.
100. **Labarrere, C., Alonso, J., Manni, J. et al.,** Immunohistochemical findings in acute atherosis associated with intrauterine growth retardation, *Am. J. Reprod. Immunol. Microbiol.,* 7, 149, 1985.

Chapter 5

OBSTETRIC MANAGEMENT OF INTRAUTERINE GROWTH RETARDATION

**Pall Agustsson and Naren Patel**

TABLE OF CONTENTS

# I. INTRODUCTION

The growth-retarded fetus with its attendant morbidity is of a major concern to obstetric and pediatric staff alike. For the proper management and optimum fetal surveillance an accurate diagnosis of intrauterine growth retardation is a prerequisite necessary to reduce the increased morbidity and mortality seen in this group of infants.[1,2]

When discussing intrauterine fetal growth, standard reference curves for the distribution of birthweight appropriate to the area in question need to be employed to account for regional differences in birthweight.[3-5] This helps to accurately assess fetal growth and to avoid misinterpretation when results from different centers are being compared. Small-for-gestational-age infants are most commonly defined as infants born with a birthweight less than the tenth percentile for gestational age or of a birthweight less than 2500 g.[6,7] Some authorities are more strict in their definition and use the fifth or third percentile but others prefer to use standard deviations from the mean and consider fetuses of a birthweight less than the mean $-2$ SD as the major risk group, a cutoff level which corresponds to the third percentile for gestational age.[8-10] Defined in such a way, not all small-for-gestational-age infants are growth retarded; many are constitutionally small, healthy, and not at increased risk of subsequent neuro-developmental sequelae.[11] On the other hand, many infants with a birthweight greater than 2500 g or a birthweight above the tenth percentile for gestational age, have not fulfilled their growth potential and are, therefore, to be regarded as small for gestational age.[12,13] These infants are usually not diagnosed antenatally and few reports have been published of their subsequent outcome.[12]

The most serious threat facing the growth-retarded fetus is hypoxia and acidosis which if it occurs antenatally becomes chronic in nature and can cause fetal demise or damage.[14] These fetuses may not tolerate the additional stress labor imposes, often severe enough to exhaust whatever reserve is left, and can lead to severe birth asphyxia.[15] Acute hypoxia and acidosis may also initially arise during the course of labor and the precarious metabolic balance of the compromised but still compensated fetus can be disturbed with adverse consequences. This increased risk of perinatal asphyxia is the main determinant, apart from social class, of the future neuro-developmental progress of the growth-retarded infant.[16-18]

Recent advances in perinatal medicine, conducting research on the fetus *in utero* by cordocentesis, support the original hypothesis that antenatal, perinatal, and postnatal factors may play a continuous sequence in the pathogenesis of the sequelae sustained by the growth-retarded infant.[19,20] Modern obstetric management must, therefore, concentrate on applying appropriate investigations and treatment during the antenatal and perinatal period, in order to prevent fetal asphyxia and subsequent handicap. The identification of the infant at risk is imperative, but the diagnosis is fraught with difficulty and only 40 to 50% of growth-retarded infants are detected antenatally by conventional clinical methods.[21,22] Other measures must therefore be employed. Primary tests to identify the at-risk group, supplemented by secondary tests to ensure proper antenatal surveillance and adequate care during labor, are the mainstay of present day obstetric management.

# II. ETIOLOGY

Various factors are known to influence the growth potential, and thereby the birthweight, of the individual fetus.[23-28] Small-for-gestational-age fetuses, a subgroup of whom is suffering from retarded intrauterine growth, form a heterogeneous group.

Genetic factors, both maternal and fetal, account for approximately 40% of the normal variation seen in the distribution of birthweight.[23,24] The uterine environment constrains fetal growth, and this effect is clearly seen in primiparous women whose infants have a lower average birthweight than infants born to parous women.[28] These variables have however,

**Table 1**
## FACTORS CAUSING OR ASSOCIATED WITH INTRAUTERINE GROWTH RETARDATION

Fetal origin:
  Idiopathic
  Chromosomal abnormalities
Feto-maternal:
  Intrauterine infection: rubella
  Cytomegalovirus, toxoplasmosis, ?HIV
  Pre-eclampsia
Maternal origin:
  Medical
    Cardiovascular disease
    Renal disease
  Obstetric
    Previous stillbirth
    Previous infant with intrauterine growth retardation
    Low prepregnancy weight
    Low weight gain during pregnancy
    Vaginal bleeding during pregnancy
    High alphafetoprotein in maternal blood in the early second trimester
  Social
    Smoking
    Alcohol abuse
    Drug abuse

not been associated with subsequent neuro-developmental deficit. Several factors adversely affect the fetus *in utero* and constrict its inborn growth potential (Table 1). Chromosomal and congenital abnormalities commonly lead to retarded intrauterine growth, and some forms of congenital infection such as rubella and cytomegalovirus can have the same effect.[23,25,29–31] Low prepregnancy weight and lack of weight gain during the pregnancy, maternal smoking, alcohol abuse, and certain drugs are also associated with and adversely affect birthweight.[32–36] Maternal cardiovascular disease and incompatible feto-maternal relationship causing utero-placental insufficiency, such as is seen in pre-eclampsia, includes one of the best-known examples of a condition which may cause retarded intrauterine growth.[37,38]

Two distinct forms of intrauterine growth retardation have been described with the aid of ultrasound.[39] Symmetrically small-for-gestational-age fetuses constitute one of those groups. These fetuses have a slower intrauterine growth rate than average, but body proportions are normal, which is reflected in an appropriate head-abdominal area ratio seen on ultrasound examination. When these effects are due to a pathological process the fetus is supposed to have sustained some form of intrauterine insult in early pregnancy, or to suffer from an abnormal chromosomal or genetic constituent.[40] Liver glycogen stores are, however, appropriate for body size, and the fetus is not particularly susceptible to antenatal or intrapartum asphyxia.[41] The other group comprises the asymmetrically growth retarded fetuses. According to Campbell and others these constitute 70% of all infants with pathologically constrained intrauterine growth.[42,43] These infants, of normal body length for gestation, have a disproportionate growth structure mainly due to decreased liver size and a lack of subcutaneous fat tissue.[44,45] Redistribution of blood flow in favor of vital organs, in particular the brain, heart, and adrenals at the expense of the liver, viscera and lower extremities results in the typical external appearance, with ''brain sparing'' and an increased head-abdominal area ratio.[46] Glycogen stores are deficient, and chronic hypoxia and acidosis are often present antenatally.[19,20,47,48] Energy reserve is minimal, and the additional stress labor imposes can result in superimposed acute hypoxia and acidosis, for which these infants are unable to compensate.

# III. DIAGNOSIS

The prerequisite for the optimum management of the growth-retarded fetus depends on an early and accurate diagnosis. Confirmation of this diagnosis must, however, wait until the end-point is reached, i.e., after birth, when the actual birthweight is known and the external appearance of the infant can be inspected. No test employed to date has proven to be fully effective in correctly diagnosing all growth-retarded infants.[49] We still have to accept the fact that severely growth-retarded infants can be missed, despite vigilant surveillance, and that unnecessary investigations will be performed on others wrongly assumed to be growth retarded. The following section illustrates the current methods available to the clinician faced with the problem of managing an infant suspected of intrauterine growth retardation (IUGR).

# IV. ANTENATAL MANAGEMENT

## A. Primary Tests

The primary tests employed in current practice to facilitate the identification of IUGR consist of: (1) antenatal screening to define a subgroup of women at risk of delivering an infant of low birthweight, (2) clinical acumen during antenatal care, and (3) obstetric ultrasound to accurately date the pregnancy and to assess fetal growth. The combined effort of this approach is important to detect the greater proportion of fetuses at risk.

### 1. High-Risk Pregnancy

Several variables, when present during the pregnancy, have a relation with the subsequent birthweight of the infant.[29-36,50-52] These risk factors, some of which are included in Table 1, identify a subgroup of women, 2 to 3% of whom will give birth to an infant of very low birthweight.[53] The shortcomings of this approach are clearly illustrated by the fact that 30% of the pregnant population will have one or more of these risk factors present and that retarded intrauterine growth occurs much more commonly in the primiparous patient, often without any identifiable adverse factors.[53]

### 2. Clinical Diagnosis

Abdominal palpation, or symphysis-fundus height and abdominal girth tape-measurements are the conventional methods used in clinical practice.[54,55] The large biological variation in fundal height and inter- and intraobserver variability makes this method unreliable to accurately detect the small-for-gestational-age fetus.[56,57] Only about one-half of growth-retarded fetuses are detected when this method is used, and for every one infant diagnosed correctly, three are falsely identified as growth retarded.[21,22] The predictive value of this method consequently suffers, but Bagger et al. pointed out that the sensitivity of the test could be increased if the antenatal screening of the individual pregnancy was performed by the same person.[57]

### 3. Ultrasound

The introduction of ultrasound into obstetrics has made the correct diagnosis of IUGR possible. It must however be emphasized that fetal growth pattern does not necessarily reflect fetal condition and to assess fetal well-being a different approach is necessary. Accurate dating of the pregnancy is a prerequisite for the precise and early diagnosis of IUGR. As 25 to 30% of pregnant women have an unreliable menstrual history, assessment of gestational age by ultrasound has become an essential part of modern obstetric care.[58,59]

The rapid fetal growth rate which characterizes the first half of pregnancy is well suited for accurate dating to be made. Crown-rump-length in the first trimester and the biparietal diameter (BPD) in the second trimester are the measurements most frequently employed to estimate gestational age.[60,61] Crown-rump-length has a demonstrated accuracy of ±5 d, and measurements of the BPD before the 24th week of pregnancy can be expected to confirm gestational length to within 6 d.[60,62] Femur length in the second trimester has, likewise, a good correlation with gestational age but shows no superiority to BPD assessment.[63] This early dating scan establishes a baseline which is mandatory for the interpretation of subsequent ultrasound examinations performed later in pregnancy.

Many obstetric centers have now organized a standard regimen, consisting of a two-step ultrasound screening during pregnancy, in order to increase the efficacy of detecting IUGR.[64] The first ultrasound scan is to date the pregnancy in the mid-trimester, and the second is to identify fetuses thought to be small for gestational age. Most centers perform this second examination in the early third trimester, at 32 to 34 weeks, but, the nearer term this examination is performed, the greater is the sensitivity of the method, and thereby the detection rate.[64-66]

### B. Secondary Tests

When IUGR is suspected by the primary tests mentioned above, the course of action usually taken consists of (1) admission to the antenatal ward for observation and assessment and (2) the employment of various biophysical and biochemical tests to ensure continuing fetal growth and well-being, and to detect deterioration in fetal health necessitating delivery.

### C. Biophysical Tests

*1. Ultrasound — Fetal Growth*

Serial ultrasound examinations performed to assess continuing fetal growth, complemented by antenatal cardiotocography, constitute the mainstay in the management of the small for gestational age fetus.[67,68] Most cases of retarded fetal growth occur in the third trimester, when the growth rate of the fetus is at its slowest. During this period of gestation the biparietal diameter increases on average by 1.5 mm, and the abdominal diameter by 3 mm per week.[69,70] Too frequent examinations by ultrasound are, therefore, inaccurate, and serial scanning of at least two-weekly intervals is recommended.[71]

**Biparietal diameter measurements** — A great variance in fetal head size is seen in the third trimester of pregnancy, and this makes BPD measurements unreliable as a single test to predict IUGR.[72,73] In fetuses suffering from asymmetrical growth retardation, where "brain sparing" commonly occurs, the fetal head size can remain within normal limits for a long time.[74] These high-risk fetuses may consequently go undetected until late in the pathological process when this method is used. Campbell has reported that static head growth for 3 weeks is compatible with intrauterine survival, but this may be at the expense of increased morbidity in this group of infants.[74,75] In order to detect symmetrical growth retardation, serial scanning is necessary to observe the slow growth rate characteristic of this type of growth retardation, and an earlier diagnosis can be made if a dating ultrasound scan was performed in the first half of the pregnancy.

**Abdominal measurements** — The size of the fetal abdomen is a much more sensitive predictor of fetal growth than head size.[64] The liver is the main determinant, being the organ most severely affected when retarded intrauterine growth occurs.[44,45] Abdominal diameters, circumference, and area have all been used for growth assessment, and the abdominal circumference seems to be the parameter most commonly used.[70,76-79] The highest reproducibility is obtained when a transverse section of the fetal trunk, where the umbilical vein traverses the fetal liver, is employed to perform the measurements.[80] Expression of the abdominal measurement as a ratio with the fetal head size is sometimes employed, but symmetrically small fetuses will be missed if the individual measurements are not analyzed separately.[81]

**Uterine volume measurements** — The total uterine volume as measured by the parallel planimetric method and the prolate ellipsoid method has a significant relationship with reduced intrauterine growth and can be used as an alternative to other methods.[82,83] They show, however, no superiority and have the disadvantage of being time consuming and require static ultrasound equipment. Their use in clinical practice remains, therefore, limited.

**Fetal weight estimation** — Fetal weight estimation is not commonly used but can be of value in the management of the growth-retarded fetus when early delivery is contemplated. Several fetal parameters have been employed to calculate fetal weight, but opinion differs as to which parameter is the most reliable. Abdominal circumference, used as a single test, has been demonstrated to predict birthweight to within 160 g/kg and when used in conjunction with the biparietal diameter an even smaller error has been recorded (106 g/kg).[84,85]

**Fetal abnormalities** — The incidence of fetal abnormalities, either chromosomal or structural, is higher in fetuses with IUGR than in the normal population.[86,87] This applies especially to fetuses with symmetrically retarded growth, and can have an important bearing on further management. Various markers exist for chromosomal derangements and these need to be looked for when a fetus with retarded intrauterine growth is being assessed by ultrasound.[88] Chromosomal analysis may be considered an appropriate option. If an abnormality is detected, a decision has to be made about how to manage the patient's intrapartum care.

### 2. Nonstressed Test (NST) — Cardiotocography

Fetal heart rate pattern recognition remains the method most widely used to assess fetal well-being. No universally accepted scoring system exists, and interpretation is subject to interobserver variation.[89] This reflects the lack of understanding of basic fetal physiology and explains the limitations of the test.

Evaluation of fetal heart rate takes into account baseline heart rate, variability, periodic changes, and decelerations. Several of the available scoring systems are illustrated in Table 2, but the simple approach of dividing fetal heart rate patterns into a "reactive" and a "nonreactive" test has been demonstrated to be as good a predictor of fetal condition as the more complicated scoring systems and is to be preferred.[90-93] Nonstressed test, or antenatal cardiotocography, utilizes the Doppler technique to record fetal heart movements from the mother's abdomen. A test is described as "normal" or "reactive" if the fetal baseline heart rate and variability are within normal limits;[93] and the fetal heart responds, with accelerations of at least 15 beats per min, to fetal movements or uterine contractions. This type of heart rate pattern has been considered a reliable indication of fetal well-being, and fetal demise within a week of a reactive test is considered uncommon.[94,95]

A "nonreactive" fetal heart rate pattern is a worrying sign when the growth-retarded fetus is being monitored.[96,97] Apart from being an indicator of fetal compromise, this pattern can be due to innocuous factors like fetal sleep state or maternal sedation. If a nonreactive fetal heart rate pattern is demonstrated on testing, intensive monitoring of the growth retarded fetus by *daily* cardiotocography is to be recommended.[98] When persistent, and especially if accompanied by decelerations, a nonreactive trace is usually an ominous sign signifying deterioration in fetal health, and warrants immediate delivery in fetal interest. Recent research by Doppler ultrasound into the feto-placental circulation suggests that fetal heart rate changes present as a late component in the deterioration of the growth-retarded fetus, but this needs further evaluation.[99,100]

### 3. Oxytocin Challenge Test (OCT)

The contraction-stress test has mainly gained popularity in America and on the continent of Europe, but is hardly ever used in the U.K. It is essentially an extension of the nonstressed test but is unphysiological as oxytocics are employed to stimulate uterine contractions.[101]

**Table 2**
**CARDIOTOCOGRAPH SCORING SYSTEMS**

I. A Six-Point Scoring System for Antenatal Cardiotocographs[90] ("Cardiff Scoring System")

| | Score | | |
|---|---|---|---|
| **Details** | **0** | **1** | **2** |
| Baseline FHR (beats/min) | <100 or >180 | 100—200 or 160—180 | 120—160 |
| Movements | None | Present | Absent |
| FHR change[a] | | No change | Accelerations |
| Contractions + FHR change[a] | Decelerations | No change | Accelerations |

II. Modified Myer-Menk/Ficher Scoring System[89,91,92]

| | Score | | |
|---|---|---|---|
| **Details** | **0** | **1** | **2** |
| Baseline FHR (beats/min) | >180 or <100 | 100—119 or 161—180 | 120—160 |
| Baseline variability (beats/min) | 2 or sinusoidal | 3—5 | 5—20 |
| Oscillatory frequency (cycles/min) | <2 | 2—6 | >6 |
| Accelerations of fetal heart to fetal movements (beats/min) | None | <15 | >15 |
| Decelerations | Late | Broad variable | None |

III. Reactive — Nonreactive[93]

Reactive
1. Accelerations in FHR of >15 beats per min in response to fetal movements (four such responses in 20 min).
2. A baseline variability of 5 to 20 beats per min
3. A baseline FHR of 120—160 beats per min

[a]  FHR — fetal heart rate.

*Note:* Nonreactive — FHR does not show these features.

The test is time consuming and can also cause uterine hyperstimulation and may provoke preterm labor. Opponents of the test point out that uterine contractions produce a transient hypoxic insult in the fetus by compromising the utero-placental circulation. Healthy fetuses can compensate for this, but the growth-retarded fetus with minimal functional reserve is predisposed to superimposed hypoxia and acidosis which, in severe cases, may add to the already increased risk of subsequent morbidity.

To perform the test, a diluted solution of Syntocinon is given intravenously to the mother by a standard regimen to provoke uterine contractions. Three contractions per 10 min are required for valid interpretation of the test by fetal heart rate pattern analysis. The test is considered "normal", or "negative", if fetal heart rate accelerations occur in response to uterine contractions. A negative OCT is a good predictor of fetal well-being, and fetal demise within a week of a negative OCT is a rare occurrence.[102,103] Late decelerations in the fetal heart rate pattern signify an "abnormal", or "positive", OCT, and delivery of the fetus is recommended.[104] The sensitivity of the test is disappointing as the false positive rate of an abnormal OCT has been recorded as high as 57%, as judged by the fetal heart rate pattern in labor, or the infant's condition at birth.[105-107] Unequivocal results are not infrequently encountered and the test is then repeated within 24 h. Several studies have shown a reactive nonstressed test to be as good a predictor of fetal well-being as a negative OCT.[108,109] An OCT may, however, be a useful adjunct in patients where a persistant nonreactive NST is obtained.[108,109]

### 4. Nipple Contractions Test

The nipple contractions test is a physiological variant of the OCT.[110] Stimulation of the nipples causes endogenous release of oxytocin which provokes uterine contractions. Interpretation of the test is performed in the same way as in the oxytocin challenge test.[111]

### 5. Fetal Movements — Kick Charts

Regular rest-activity cycles characterize intrauterine existence and form an integral part of normal fetal physiology. Each cycle lasts about 40 min and most healthy fetuses move vigorously about during the activity phase but fetal quiescence of up to 70 min has been recorded as normal.[112] Approximately 85% of pregnant women have no difficulty in perceiving at least a proportion of these movements.[113,114] An assessment of fetal movements constitutes therefore, a convenient and inexpensive way of fetal surveillance.

It has been noticed that fetal movements diminish or cease 24 to 48 h before intrauterine death. Pearson and Weaver in 1976 constructed the fetal kick chart in order to detect these fetuses at risk.[115] This requires the mothers to make a daily count of the fetal movements and to record their presence on preprinted charts. The time taken to perceive the first 10 fetal movements is noted, and 10 or more movements, over a 12-h period each day, is considered to indicate continuing fetal well-being.[115,116] This chart has subsequently been modified by others, but its sensitivity to detect the fetus at risk of intrauterine death remains untested in a randomized trial.

As perinatal mortality rates fall, the morbidity sustained by surviving infants becomes all the more important. In the compromised fetus, body movements cease in order to conserve energy and maintain adequate oxygen delivery to vital organs. The cessation of fetal movements is clearly a late component in the sequence of events leading to fetal demise, and it remains uncertain if fetal kick charts are effective in preventing the adverse neuro-developmental sequelae so frequently seen in growth-retarded infants.

### 6. Biophysical Profile

Fetal intrauterine behavior and environment is an interesting and challenging subject to explore. Modern ultrasound equipment has facilitated the investigation of the various components of fetal activity and helped to create the concept of what constitutes a normal fetal behavior. Deterioration in fetal health, as can occur in IUGR, is reflected in decreased or abnormal fetal activity, and the biophysical profile score can be used to detect fetuses at risk of intrauterine demise.[117]

The biophysical profile utilizes and combines five independent variables: fetal body movements, fetal breathing movements, fetal tone, size, number of amniotic fluid pockets, and fetal heart rate pattern. Each of these variables is scored individually according to a defined system and the results are added together to form the biophysical profile scoring (Table 3).[118] When each of the variables is used as a single test, specificity is high, but the sensitivity suffers because of a high proportion of false positive cases. When all the variables are combined together in a single scoring system, the sensitivity improves and mortality rates in high-risk pregnancies have been shown to be reduced markedly when this method is employed.[118,119]

## Table 3
## THE BIOPHYSICAL PROFILE

| Parameter | Score 2 | Score 0 |
|---|---|---|
| Amniotic fluid volume | >1 cm pocket in two perpendicular planes | <1 cm pocket in two perpendicular planes |
| Fetal movements | 3 or more gross body movements in 30 min | 2 or less body movements in 30 min |
| Fetal breathing movements | At least 30 s of sustained FMB in 30 min | <30 s of FBM in 30 min |
| Fetal tone | 1 episode of limb motion from flexion to extension to flexion in a rapid motion | No evidence of flexion movements or fetal movements |
| Fetal reactivity | 2 or more FHR accelerations of 15 beats per min for 15 s with fetal movements in 40 min | <2 accelerations in 40 min |

## Table 4
## FETAL BEHAVIORAL STATES

| FHRP[a] | FEM[b] | FM[c] |
|---|---|---|
| A | Absent | Absent |
| B | Present | Present |
| C | Present | Absent |
| D | Present | Present |

*Note:* (A) Stable heart rate variability <10 beats per min, isolated accelerations in relation to FM. (B) Stable heart rate, variability >10 beats per min, numerous accelerations. (C) Stable heart rate, variability >10 beats per min, absence of accelerations. (D) Unstable heart rate, large long-lasting accelerations.

[a]  FHRB — fetal heart rate pattern.
[b]  FEM — fetal eye movements.
[c]  FM — fetal movements.

## 7. Fetal Behavioral States

The normal healthy fetus develops a distinct behavioral pattern in late gestation, which bears a striking resemblance to that observed in newborn infants.[120] Ultrasound is employed to detect fetal body movements, breathing movements, and eye movements.[121] These variables, together with cardiotocography, are used to determine the particular behavioral stage the fetus occupies at the time of examination.[122] Four different behavioral states have been described: quiet sleep (1F), active sleep (2F), quiet awake (3F), and active awake (4F), and these are illustrated in Table 4.[123] The appearance and maturation of the fetal behavioral states depend on an intact central nervous system and several studies have shown that the development of these behavioral states are incomplete in asymmetrically growth-retarded fetuses.[122,124] This may be the result of a delayed neuro-motor development or, on the other hand, an adaptive response to a hostile intrauterine environment in order to conserve energy and oxygen consumption. It has further been implied that fetal heart rate pattern recognition may be improved by taking fetal behavioral states into account, and this may help to increase the sensitivity of cardiotocography.[122]

### 8. Doppler Ultrasound

Recent developments in Doppler ultrasound techniques have enabled signals from the fetal, placental, and uterine vessels to be detected and analyzed.[125] This approach, which at present should be regarded as experimental, needs further evaluation before being applied in clinical practice. The results already obtained indicate that this noninvasive test may be valuable for fetal surveillance in high-risk pregnancies.[126-130]

In growth-retarded fetuses, blood-flow velocity waveform analysis shows a significant reduction, and often lacks in the diastolic component of the Doppler shift obtained from the fetal descending aorta and umbilical vessels.[131,132] This is thought to reflect increased placental resistance, and this new technique may considerably improve the detection rate of the small-for-gestational-age fetus at risk of perinatal asphyxia and subsequent handicap. Recent studies have also suggested that blood flow velocity waveform analysis is an earlier and more sensitive predictor of fetal compromise than conventional cardiotocography.[99] This implies that Doppler ultrasound may assist not only in reducing mortality, but, more importantly, morbidity in this group of infants and further developments in this field are awaited with interest.

### 9. Antenatal Fetal ECG

Antenatal fetal ECG transmitted from electrodes attached to the maternal abdomen have so far been of limited value in fetal assessment.[133] Bulky machinery, high background noise, and interference with maternal ECG complexes have been the main limitations and have hindered further progress in this field.[133,134]

### D. Biochemical Tests

### 1. Placental Function Tests

The placenta being the live anchor of the fetus serves several important functions.[135] Fetal oxygen and nutritional demands are met and waste products are excreted. The production of various hormones and proteins in the placenta have been employed to measure placental function.[136,137] The substances most commonly used for fetal surveillance are oestriol and human placental lactogen as they are considered to reflect best fetal condition.[138,139] The early enthusiasm, that placental function tests could reliably diagnose deterioration in fetal health, have not been borne out, and placental function tests can presently only be used as an adjunct to other means in the management of the fetus with IUGR.[140-142]

### 2. Cordocentesis — Acid-Base Balance

It has been suspected for a long time that growth-retarded fetuses might suffer from chronic intrauterine hypoxia but inaccessibility of the fetus *in utero* has, until recently, prevented research into this field. Cordocentesis, or needling of the umbilical vessels, has become possible in the last few years.[143,144] This method has been employed by Soothill et al. and others to analyze acid-base balance in fetuses with IUGR.[19,20] It was demonstrated that a porportion of this high risk group suffered from acidosis *in utero*, which has an important bearing on management and subsequent handicap. This interesting area needs to be explored further but it remains to be seen if this approach will be available except in research centers.

## V. ANTENATAL TREATMENT

### A. Bed Rest

Admission to a hospital in a pregnancy complicated by IUGR serves two purposes. Firstly, further assessment of fetal growth and well-being is possible and secondly, it has been proposed that by decreasing the physical activity of the mother fetal growth may be improved.[145] Bed rest in the left lateral recumbent position has been shown to increase uterine blood flow.[146] This may reflect a concomitant increase in placental perfusion and thereby better placental exchange of oxygen and nutrients, leading to improved fetal condition and growth. Controversy reigns as to the beneficial value of this approach.[147,148] Laurin and Persson[147] could not demonstrate a beneficial effect on birthweight from bed rest in the hospital as compared to rest at home, in two groups of women where the pregnancy was complicated by IUGR, and therapeutic rest in twin pregnancies has not been shown to increase birthweight or to prevent preterm delivery.

## B. Medical Treatment

Placental exchange of oxygen and nutrients is known to be defective in a proportion of fetuses with IUGR.[149] This may be due to maternal disease like preeeclampsia, and one approach to improve fetal condition has been to use antihypertensive drugs to lower the mother's blood pressure.[150] This is controversial as only one symptom in the pathological process is being treated and may in fact disguise other progressive features of the disease. Also, by compromising utero-placental blood flow, it may lead to deterioration in fetal health.[151]

Hyperalimentation of the mother, or directly to the fetus through the amniotic cavity has been used to improve fetal growth but is of doubtful value.[145,152] Recently, it has been claimed in a preliminary report that intensive oxygen therapy given to the pregnant woman may improve fetal growth and prevent fetal demise in severe early IUGR, but whether subsequent handicap rate will be altered remains to be seen.[153]

## VI. LABOR MANAGEMENT

## A. Caesarean Section

The Caesarean section rate in women with a pregnancy complicated by IUGR is, as expected, much higher than in the general population.[154,155] Delivery by Caesarean section frequently needs to be expedited in maternal interest, such as in pre-eclampsia, or when the fetus is not expected to tolerate trial of labor. A liberal use of Caesarean section during labor, at the earliest sign of fetal distress, is imperative to prevent fetal asphyxia. This accounts for a large proportion of the increased rate of surgical intervention seen in this group of infants. In order to ensure optimum care, a combined obstetric-pediatric approach is essential when the growth-retarded fetus requires delivery. Adequate resuscitation of the infant at birth is mandatory, and an experienced pediatrician should always be present at the delivery.

## B. Vaginal Delivery

Vigilant surveillance of the growth-retarded fetus during labor is mandatory when a vaginal delivery is contemplated. Due to the increased risk of asphyxia, modern methods of monitoring are essential to detect deterioration in fetal condition and to prevent adverse neurodevelopmental outcome.

## C. Electronic Fetal Monitoring

Continuous fetal heart rate monitoring by a fetal scalp electrode is at present the method of choice to assess fetal condition during labor. This approach is, however, subjected to the same limitations as antenatal cardiotocography and if used as a single measure, leads to an increase in Caesarean section without apparent improvement in condition at birth.[155]

A reactive fetal heart rate without decelerations is usually considered to be a sign of a good functional reserve, enabling labor to be continued without the risk of fetal compromise. The interpretation of the fetal heart rate pattern during labor, however, becomes difficult when decelerations of the fetal heart rate occur, especially when the baseline and variability are within normal limits. It has been demonstrated that up to 50% of such heart rate patterns, when compared to fetal outcome, have to be regarded as false positive.[156] This may, however, not be as innocuous in a fetus with retarded growth as in the well-grown fetus, who can sustain brief hypoxic insult during contractions without damage. Additional measures, such as fetal scalp blood sampling for blood gas analysis, are therefore imperative to complement fetal hart rate pattern recognition if vaginal delivery is to be safely conducted without an unreasonable increase in Caesarean section.

### D. Fetal Blood Gas Analysis

The intrapartum morbidity and mortality in IUGR is ten times higher than that seen when the fetus is of an appropriate weight for gestation.[157] The capacity of the growth-retarded fetus to compensate for the increased hypoxia experienced during labor is often minimal and anaerobic metabolism frequently supervenes, resulting in lactic acidosis with its adverse sequelae. Hypoxia, if severe enough, causes decelerations in the fetal heart rate but metabolic acidosis is not invariably present.[158] It has therefore been recommended that fetal scalp blood sampling should be performed, if fetal heart rate abnormality appears during labor, to assess the acid-base balance of the fetus.[159-161] Metabolic acidosis when present, as judged by a low pH and increased base deficit, requires immediate delivery in fetal interest.

### E. Fetal ECG

Recent developments in processing the ECG signal obtained from the fetal scalp during labor has suggested that the fetal ECG may hold the promise of being an earlier indicator of fetal hypoxia than internal fetal heart rate monitoring.[162] This method is still experimental but changes seen in the ECG waveform, mainly in the PR interval and the ST segment, imply that ECG waveform pattern analysis may be a valuable aid in the intrapartum management of the growth-retarded fetus.[133]

## VII. SUMMARY

The identification of the pregnancy complicated by IUGR is the key to successful management. Two-step ultrasound screening programs appear at present to be the most efficient methods available to diagnose the growth-retarded fetus antenatally and a detection rate of up to 75% has been reported.[163] As not all small-for-gestational-age fetuses are growth retarded, further tests are necessary to evaluate fetal well-being and to detect those fetuses at risk of hypoxia and acidosis *in utero* or during labor.

The biophysical tests, antenatal cardiotocography, fetal kick-charts, and the biophysical profile are currently together with serial ultrasound scanning, the methods most widely used to assess fetal condition and may considerably improve perinatal survival. Deterioration in fetal health as diagnosed by these tests is, however, a late component in the process of IUGR. Marked hypoxia, with or without acidosis, may be present before abnormal results are obtained.

This raises questions about the efficacy of these tests in significantly reducing the increased morbidity seen in growth-retarded infants and explains the difficulty encountered when deciding the optimal timing of delivery. Presently a conservative approach is usually taken and delivery only expedited after fetal movements have decreased or stopped altogether, or when significant changes are already present in the fetal heart rate pattern. The recent developments in Doppler ultrasound obtaining signals from the feto-placental circulation hold the promise of enabling deterioration in fetal health to be diagnosed earlier than is possible by the conventional methods used today. This would result in a more effective timing of the delivery and hopefully, to a decrease in damage and neuro-developmental handicap. Once a decision has been made to deliver the growth-retarded fetus, a choice has to be made between a Caesarean section or a vaginal delivery. Whichever approach is taken, it is essential to ensure optimum surveillance during labor and delivery and an adequate resuscitation of the infant at birth to prevent peripartum asphyxia from occurring.

## REFERENCES

1. **McIlwaine, G. M., Howat, R. C. L., Dunn, F., and Macnaughton, M. C.,** The Scottish perinatal mortality survey, *Br. Med. J.,* 2, 1103, 1979.
2. **Dobson, P. C., Abell, D. A., and Beisher, N. A.,** Mortality and morbidity of fetal growth retardation, *Aust. N.Z. J. Obstet. Gynaecol.,* 21, 69, 1981.
3. **Simmonds, K., Savage, W., Nicholls, B., and Rao, V.,** Fetal growth measured by ultrasound in Bengali women, *J. Obstet. Gynecol.,* 5, 233, 1985.
4. **Gairdner, D. and Pearson, J.,** A growth chart for premature and other infants, *Arch. Dis. Child.,* 46, 783, 1971.
5. **Karlberg, P., Niklason, A., Ericson, A., Fryer, J. G., Hunt, R. G., Lawrence, C. J., and Munford, A. G.,** Methodology for evaluating size of birth, *Acta Paediatr. Scand. Suppl.,* 319, 26, 1985.
6. **Lubchenko, L. O., Hansmann, C., Dressler, M., and Boyd, E.,** Intrauterine growth as estimated from live born birthweight data at 24—42 weeks gestation, *Pediatrics,* 32, 793, 1963.
7. **Thomson, A. M., Billewicz, W. Z., and Hytten, F. E.,** The assessment of fetal growth, *J. Obstet. Gynaecol. Br. Commonw.,* 75, 903, 1968.
8. **Miller, H. C. and Merritt, T. A.,** Fetal growth, in *Humans,* Year Book Medical Publishers, Chicago, 1979.
9. **Usher, R. and McLean, F. H.,** Intrauterine growth of liveborn Caucasian infants at sea level obtained from measurements of seven diameters of infants born between 25 and 44 weeks. *J. Pediatr.,* 74, 901, 1969.
10. **Laurin, J. and Persson, P. H.,** Ultrasound screening for detection of intrauterine growth retardation, in *Intrauterine Growth Retardation: A Clinical and Ultrasonic Investigation of Diagnosis and Fetal Surveillance,* Laurin, J., Ed., University of Lund, Malmo, Sweden, 1987.
11. **Wilcox, A. J.,** Intrauterine growth retardation: beyond birthweight criteria, *Early Hum. Dev.,* 8, 189, 1983.
12. **Daikoku, N. H., Johnson, J. W. C., Graf, C., Kearney, K., Tyson, J. E., and King, T. M.,** Patterns of intrauterine growth retardation, *Obstet. Gynecol.,* 54, 211, 1979.
13. **Hull, D., Dobbing, J., Miller, R. W., Naftolin, F., Ounsted, M., Rehder, H., Robinson, J. S., Tudge, C., and Usher, R. H.,** Definition, epidemiology, identification of abnormal fetal growth, in *Abnormal Fetal Growth,* Naftolin, D., Ed., Dahlem, Konferenzen, Berlin, 1978.
14. **Pearson, J. F.,** The value of antenatal fetal monitoring, *Prog. Obstet. Gynaecol.,* 1, 105, 1981.
15. **Jones, R. A. K. and Robertson, N. R. C.,** Problems of the small-for-dates baby, *Clin. Obstet. Gynaecol.,* 11, 499, 1984.
16. **Westwood, M., Kramer, M. S., Munz, D., Lowett, J. M., and Watters, G. V.,** Growth and development of full-term non-asphyxiated small-for-gestational age newborns. Follow-up through adolescence, *Pediatrics,* 71, 376, 1983.
17. **Low, J. A., Galbraith, R. S., Muir, D., Killen, H., Pater, B., and Karchmar, J.,** Intrauterine growth retardation. A study of long-term morbidity, *Am. J. Obstet. Gynecol.,* 142, 670, 1982.
18. **Babson, S. G. and Henderson, N. B.,** Fetal undergrowth: relation of head growth to later intellectual performance, *Pediatrics,* 53, 890, 1974.
19. **Pearce, J. M. and Chamberlain, G. V. P.,** Ultrasonically guided precutaneous umbilical blood sampling in the management of intrauterine growth retardation, *Br. J. Obstet. Gynaecol.,* 94, 318, 1987.
20. **Soothill, P. W., Nicolaides, K. H., and Campbell, S.,** Prenatal asphyxia, hyperlacticaemia, hypoglycaemia and erythroblastosis in growth retarded fetuses, *Br. Med. J.,* 294, 1051, 1987.
21. **Hall, M., Chng, P. K., and MacGillivray, I.,** Is routine antenatal care worth while? *Lancet,* 2, 78, 1980.
22. **Rosenberg, K., Grant, J. M., and Hepburn, M.,** Antenatal detection: actual practice in a large maternity hospital, *Br. J. Obstet. Gynaecol.,* 89, 12, 1982.
23. **Polani, P. E.,** Chromosomal and other genetic influences on birthweight variation, in *Size at Birth,* Elliott, K. and Knight, J., Eds., Ciba Foundation Symposium 27, Associated Scientific Publishing, Amsterdam, 1974. 127.
24. **Jones, O. W.,** Genetic factors in the determination of fetal size, *J. Reprod. Med.,* 21, 305, 1978.

25. **Lechtig, A., Delgado, H., Irwin, M., Klein, R. E., Martorell, R., and Yarbrough, C.,** Intrauterine infection, fetal growth and mental development, *J. Trop Pediatr.,* 25, 127, 1979.

26. **Cohen-Overbeck, T., Pearce, J. M. F., and Campbell, S.,** The antenatal assessment of utero-placental and fetal-placental blood flow using Doppler ultrasound, *J. Ultrasound Med. Biol.,* 11, 329, 1985.

27. **Brosens, I., Robertson, W. B., and Dixon, H. G.,** The role of the spiral arteries in the pathogenesis of pre-eclampsia, in *Obstetrics and Gynecology Annals,* Wynn, R. M., Ed., Appleton-Century-Crofts, New York, 1972.

28. **Gluckman, P. D. and Liggins, G. C.,** Regulation of fetal growth, in *Fetal Physiology and Medicine,* Beard R. W. and Nathaniels, P. W., Eds., Marcel Dekker, New York, 1984.

29. **Primhac, R. A. and Simpson, R. M.,** Screening small for gestational age babies for congenital infection, *Clin. Pediatr.,* 21, 417, 1982.

30. **Chen, A. T. and Falek, A.,** Chromosome aberrations in full-term low birthweight neonates, *Hum. Genet.,* 21, 13, 1974.

31. **Anderson, N. G.,** A five year survey of small for dates infants for chromosome abnormalities, *Aust. Paediatr. J.,* 12, 19, 1976.

32. **Adelstein, P. H. and Fredrick, J.,** Antenatal identification of women at increased risk of being delivered of a low birth weight infant at term, *Br. J. Obstet. Gynaecol.,* 85, 8, 1978.

33. **Galbraith, R. S., Karchmar, B. A., Piercy, W. N., and Low, J. A.,** The clinical prediction of intrauterine growth retardation, *Am. J. Obstet. Gynecol.,* 133, 281, 1979.

34. **Miller, H. C., Hassanein, K., and Hensleigh, P. A.,** Fetal growth retardation in relation to maternal smoking and weight gain in pregnancy, *Am. J. Obstet. Gynecol.,* 125, 55, 1976.

35. **Redmond, G. P.,** Effects of drugs on intrauterine growth, *Clin. Perinatol.,* 6, 5, 1979.

36. **Tennes, K. and Blackard, C.,** Maternal alcohol consumption, birthweight and minor physical anomalies, *Am. J. Obstet. Gynecol.,* 138, 774, 1980.

37. **Moore, M. P. and Redman, C. W. G.,** Case-control study of severe pre-eclampsia of early onset, *Br. Med. J.,* 287, 580, 1983.

38. **Long, P. A., Abell, D. A., and Beischer, N. A.,** Fetal growth retardation and pre-eclampsia, *Br. J. Obstet. Gynaecol.,* 87, 13, 1980.

39. **Campbell, S.,** Fetal growth, *Clin. Obstet. Gynaecol.,* 1, 41, 1972.

40. **Pearce, J. M. F. and Campbell, S.,** Ultrasonic monitoring of normal and abnormal fetal growth, in *Modern Management of High Risk Pregnancy,* Laurensen, N. H., Ed., Plenum Press, New York, 1983, 57.

41. **Pearce, J. M. F. and Campbell, S.,** Intrauterine growth retardation, in *The Management of Labour,* Studd, J., Ed., Blackwell Scientific, Oxford, 1985, 68.

42. **Campbell, S. and Thoms, A.,** Ultrasound measurement of the fetal head to abdominal circumference ratio in the assessment of growth retardation, *Br. J. Obstet. Gynaecol.,* 84, 165, 1977.

43. **Brandt, I. and Hansmann, M.,** Catch-up growth after intrauterine growth retardation under favourable nutritional conditions, in *Poor Intrauterine Fetal Growth,* Salvadori, B. and Bocchi-Modena, A., Eds., Edizioni Minerva Medica, Parma, Italy, 1977, 527.

44. **Brooke, O. G., Wood, C., and Butters, F.,** The body proportions for small for dates infants, *Early Hum. Dev.,* 10, 85, 1984.

45. **Shelley, H. J. and Neligan, G. A.,** Neonatal hypoglycaemia, *Br. Med. Bull.,* 22, 34, 1966.

46. **Wladimiroff, J. W., Tonge, H. M., and Stewart, P. A.,** Doppler ultrasound assessment of cerebral blood flow in the human fetus, *Br. J. Obstet. Gynaecol.,* 93, 471, 1986.

47. **Illingworth, R. S.,** Why blame the obstetrician? A review, *Br. Med. J.,* 1, 797, 1979.

48. **Symonds, E. M.,** Antenatal, perinatal or postnatal brain damage, *Br. Med. J.,* 294, 1046, 1987.

49. **Simpson, G. F. and Creasy, R. K.,** Obstetric management of the growth retarded baby, in *Clinical Obstetrics and Gynaecology,* Vol. 11, Howie, P. W. and Patel, N. B., Eds., W. B. Saunders, London, 1984, 481.

50. **Brock, D. J. H., Barrow, J., Jelen, P., Watt, M., and Scrimgeour, J. B.,** Maternal serum alphafetoprotein measurements as an early indicator of low birthweight, *Lancet,* 2, 267, 1977.

51. **Tejani, N. and Mann, C. I.,** Diagnosis and management of the small-for-gestational age fetus, *Clin. Obstet. Gynaecol.,* 20, 943, 1977.

52. **Wennergen, M. and Karlsson, K.,** A scoring system for antenatal identification of fetal growth retardation, *Br. J. Obstet. Gynaecol.,* 89, 520, 1982.

53. **Cnattingius, S., Axelsson, O., Eklund, G., Lindmark, G., and Meirik, O.,** Factors influencing birthweight for gestational age with special respect to risk factors for intrauterine growth retardation, *Early Hum. Dev.,* 10, 45, 1984.

54. **Calvert, J. P., Crean, E. E., Newcombe, R. G., and Pearson, J. F.,** Antenatal screening by measurement of symphysis-fundus height, *Br. Med. J.,* 285, 846, 1982.

55. **Westin, B.,** Gravidogram and fetal growth, *Acta Obstet. Gynecol. Scand.,* 56, 273, 1977.

56. **Beazly, J. M. and Underhill, R. A.,** Fallacy of the fundal height, *Br. Med. J.,* 2, 404, 1970.
57. **Bagger, P. V., Sindberg-Eriksen, P., Secher, N. J., Thisted, J., and Westergaard, L.,** The precision and accuracy of symphysis-fundus distance measurements during pregnancy, *Acta Obstet. Gynecol. Scand.,* 64, 371, 1985.
58. **Grennert, L., Persson, P. H., and Gennser, G.,** Benefits of ultrasonic screening of a pregnant population, *Acta Obstet. Gynecol. Scand. Suppl.,* 78, 5, 1978.
59. **Campbell, S.,** The assessment of fetal development by diagnostic ultrasound, *Clin. Perinatol.,* 1, 507, 1974.
60. **Robinson, H. P. and Flemming, J. E. E.,** A critical evaluation of sonar crown-rump length measurements, *Br. Med. J.,* 4, 28, 1975.
61. **Shepard, M. and Filly, R. A.,** A standard plane for biparietal diameter measurement, *J. Ultrasound Med. Biol.,* 1, 145, 1982.
62. **Campbell, S.,** Fetal growth, in *Fetal Physiology and Medicine,* Beard, Nathaniels, Ed., W. B. Saunders, London, 1974, 271.
63. **Jeanty, P.,** Estimation of fetal age by long bone measurement, *J. Ultrasound Med.,* Suppl. 1, 189, 1982.
64. **Nielson, J. P., Whitfield, C. R., and Aitchison, T. C.,** Screening for the small-for-dates fetus: a two-stage ultrasonic examination schedule, *Br. Med. J.,* 280, 1230, 1980.
65. **Kullander, S., Marsal, K., and Persson, P. H.,** Human placental lactogen and ultrasonic screening for the detection of placental insufficiency, in *Contributions to Gynecology and Obstetrics,* Vol. 9, Keller, P. J., Ed., S. Karger, Basel, 1982, 129.
66. **Kullander, S., Marsal, K., and Persson, P. H.,** Human placental lactogen and ultrasound screening for the detection of placental insufficiency, *Cantr. Cynec. Obstet.,* 9, 129, 1982.
67. **Flynn, A. M., Kelly, J., and O'Connor, M.,** Unstressed antepartum cardiotocography in the management of the fetus suspected of growth retardation, *Br. J. Obstet. Gynaecol.,* 86, 106, 1979.
68. **Geirsson, R. T. and Persson, P. H.,** Diagnosis of intrauterine growth retardation using ultrasound, in *Clinical Obestetrics and Gynaecology,* Vol. 11, Howie, P. W. and Patel, N. B., Eds., 1984, 457.
69. **Davidson, J. M., Lind, T., Farr, V., and Whittingham, T. A.,** The limitations of ultrasonic fetal cephalometry, *J. Obstet. Gynaecol. Br. Commonw.,* 80, 769, 1973.
70. **Eriksen, P. S., Secher, N. J., and Weis-Bentzon, M.,** Normal growth of the fetal biparietal diameter and the abdominal diameter in a longitudinal study, *Acta Obstet. Gynecol. Scand.,* 64, 65, 1985.
71. **Deter, R. L., Hadlock, F. P., and Harrist, R. B.,** Evaluation of normal fetal growth and the detection of intrauterine growth retardation, in *Ultrasonography in Obstetrics and Gynaecology,* Callen, P. W., Ed., W. B. Saunders, London, 1983, 7.
72. **Persson, P. H., Grennert, L., and Gennser, G.,** Diagnosis of intrauterine growth retardation by serial ultrasonic cephalometry, *Acta Obstet Gynecol. Scand. Suppl.,* 78, 40, 1978a.
73. **Hadlock, F. P., Deter, R. L., Harrist, R. B., and Park, S. E.,** Fetal biparietal diameter. Rational choice of plane of section for sonographic measurement, *Am. J. Roentgenol.,* 138, 871, 1982.
74. **Pearce, J. M. and Campbell, S.,** Intrauterine growth retardation, in *Mangement of Labour,* Studd, J., Ed., Blackwell Scientific, Oxford, 1985, 68.
75. **Fancourt, R., Campbell, S., Harvey, D., and Norman, A. P.,** A follow up study of small for dates babies, *Br. Med. J.,* 1, 1435, 1976.
76. **Deter, R. L., Harrist, R. B., Hadlock, F. P., and Carpenter, J.,** The use of ultrasound in the assessment of normal fetal growth: a review, *J. Clin. Ultrasound,* 9, 481, 1981.
77. **Campbell, S. and Wilkin, D.,** Ultrasonic measurement of fetal abdominal circumference in the estimation of fetal weight, *Br. J. Obstet. Gynaecol.,* 82, 689, 1975.
78. **Neilson, J. P., Murjanja, S. P., and Whitfield, C. R.,** Product of fetal crown-rump length and trunk area: ultrasound measurement in high risk pregnancies, *Br. J. Obstet. Gynaecol.,* 91, 756, 1984a.
79. **Warsof, S. L., Cooper, D. J., Little, D., and Campbell, S.,** Routine ultrasound screening for antenatal detection of intrauterine growth retardation, *Obstet. Gynecol.,* 67, 33, 1986.
80. **Chudleigh, P. and Pearce, J. M.,** Normal and abnormal growth, in *Obstetric Ultrasound, How, When, Why,* Chudleigh, P. and Pearce, J. M., Eds., Churchill Livingstone, 1986, 131.
81. **Campbell, S. and Thoms, A.,** Ultrasound measurement of the fetal head to abdomen circumference ratio in the assessment of growth retardation, *Br. J. Obstet. Gynaecol.,* 84, 165, 1977.
82. **Geirsson, R. T., Christie, A. D., and Patel, N. B.,** Ultrasound volume measurements comparing the prolate ellipsoid method with a parallel planimetric area method against a known volume, *J. Clin. Ultrasound.,* 10, 329, 1982.
83. **Gohari, P., Berkowitz, R. L., and Hobbins, J. C.,** Prediction of intrauterine growth retardation by determination of total intrauterine volume, *Am. J. Obstet. Gynecol.,* 127, 255, 1977.
84. **Warsof, S. L., Pearce, J. M., and Campbell, S.,** Routine ultrasound screening, *Clin. Obstet. Gynaecol.,* 10, 445, 1983.
85. **Campbell, S. and Wilkin, D.,** Ultrasonic measurement of fetal abdominal circumference in the estimation of fetal weight, *Br. J. Obstet. Gynaecol.,* 84, 165, 1975.

86. **Van den Berg, B. J. and Yerushalmy, J.,** The relationship of the rate of intrauterine growth of infants of low birth weight to mortality, morbidity and congenital abnormalities, *J. Pediatr.*, 69, 531, 1966.
87. **Chen, A. T. L. and Falec, A.,** Chromosome aberrations in full-term low birthweight neonates, *Hum. Genet.*, 21, 13, 1974.
88. **Smith, P. A., Chudleigh, P., and Campbell, S.,** Prenatal diagnosis: ultrasound, *Br. J. Hosp. Med.*, 31, 421, 1984.
89. **Flynn, A. M., Kelly, J., Matthews, K., O'Connor, M., and Viegas, O.,** Predictive value of an observer variability in several ways of reporting of antepartum cardiotocography, *Br. J. Obstet. Gynaecol.*, 89, 434, 1982.
90. **Pearson, J. F. and Weaver, J. B.,** A six-point scoring system for antenatal cardiotocographs, *Br. J. Obstet. Gynaecol.*, 85, 321, 1978.
91. **Fischer, W. M., Stude, I., and Brandt, H.,** Ein vorschlag zur Beurteilung des antepartualen kardiotokograms, *Z. Geburtshilfe Perinatol.*, 180, 117, 1976.
92. **Myer-Menk, W., Ruttgers, H., Boos, R., Wurth, G., Adis, B., and Kubli, F.,** A proposal for a new method of CTG evaluation, in *Abstracts of Free Communications*, 5th European Congr. Perinatal Medicine, Almquist and Wiksell Int., Stockholm, 1976, 138.
93. **Flynn, A. M. and Kelly, J.,** Evaluation of fetal wellbeing by antepartum fetal heart monitoring, *Br. Med. J.*, 1, 936, 1977.
94. **Flynn, A. M., Kelly, J., and O'Connor, M.,** Unstressed antepartum cardiotocography in the management of the fetus suspected of growth retardation, *Br. J. Obstet. Gynaecol.*, 86, 106, 1979.
95. **Lin, C., Devoe, L. D., River, L., and Moawad, A. H.,** Oxytocin challenge test and intrauterine growth retardation, *Am. J. Obstet. Gynecol.*, 140, 282, 1981.
96. **Varma, T. R.,** Unstressed antepartum cardiotocography in the management of pregnancy complicated by intrauterine growth retardation, *Acta Obstet. Gynecol. Scand.*, 63, 129, 1984.
97. **Lenstrup, C. and Haase, N.,** Predictive value of antepartum fetal heart rate non-stress test in high risk pregnancy, *Acta Obstet. Gynecol. Scand.*, 64, 133, 1985.
98. **Schifrin, B. S., Foye, G., Amato, J., Kates, R., and MacKenna, J.,** Routine fetal heart rate monitoring in the antepartum period, *Obstet. Gynecol.*, 54, 21, 1979.
99. **Trudinger, B. J., Cook, C. M., Jones, L., and Giles, W. B.,** A comparison of fetal heart rate monitoring and umbilical artery waveforms in the recognition of fetal compromise, *Br. J. Obstet. Gynaecol.*, 93, 171, 1986.
100. **Jouppila, P. and Kirkinen, P.,** Increased vascular resistance in the descending aorta of the human fetus in hypoxia, *Br. J. Obstet. Gynaecol.*, 91, 853, 1984a.
101. **Kubli, F. W., Kaeser, O., and Hinselmann, M.,** Diagnostic management of chronic placental insufficiency, in *The Fetal Placental Unit*, Exerpta Medica, Amsterdam, 1968.
102. **Ray, M., Freeman, R. K., and Pine, S.,** Clinical experience with the oxytocin challenge test, *Am. J. Obstet. Gynecol.*, 114, 1, 1972.
103. **Garite, T. J. and Freeman, R. K.,** Antepartum stress monitoring, *Clin. Obstet. Gynecol.*, 6, 295, 1979.
104. **Cetrulo, C. L. and Freeman, R. K.,** Bioelectric evaluation in intrauterine growth retardation, *Clin. Obstet. Gynecol.*, 20, 979, 1977.
105. **Weingold, A. B., De Jesus, T. P. S., and O'Keeffe, J.,** Oxytocin challenge test, *Am. J. Obstet. Gynecol.*, 123, 466, 1975.
106. **Garite, T. J., Freeman, R. K., and Hachleutner, I.,** Oxytocin challenge test: achieving the desired goals, *Obstet. Gynecol.*, 57, 614, 1978.
107. **Freeman, R. K., Coelbelsmann, U., and Nachimson, D.,** An evaluation of the significance of a positive oxytocin challenge test, *Obstet. Gynecol.*, 47, 8, 1986.
108. **Solum, T., Ingimarsson, I., and Sjoberg, N.-O.,** Selection criteria for oxytocin stress test, *Z. Geburtshilfe Perinatol.*, 184, 200, 1980.
109. **Keegan, K. A. and Paul, R. H.,** Antepartum fetal heart rate testing, IV. The non-stress test as a primary approach, *Am. J. Obstet. Gynecol.*, 136, 75, 1980.
110. **Copel, J. A., Otis, C. S., Stewart, I., Rosetti, C., and Weiner, S.,** Contraction stress testing with nipple stimulation, *J. Reprod. Med.*, 30, 465, 1985.
111. **Huddleston, J. F., Sutcliffe, G., and Robinson, D.,** Contraction stress test by intermittent nipple stimulation, *Obstet. Gynecol.*, 63, 669, 1984.
112. **Ritchie, J. W. K.,** Fetal surveillance, in *Dewhurst's Textbook of Obstetrics and Gynaecology for Postgraduates*, Whitfield, C. R., Ed., Blackwell Scientific, Oxford, 1986, 442.
113. **Sadovski, E. and Polishuk, W. Z.,** Fetal movements *in utero, Obstet. Gynecol.*, 50, 49, 1977.
114. **Wood, C., Walters, W. A. W., and Trigg, P.,** Methods of recording fetal movement, *Br. J. Obstet. Gynaecol.*, 84, 561, 1977.
115. **Pearson, J. F. and Weaver, J. B.,** Fetal activity and fetal wellbeing: an evaluation, *Br. Med. J.*, 1, 1305, 1976.
116. **Liston, R. M., Cohen, A. W., Mennuti, M. T., and Gabbe, S. G.,** Antepartum fetal evaluation by maternal perception of fetal movement, *Obstet. Gynecol.*, 60, 424, 1982.

117. **Manning, F. A., Platt, L. D., and Sipos, L.,** Antepartum fetal evaluation. Development of a fetal biophysical profile, *Am. J. Obstet. Gynecol.,* 136, 787, 1980.

118. **Manning, F. A., Baskett, T. F., Morrison, I., and Lange, I.,** Fetal biophysical profile scoring: a prospective study in 1184 high-risk patients, *Am. J. Obstet. Gynecol.,* 140, 289, 1981.

119. **Vintzileos, A. M., Campbell, W. A., Ingardia, C. J., and Nochimson, D. J.,** The fetal biophysical profile and its predictive value, *Obstet. Gynecol.,* 62, 271, 1983.

120. **Prechtl, H. F. R.,** Ultrasound studies of human fetal behaviour, *Early Hum. Dev.,* 12, 91, 1985.

121. **von Vliet, M. A. T., Martin, G. B., Jr., Nijhuis, J. G., and Prechtl, H. F. R.,** Behavioural states in the fetusus of nulliparous women, *Early Hum. Dev.,* 12, 121, 1985.

122. **Rizzo, G., Arduini, D., Pennestri, F., Romanini, C., and Mancuso, S.,** Fetal behaviour in growth retardation: its relationship to fetal blood flow, *Prenat. Diagn.,* 7, 229, 1987.

123. **Nijhuis, J. G., Prechtl, H. F. R., Martin, C. B., Jr., and Bots, R. S. G. M.,** Are there behavioural states in the human fetus? *Early Hum. Dev.,* 6, 177, 1982.

124. **von Vliet, M. A. T., Martin, G. B., Jr., Nijhuis, J. G., and Prechtl, H. F. R.,** Behavioural states in growth-retarded human fetuses, *Early Hum. Dev.,* 12, 183, 1985.

125. **Fitzgerald, B. E. and Drumm, J. E.,** Non-invasive measurement of human fetal circulation using ultrasound: a new method, *Br. Med. J.,* ii, 1450, 1977.

126. **Eik-Nes, S. H., Brubakk, H. C., and Ulstein, M. K.,** Measurement of fetal blood flow, *Br. Med. J.,* 280, 283, 1980a.

127. **Gill, R. W., Trudinger, B. J., Garrett, W. J., Kossoff, G., and Warren, P. S.,** Fetal umbilical venous flow measured *in utero* by pulsed Doppler and B mode ultrasound. I. Normal pregnancies, *Am. J. Obstet. Gynecol.,* 139, 720, 1981.

128. **Hackett, G. A., Campbell, S., Gamsu, M., Cohen-Overbeck, T., and Pearce, J. M. F.,** Doppler studies in the growth retarded fetus and prediction of neonatal necrotizing enterocolitis, haemorrhage and neonatal morbidity, *Br. Med. J.,* 294, 13, 1987.

129. **Erskine, R. L. A. and Ritchie, J. W. K.,** Umbilical artery blood flow characteristics in normal and growth-retarded fetuses, *Br. J. Obstet. Gynaecol.,* 92, 605, 1985.

130. **Giles, W. B., Trudinger, B. J., and Baird, P. J.,** Fetal umbilical artery flow velocity waveforms and placental resistance: pathological correlation, *Br. J. Obstet. Gynaecol.,* 92, 31, 1985.

131. **Griffin, S., Bilardok, K., Masini, L., Diaz-Recasens, J., Pearce, J. M., Willson, K., and Campbell, S.,** Doppler blood flow waveforms in the descending thoracic aorta of the human fetus, *Br. J. Obstet. Gynaecol.,* 91, 997, 1984.

132. **Giles, W. B., Trudinger, B. J., and Cook, C. M.,** Fetal umbilical artery waveforms, *J. Ultrasound Med.,* Suppl. 1, 98, 1982.

133. **Greene, K. R.,** The ECG waveform, in *Bailliers Clinical Obstetrics and Gynaecology,* Vol. 1, Whittle, M. J., Ed., Bailliere Tindal, London, 1987, 131.

134. **Hon, E. H. and Lee, S. T.,** The fetal electrocardiogram. I. The electrocardiogram of the dying fetus, *Am. J. Obstet. Gynecol.,* 87, 804, 1963a

135. **Diczfalusy, E.,** Endocrine functions of the human placenta, *Am. J. Obstet. Gynacol.,* 119, 419, 1974.

136. **Chard, T. and Klopper, A.,** Steroid hormones, in *Placental Function Tests,* Chard, T. and Klopper, A., Eds., Springer-Verlag, Berlin, 1982, 39.

137. **Chard, T. and Klopper, A.,** Placental protein hormones, in *Placental Function Tests,* Chard, T. and Klopper, A., Eds., Springer-Verlag, Berlin, 1982, 56.

138. **Gerhard, I., Fitzer, C., Klinga, K., Rahmon, N., and Runnebaum, B.,** Estrogen screening in evaluation of fetal outcome and infant's development, *J. Perinat. Med.,* 14, 279, 1986.

139. **Spellacy, W. N., Buhi, W. C., and Birk, S. A.,** Human placental lactogen and IUGR, *Obstet. Gynecol.,* 47, 446, 1976.

140. **Duenhoelter, J. H., Whalley, P. J., and MacDonald, P.,** An analysis of plasma immunoreactive estrogen measurements in determining delivery time with a fetus considered at high risk, *Am. J. Obstet. Gynecol.,* 125, 889, 1976.

141. **Aickin, D. R., Duff, G. B., Evans, J. J., and Legge, M.,** Antenatal biochemical screening to predict low birthweight infants, *Br. J. Obstet. Gynaecol.,* 90, 129, 1983

142. **Persson, P. H., Grennert, L., Gennser, G., and Eneroth, P.,** Fetal biparietal diameter and maternal plasma concentration of placental lactogen, chorionic gonadotrophin oestriol and alphafetoprotein in normal and pathological pregnancies, *Br. J. Obstet. Gynaecol.,* 87, 25, 1980.

143. **Dafflos, F., Capella-Pavloski, M., and Forestier, F.,** Fetal blood sampling via the umbilical cord using a needle guided by ultrasound: report of 66 cases, *Prenat. Diagn.,* 3, 271, 1983.

144. **Nicolaides, K. H., Soothill, P. W., Rodeck, C. H., and Campbell, S.,** Ultrasound guided sampling of umbilical cord and placental blood to assess fetal wellbeing, *Lancet,* 1, 1065, 1986.

145. **Beischer, N. A.,** Treatment of fetal growth retardation, *Aust. N.Z. J. Obstet. Gynaecol.,* 18, 28, 1978.

146. **Morris, N., Osborn, S. B., and Wright, H. P.,** Effective uterine blood flow during exercise in normal and pre-eclamptic pregnancies, *Lancet,* 2, 481, 1956.

147. **Laurin, J. and Persson, P. H.,** The effect of bedrest in hospital on fetal outcome in pregnancies complicated by intrauterine growth retardation, in *Intrauterine Growth Retardation: A Clinical and Ultrasonic Investigation of Diagnosis and Fetal Surveillance,* Vol. 4, Laurin, J., Ed., Department of Obstetrics and Gynecology, University of Lund, Malmo, Sweden, 1987, 1.

148. **Saunders, M. C., Dick, J. S., and Brown, I. M.,** The effects of hospital admission for bed rest on the duration of twin pregnancy: a randomized trial, *Lancet,* 2, 793, 1985.

149. **Sheppard, B. L. and Bonnar, J.,** The effect of hypertension on the uteroplacental vasculature, in *Perinatal Medicine,* Clinch, J. and Matthews, T., MTP Press, Lancaster, England, 1984, 127.

150. **Naden, R. P. and Redman, C. W.,** Antihypertensive drugs in pregnancy, *Clin. Perinatol.,* 12, 521, 1985.

151. **Davey, D. A., Dommisse, J., and Garden, A.,** The investigation of labetalol in the management of hypertension in pregnancy, *Amsterdam Excerpta Medica,* 51, 1982.

152. **Renaud, R., Kirstetter, L., Koehl, C., Boog, G., Brettes, J. P., Schumacher, J. C., Vincedon, G., Willard, D., and Gandar, R.,** Intra-amniotic amino-acid injections, in *Therapy of Feto-Placental Insufficiency,* Salvadori, B., Ed., Springer-Verlag, Berlin, 1975, 265.

153. **Nicolaides, K. H., Campbell, S., Bradley, R. J., Bilardo, C. M., Soothill, P. W., and Gibb, D.,** Maternal oxygen therapy for intrauterine growth retardation, *Lancet,* 2, 942, 1987.

154. **Banta, D. H. and Thacker, S. B.,** Costs and benefits of electronic fetal monitoring, *Obstet. Gynaecol. Surv.,* 34, 627, 1979.

155. **Haverkamp, A. D., Orleans, M., Langendoerfer, S., McFee, J., Murphy, J., and Thompson, H. E.,** A controlled trial of the differential effects of intrapartum monitoring, *Am. J. Obstet. Gynecol.,* 134, 399, 1979.

156. **Hutchison, R. S. and Crawford, J. W.,** Intrapartum fetal monitoring: present status, in *The Management of Labour,* Studd, J., Ed., Blackwell Scientific, Oxford, 1985, 195.

157. **Dobson, P. C., Abell, D. A., and Beischer, N. A.,** Mortality and morbidity of fetal growth retardation, *Aust. N.Z. J. Obstet. Gynaecol.,* 21, 69, 1981.

158. **Beard, R. W., Filshie, G. M., Knight, C. A., and Roberts, G. M.,** The significance of the changes in the continuous fetal heart rate in the first stage of labour, *J. Obstet. Gynaecol. Br. Commonw.,* 78, 865, 1971.

159. **Smith, N. C., Soutter, W. P., Sharp, F., McColl, J., and Ford, I.,** Fetal scalp blood lactate as an indicator of intrapartum hypoxia, *Br. J. Obstet. Gynaecol.,* 90, 821, 1983.

160. **Lin, C. C., Moawad, A. H., Rosenow, P. J., and River, P.,** Acid base characteristics of fetuses with intrauterine growth retardation during labor and delivery, *Am. J. Obstet. Gynecol.,* 137, 533, 1980.

161. **Katz, M., Meizner, I., Maxor, M., and Jasler, V.,** Fetal heart rate pattern and scalp blood pH as predictors of fetal distress, *Isr. J. Med. Sci.,* 17, 260, 1981.

162. **Lilja, H., Greene, K. R., Karlsson, K., and Rosen, K. G.,** ST waveform changes of the fetal electrocardiogram during labour — a clinical study, *Br. J. Obstet. Gynaecol.,* 92, 611, 1985.

163. **Holmqvist, P., Ingemarsson, I., and Sjoberg, N.-O.,** Intrauterine growth retardation and gestational age, *Acta Obstet. Gynecol. Scand.,* 65, 633, 1986.

Chapter 6

# THE CREATION OF A PERINATAL GROWTH CHART FOR INTERNATIONAL REFERENCE

## Peter M. Dunn

Nomenclature, definitions, and classification are the bedrock on which scientific progress is built. Lacking a common language, much time and effort will be wasted. As chairman of the International Federation of Gynecology and Obstetrics (FIGO) Sub-Committee on Perinatal Epidemiology and Health Statistics, I organized a workshop in Cairo in November 1984 with the aim of making recommendations on the methodology of the measurement and recording of infant growth in the perinatal period. Participants were invited from all parts of the world and from all the main international organizations with a major interest in the subject, including the World Health Organization, the International Pediatric Association, and the International Association for Maternal and Neonatal Health. Care was also taken to see that the disciplines of growth and nutrition, pediatrics, obstetrics, perinatal pathology, epidemiology, community medicine, and public health were all represented. The working papers of the participants were published as a Supplement of Acta Paediatrica Scandinavica,[1] while the Workshop Report was submitted to the President and Executive Board of FIGO at its meeting in Berlin in September 1985. It was warmly received and was formally published by FIGO in May 1986.[2]

The report makes recommendations on the methodology of maternal, placental, and infant anthropometry, on the measurement of gestational age, and on the assessment of fetal growth. Agreement was also reached on an internationally acceptable reference for growth throughout late fetal and early postnatal life. The remainder of this chapter discusses the philosophy on which this latter FIGO recommendation was based.[3]

The need for an international reference chart to represent normal growth throughout late fetal and early postnatal life has long been recognized.[4] Many charts, like that of Lubchenco and her colleagues,[5] have been advanced during the last two decades. Such charts have usually been created from cross-sectional measurements of birthweight following delivery at different gestational ages. Typically they show a number of curves representing the distribution of birthweight between 26 and 43 weeks' gestation. While some charts show a normal distribution over all or part of the gestational age range, others do not. In many, the curves have been smoothed. Any effort to superimpose these charts on each other reveals how dissimilar they are, especially in the lower gestational age range.[6,7] This should not surprise us in view of the inherent problems involved: the difficulty of determining gestational age accurately; the fact that pre- and postterm delivery is itself deviant and infants born early or late may well reflect aberrant growth; the ethnic, socioeconomic, and other variations between the different populations studied; and the lack of uniformity in arbitrarily excluding groups of babies whose prenatal growth was suspected of being abnormal.

My own search for a perinatal growth chart that was versatile enough to serve as an international reference and at the same time simple to understand, to reproduce, and to use, was undertaken between 1962 and 1966. Previous accounts may be found elsewhere.[8-14] At this time it will only be possible to sketch an outline of the arguments and hypotheses on which the chart is based.

A study of the various fetal growth charts that were available revealed a number of shared characteristics: a linearity for mean weight between 28 and 38 weeks' gestation indicating a steady incremental weight gain; a slope of the line which appeared remarkably constant; and a curved flattening of the line as term was reached and passed.[6] Moreover, a study of

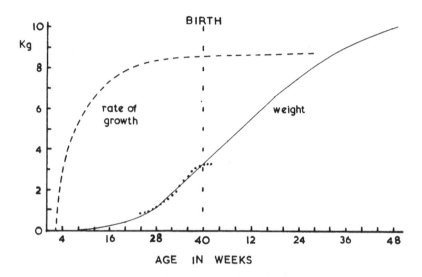

FIGURE 1.   Normal weight gain and rate of growth (see text) during prenatal and early postnatal life. The median from the chart of Lubchenco et al. has been superimposed on the weight line (24 to 43 weeks' gestation). (Adapted from Lubchenco, L. O., Hansman, C., Dressler, M., and Boyd, E., *Pediatrics*, 37, 793, 1963.)

postnatal growth charts based on longitudinal studies showed that for the first 18 weeks after term delivery, the infant resumed a linear incremental weight gain very similar to that maintained between 28 and 38 weeks' gestation.[15] Prior to 28 weeks' gestation and after 18 weeks' postnatal age the line gradually flattened to produce a gentle S-shaped curve (Figure 1). This observation, first recorded by McKeown and Record[15] and since confirmed by others,[16] suggested that the flattening of the growth line at and after term with singleton infants, and before term with multiple births,[17] was due to maternal/placental constraint of normal fetal growth.[6] Support for this hypothesis comes from the observation that when very normal populations are studied, the linear period of growth in the 3rd trimester is maintained until 40 or even 41 weeks.[18-20] As in the case of an individual infant, it is a matter of chance whether or not he or she remains *in utero* long enough to experience this period of terminal growth constraint and, as the intention was to base the reference line on normal unconstrained growth throughout the perinatal period, it seemed reasonable and indeed necessary to ignore this late-term and postterm flattening of the growth curve. The same applied to the short pause in growth that typically follows birth while feeding is becoming established. There remained then the task of determining the position and slope of a line representing normal weight gain over the period being discussed. While the final precise position and slope might be determined arbitrarily, it was necessary that it should closely reflect normal observed weight gain over the whole period. In this sense "normal" was equated with "average", since it is known that both growth acceleration and retardation may be associated with increased perinatal mortality and morbidity. The reference line that was ultimately chosen commenced at 1.1 kg at 28 weeks, and demonstrated a steady incremental weight gain of 1.1 kg every 6 weeks until reaching a weight of 6.6 kg at 18 weeks' postnatal age. It is thus easy to remember as well as to reproduce (Figure 2).

The average weight for age of the fetus and of the infant soon after birth is shown in Figure 1. Also shown is the rate of growth as judged by the time taken to successively double body weight (see also Figure 3). Note that while incremental weight gain is proceeding rapidly in the perinatal period, the rate of growth at that time has greatly slowed as compared with the rate in early pregnancy (see also Figure 2). It is possible to explain the whole normal distribution of weight-for-age observed throughout the period in terms of a very

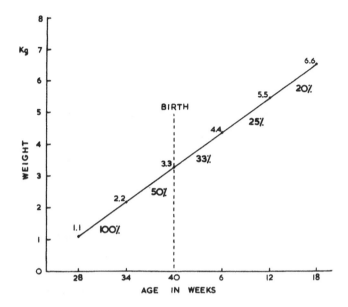

FIGURE 2. Line representing the normal weight gain of the average. Caucasian infant during the period before and after birth. The weights are given at 6-week intervals from 28 weeks' gestation to 18 weeks' postnatal age. The percentages indicate the steady deceleration in the rate of growth expressed as the ability to double weight during each period.

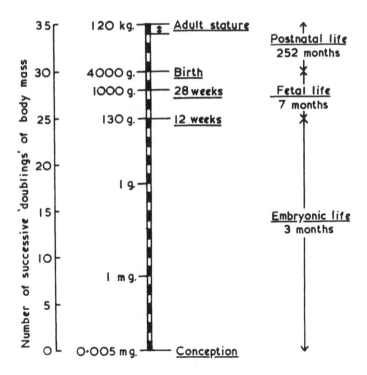

FIGURE 3. Between conception and the attainment of adult stature the human body successively doubles its weight some 34 to 35 times. No less than 30 of these successive doublings occur before birth, 25 during the first trimester, 3 during the second, and 1 to 2 during the third.

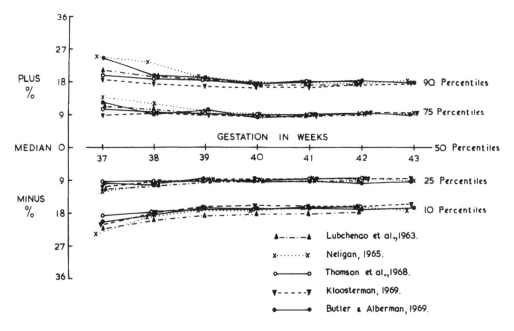

FIGURE 4. The 10th, 25th, 75th, and 90th percentiles of birthweight-for-gestational age (37 to 43 weeks) from five studies in the 1960s are shown plotted as plus or minus percentages of their own median weight curves.

small variation ($\pm 1.5\%$) in the growth velocity from conception onwards.[8] When this knowledge is combined with the fact that about 95% of all relative prenatal growth has taken place by 28 weeks' gestation,[8,10] then we can afford to assume that, for all practical purposes, normally growing fetuses have almost identical potential growth velocities during the last trimester and differ significantly from each other only in the weight they have achieved at the start of that period. Again, one can argue that within any population there must be *"normal"* subgroups, as for instance males and females, with growth lines balanced above and below the central tendency. The lines for these subgroups would tend to diverge progressively from each other as time went on.[21,22] The same applies to postnatal weight charts.[23,24] If these observations are applied, it should be possible to construct diverging lines relating to the original reference line and embracing the area of observed weight-for-age. Unfortunately, as has already been said, the distributions of the various published fetal growth charts vary enormously from each other. However, when in 1969 the various centiles of birthweight-for-gestation of five well-known fetal growth charts for Caucasian infants[5,22,25-27] were plotted as a plus or minus percentage of their own medians, a remarkable correspondence was revealed (Figure 4). Thus, the 25th and 75th centiles for infants 37 to 43 weeks gestation lay at $\pm 9.1\%$ of the median value, while the 10th and 90th centiles lay at $\pm 18.2\%$.[13] This knowledge was used to help construct the Bristol Perinatal Growth Chart. (1.1 kg plus 18.2% at 28 weeks is exactly 1.3 kg, while 1.1 kg minus 18.2% is 0.9 kg.) If lines are now constructed $\pm 18.2\%$ from the reference line, they will be found to diverge steadily. Infants growing along them will again show an incremental weight gain every 6 weeks equal to their initial weight at 28 weeks (e.g., 1.3 kg $\rightarrow$ 2.6 $\rightarrow$ 3.9 $\rightarrow$ (term) $\rightarrow$ 5.2 $\rightarrow$ 6.5 $\rightarrow$ 7.8 kg at 18 weeks postnatal age; and 0.9 kg $\rightarrow$ 1.8 $\rightarrow$ 2.7 $\rightarrow$ (term) $\rightarrow$ 3.6 $\rightarrow$ 4.5 $\rightarrow$ 5.4 kg at 18 weeks postnatal age). Once again, these lines are easy to remember, to reproduce, and to use (Figure 5). In Figure 6 the 10th, 50th, and 90th centiles of the Lubchenco chart[5] have been superimposed on the Bristol Chart up to 40 weeks' gestation, while those of Tanner[23] are shown for the early postnatal period. The close correspondence is striking. It is important to appreciate that while the incremental weight gain ranges from

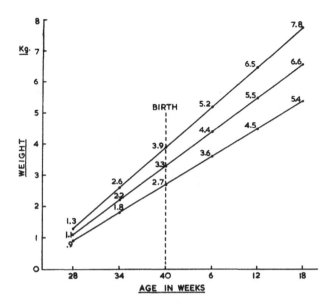

FIGURE 5. The Bristol Perinatal Growth Chart with fetal and infant weights shown at 6-week intervals.

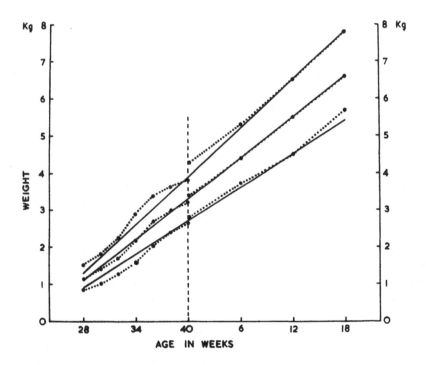

FIGURE 6. The fetal growth curves (10th, 50th, and 90th percentiles) of Lubchenco et al. and the early postnatal growth curves for boys and girls combined (10th, 50th and 90th percentiles) of Tanner are shown superimposed on the Bristol Perinatal Growth Chart. (Adapted from Lubchenco, L. O., Hansman, C., Dressler, M., and Boyd, E., *Pediatrics,* 32, 793, 1963; Tanner, J. M., *Modern Trends in Paediatrics,* 2nd series, Hozel, A. and Tizard, J. P. M., Eds., Butterworths, London, 1968, 325.)

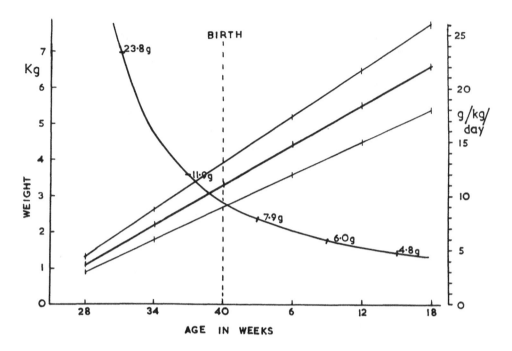

FIGURE 7.   The perinatal growth reference line and two related lines at ±18.2%. The incremental weight gain of a fetus growing along the lowest line would be 21.4 g/d, along the central line 26.2 g/d and along the upper line 31.0 g/d. Yet all three fetuses have an identical decreasing rate of growth expressed in g/kg/d and shown by the falling, curved slope.

21.4 g/d for infants on the lower line, through 26.2 g/d for the reference line, to 31.0 g/d for the upper line, the rate of growth expressed as g/kg/d is identical for all three lines, slowing from 23.8 g/kg/d in the first 6-week period to 4.8 g/kg/d in the last (Figure 7).

The Bristol Perinatal Growth Chart has many uses in addition to that as a standard against which other charts may be compared. For example, if the assumption of a normal distribution of weight-for-gestational-age proves correct (as appears to be the case for monkeys[28] and for infants after birth[23,24]), then the chart may be used to categorize infants that are heavy, appropriate, or light for their gestational age (Figure 8), (note that lines drawn at ±25% approximate to ±2 SD). Then it may be used to study special groups of infants as, for example, those born, without malformation, to women with polyhydramnios (Figure 9).[11,12] The chart may also be used to study the longitudinal growth of individual infants (Figure 10).[12] Its nature and symmetry also permit allowance to be made for biological variables influencing growth. For example, boys weigh on average 6% more than girls throughout the perinatal period.[21] It is thus possible to make a ±3% allowance according to the sex of the infants under study (Figure 11). Allowance may also be made for other biologic variables such as maternal height.[11,21,27]

The mathematical simplicity and symmetry of the Bristol Chart makes it a convenient tool with which to study the metabolic requirements of the fetus/placenta or infant in relation to its growth. We have already noted that the average infant has a steady incremental weight gain of 1.1 kg every 6 weeks throughout the perinatal period. This, of course, does *not* indicate a steady rate of growth. Rather it indicates a steady and rapid deceleration in the rate of growth throughout this period. Thus, during the first 6-week period from 28 to 34 weeks the fetus doubles its weight from 1.1 to 2.2 kg. If we call this + 100%, then the figures for the following 6-week periods are + 50%, + 33%, + 25% and + 20% (Figure 2). Let us focus on the fetus of 28 to 34 weeks' gestation. It is true that he is growing much less rapidly than he did during his embryonic days but he is still growing some 52 times

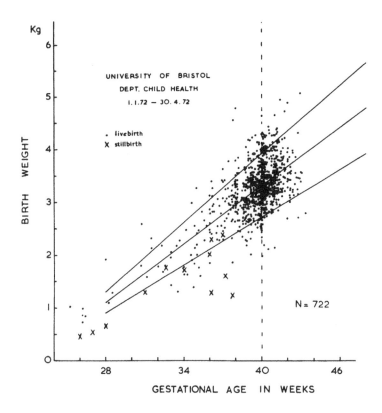

FIGURE 8. Birthweight-for-gestation of 722 consecutively born British infants plotted on the Bristol Perinatal Growth Chart. Of the infants, 10% fall below the lower line and 10% above the upper line.

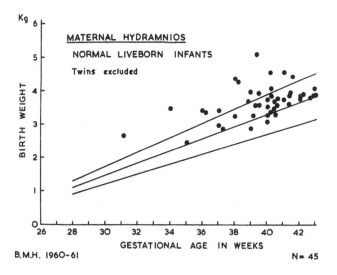

FIGURE 9. Birthweight and gestational age of 45 normal liveborn singleton infants born to women with hydramnios at the Birmingham Maternity Hospital, 1960 to 61, superimposed on the Bristol Perinatal Growth Chart (28 to 43 weeks). (Adapted from Dunn, P. M., *Acta Medica Auxol.*, 7, 63, 1975.)

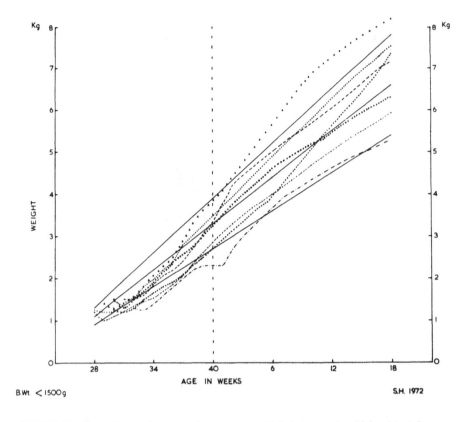

FIGURE 10.   Postnatal growth curves of seven consecutively born very low birthweight infants superimposed on the Bistol Perinatal Growth Chart. (Adapted from Dunn, P. M., Perinatal Medicine, 6th European Congr. Perinatal Medicine, Vienna (1978), Thalhammer, O., Baumgarten, K., and Pollak, A., Eds., Georg Thieme Verlag, Stuttgart, 1979, 1.)

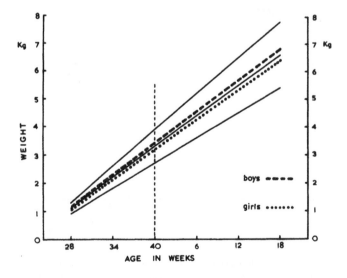

FIGURE 11.   Mean fetal growth lines for boys and girls ( ± 3%) in relation to the Bristol Perinatal Growth Chart.

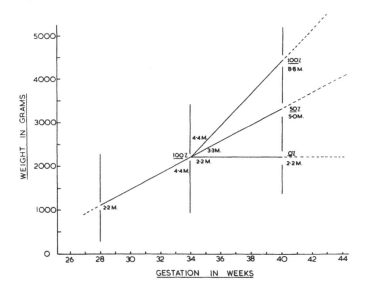

FIGURE 12. The hypothetical metabolic requirements (M) of a fetus in relation to its rate of growth and size during the last trimester (see text).

faster than a child of 5 to 11 years of age. It can be calculated that if such a fetus maintained its rate of growth unaltered until the age of 3 years, it would then weigh 148 million kg or 145,000 tons and be the size of St. Paul's Cathedral. What work does a fetus of this gestational age have to do in his uterine incubator? He may occasionally kick and breathe and, of course, his heart has to keep pumping. However, apart from this he really has very little to do, except to grow and grow and grow. It seems not unreasonable to speculate that the metabolic requirements to maintain the growth of a fetus that doubles its weight in 6 weeks are likely to be at least equal to those required to maintain its basal metabolic rate. It would appear from the work of Brooke[29] that this speculation falls within the bounds of calculated probability.

The next step was to invent a unit of metabolic requirement called "M". A single "M" was defined as the metabolic requirement needed to maintain the basal metabolic rate of 1 kg of fetus. It was also, according to the speculative assumption already mentioned, the metabolic requirement per kg of fetus needed to maintain growth when the fetus was doubling its weight in 6 weeks, what has been referred to as "100% growth".

Figure 12 demonstrates the number of "M" required by a fetus during the last trimester of pregnancy in relation to its weight and rate of growth. Thus, a fetus of 1.1 kg with "100% growth" will require 2.2 M at 28 weeks gestation and 4.4 M at 34 weeks when its weight has doubled to 2.2 kg. If the same rate of growth is maintained during the second half of the last trimester, the weight of the fetus will have risen to 4.4 kg and the metabolic requirement to 8.8 M. If, on the other hand, the rate of growth has slowed to 50%, as it usually does (Figure 2), then the infant will weigh 3.3 kg at 40 weeks and will require only 5.0 M to maintain basal metabolism and growth. Finally, let us suppose that at 34 weeks fetal growth is abruptly switched off. Then the metabolic requirements will immediately fall to 2.2 M and will still be at that figure 6 weeks later at term. Thus, we see from this model that the larger rapidly growing fetus may require four times the metabolic resources of the smaller fetus that is not growing.

But another factor must also be examined, which is the ability of the utero-placental circulation to process and transfer the metabolic requirements from mother to fetus. Now, this ability may be excellent, average, or poor, but whichever it is, it is likely to deteriorate as term is reached and passed, and the utero-placental vasculature "ages". In the model

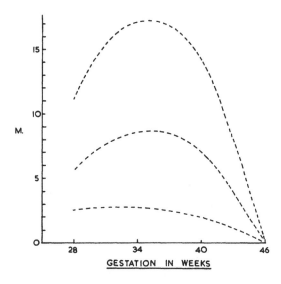

FIGURE 13.   The hypothetical potential of three types of utero-placental circulation with good, average or poor function, to transfer metabolic requirements to the fetus. The assumption is made that, due to the ageing of the vasculature, utero-placental function will fall to zero in each case at 46 weeks' gestation.

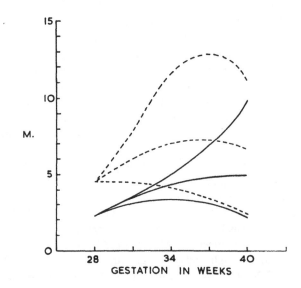

FIGURE 14.   The hypothetical dynamic interplay between the fetal metabolic requirements in relation to rate of growth and size (unbroken line, see Figure 12), and the ability of the utero-placental circulation to provide this metabolic requirement in relation to its functional capacity and age (interrupted line, see Figure 13).

seen in Figure 13 which shows the functional capacity of three hypothetical utero-placental circulations — very good, average, and poor, it has been assumed in each case that the utero-placental vasculature finally completely "fails" at 46 weeks gestation. If this.is the case then the functional capacity of the "very good" utero-placental circulation will fall much more rapidly as it ages than will that of the "poor" utero-placental circulation.

In Figure 14 the dynamic interreaction of the two sets of models which we have just considered are examined, namely the fetal metabolic requirements and the utero-placental

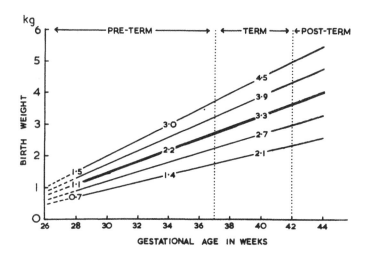

FIGURE 15. A shortened version of the Bristol Perinatal Growth Chart (28 to 44 weeks).

functional capacity. If we take the lower pair of lines representing poor utero-placental function and a small fetus that is not growing, we see that the two curves both fall gradually together, approaching but not crossing each other. The middle pair of curves representing the normal fetus and utero-placental circulation are beginning to converge at term but are still comfortably apart. In contrast, the upper pair of curves representing excellent utero-placental function and the large fetus that is still growing rapidly as term approaches show how acutely the metabolic demands of the fetus increase, while at the same time the functional capacity of the utero-placental circulation is falling rapidly. If these curves are extended, a head-on clash is inevitable. The fetus has not time to adapt by switching off its growth. It must either be delivered or die.

These models may help to explain clinical observations and experience which might otherwise seem mysterious and paradoxical; how, on the one hand, a malnourished and growth retarded infant with a cobweb thin and tiny placenta may be born alive at 44 weeks gestation weighing perhaps only 1.8 kg; and, on the other hand, how a great big obese infant born to a woman with diabetes and weighing 5 kg at 36 weeks gestation and with a large fleshy placenta, may die suddenly in late pregnancy or during labor. In brief, it is suggested that the curtailment of the rate of fetal growth at term may serve the fetus well by protecting him from intrapartum asphyxia as well as from the more obvious danger of disproportion.

Before leaving discussion of the uses to which the Bristol Chart may be put, it is worth pointing out that for the study of the immediate perinatal period, a truncated version may be more convenient (Figure 15). It will be seen that for gestational ages of less than 28 weeks, interrupted lines have been used to indicate that linearity is progressively lost as gestational age falls to 20 weeks (Figure 1). Information on birthweight distribution in the second trimester is accumulating[30,31] and it should soon be possible to construct a standard for reference for this period too. In the same way standards for other parameters such as height and head circumference are also required for international reference.[32]

Pecorari and his colleagues[33,34] have demonstrated the use of the Bristol Perinatal Growth Chart as an international standard for reference in respect to Caucasian populations. While more non-Caucasian data is still awaited it does appear as though the normal unconstrained growth in the perinatal period of other ethnic groups is very similar, observed differences being explained either by maternal size (for which allowance can be made) or by pathological or environmental influences (which are the factors requiring study). Thus, Bhargava and

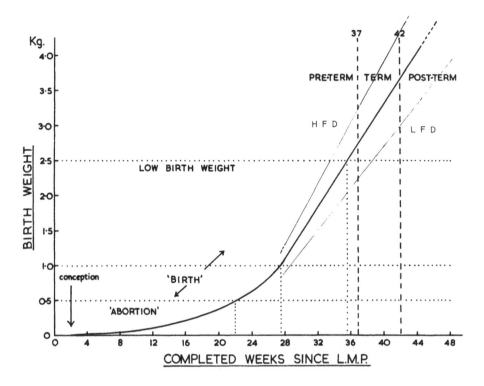

FIGURE 16.   Definitions relating to birthweight and gestational age (H.F.D. = heavy-for-dates; L.F.D. = light-for-dates).

colleagues[35] have demonstrated that the fetal growth curve of a privileged Indian population is very similar to that of Caucasian populations in developed countries, and Hendrickse[36] has written: "Studies in Nigeria have provided conclusive proof that adverse environmental factors are the key determinants of the poor growth attainment of children in West Africa when compared with European counterparts. Comparisons between an "elite" cohort of Nigeria-Yoruba children, who enjoyed good living standards, with the U.S. international reference population,[37] show essentially similar growth and development in the preschool and primary age groups . . . " He then rightly warned of the danger of judging the growth achievement of infants and children in developing countries against local standards based on populations whose growth has been profoundly influenced by their poor environment.

The possession of a perinatal reference chart for weight does not obviate the need to collect information on different populations. Indeed, this is essential in order to discover how the various populations relate to the reference standard. This may best be achieved by studying the birthweight (and subsequent growth) of healthy, normal, singleton infants born normally after a spontaneous onset of labor at 38 to 40 weeks to healthy, adequately nourished, nonsmoking, multigravid women whose pregnancies have been free of complications. Even the study of as few as 100 such infants should be sufficient to determine a relationship. To give an example, it appears that the mean birthweight at 40 weeks' gestation for Scandinavian populations is approximately 3.6 kg,[18,19] which is plus 9.1% on the reference line.

In conclusion, a versatile perinatal weight chart, based on the concept of normal unconstrained growth, has been created to serve as an international standard for reference purposes. It permits allowance to be made for biologic variables such as sex and maternal height, and appears to be applicable to differing ethnic groups. It is extremely easy to remember, to construct, and to use (Figure 16).

# ACKNOWLEDGMENT

I wish to thank the Van Neste Foundation for their support during the period when the ideas in this paper were formulated.

# REFERENCES

1. **Wharton, B. and Dunn, P. M., Eds.,** *Perinatal Growth: The Quest for an International Standard for Reference,* Acta Paediatrica Scandinavica Supplement 319, Almqvist & Wicksell, Stockholm, 1985.
2. Report of the FIGO Sub-Committee on Perinatal Epidemiology and Health Statistics following a Workshop on the Methodology of Measurement and Recording of Infant Growth in the Perinatal Period, Cairo, November 11 to 18, 1984, International Federation of Gynecology and Obstetrics (FIGO), London, 1986; *Int. J. Gynaecol. Obstet.,* 24, 483, 1986; *Bull. Int. Pediatr. Assoc.,* 8, 107, 1987.
3. **Dunn, P. M.,** A perinatal growth chart for international reference, in *Perinatal Growth: The Quest for an International Standard for Reference,* Acta Paediatrica Scandinavica Supplement 319, Wharton B. and Dunn, P. M., Eds., Almqvist & Wicksell, Stockholm, 1985, 180.
4. **Dunn, P. M.,** The search for perinatal definitions and standards, in *Perinatal Growth: The Quest for an International Standard for Reference,* Acta Paediatrica Scandinavica Supplement 319, Wharton B. and Dunn, P. M., Eds., Almqvist & Wicksell, Stockholm, 1985, 7.
5. **Lubchenco, L. O., Hansman, C., Dressler, M., and Boyd, E.,** Intrauterine growth as estimated from liveborn birthweight data at 24 to 42 weeks of gestation, *Pediatrics,* 32, 793, 1963.
6. **Gruenwald, P.,** Growth of the human fetus. I. Normal growth and its variations, *Am. J. Obstet. Gynecol.,* 94, 1112, 1966.
7. **Battaglia, F. C., Frazier, T. M., and Hellegers, A. E.,** Birth weight, gestational age, and pregnancy outcome with special reference to high birth weight — low gestational age infant, *Pediatrics,* 37, 417, 1966.
8. **Dunn, P. M. and Butler, N. R.,** Interuterine Growth. A discussion of some of the problems besetting its measurement, in *Symposia of the Society for the Study of Human Biology, 10: Biological Aspects of Demography,* Brass, W., Ed., Taylor & Francis, London, 1971, 147.
9. **Dunn, P. M.,** The gestogram — a new standard perinatal growth chart, in *Proc. 3rd German Congr. Perinatal Medicine,* Thieme Verlag, Stuttgart, Germany, 1972, 242.
10. **Dunn, P. M.,** The Bristol Perinatal Growth Chart: a simple flexible standard based on normal growth velocity, Working paper for WHO Consultation on Reporting and Analysis of Perinatal and Maternal Morbidity, Bristol, September 25 to 27, 1972, 1.
11. **Dunn, P. M.,** Late fetal growth of Caucasian infants based on weight, head circumference and length at birth, Working paper for WHO Consultation on Reporting and Analysis of Perinatal and Maternal Morbidity and Mortality, Bristol, September 25 to 27, 1972, 1.
12. **Dunn, P. M.,** Growth retardations of infants with congenital postural deformities, *Acta Medica Auxol.,* 7, 63, 1975.
13. **Dunn, P. M.,** Perinatal terminology, definitions and statistics, in *Perinatal Medicine, 6th European Congr. Perinatal Medicine, Vienna (1978),* Thalhammer, O., Baumgarten, K., and Pollak, A., Eds., Georg Thieme Verlag, Stuttgart, 1979, 1.
14. **Dunn, P. M.,** Variations in fetal growth: some causes and effects, in *Fetal Growth Retardation,* Van Assche, F. A., Robertson, W. B., and Renaer, M., Eds., Churchill Livingstone, Edinburgh, 1981, 79.
15. **McKeown, R. and Record, R. G.,** The influence of placental size on fetal growth in man, with special reference to multiple pregnancy, *J. Endocrinol.,* 9, 418, 1953.
16. **Kloosterman, G. J.,** The obstetricians and dysmaturity, in *Nutricia Symposium: Aspects of prematurity and dysmaturity,* Jonxis, J. H. P., Visser, H. K. A., and Troelstra, J. A., Eds., H. E. Stenfert Kroese, N V Leiden, 1978, 263.
17. **McKeown, T. and Record, R. G.,** Observations on foetal growth in multiple pregnancy in man, *J. Endocrinol.,* 8, 386, 1952.
18. **Biering, G., Snaedal, G., Sigvaldason, H., Ragnarsson, J., and Geirsson, R. T.,** Size at birth in Iceland, in *Perinatal Growth,* Wharton, B. A. and Dunn, P. M., Eds.; *Acta Paediatr. Scand. Suppl.,* 319, 68, 1985.
19. **Karlberg, P., Fryer, J., Ericson, A., and Niklasson, A.,** Analysis of the size at birth by gestational age, in *Perinatal Growth,* Wharton, B. A. and Dunn, P. M., Eds.; *Acta Paediatr. Scand. Suppl.,* 319, 26, 1985.

20. **Stembera, Z., Kavarik, J., and Jungmannova, C.,** Frequency of fetal growth deviations diagnosed by ultrasonic measurement and analysis of their causes, in *Perinatal Growth,* Wharton, B. A. and Dunn, P. M., Eds.; *Acta Paediatr. Scand. Suppl.,* 319, 48, 1985.

21. **Kloosterman, G. J.,** Prevention of prematurity, *Meded T Verlosk,* 66, 361, 1966.

22. **Kloosterman, G. J.,** Birthweight and maturity, WHO Seminar on the prevention of perinatal morbidity and mortality, Tours, France, April 22 to 26, 1969.

23. **Tanner, J. M.,** The evaluation of physical growth and development, in *Modern Trends in Paediatrics,* 2nd series, Holzel, A. and Tizard, J. P. M., Eds., Butterworths, London, 1968, 325.

24. **Scott, A., Moar, V., and Ounsted, M.,** Growth in the first four years. I. The relative effects of gender and weight for gestational age at birth, *Early Hum. Dev.,* 7, 17, 1982.

25. **Neligan, G.,** A community study of the relationship between birthweight and gestational age, in *Gestational Age, Size and Maturity, Clinics of Developmental Medicine, 19,* Hawkins, M. J. R. and MacGregor, W. G., Eds., William Heinemann, London, 1965, 28.

26. **Thomson, A. M., Billewicz, W. Z., and Hytten, F. E.,** The assessment of fetal growth, *J. Obstet. Gynaecol. Br. Commonw.,* 75, 903, 1968.

27. **Butler, N. R. and Alberman, E. D.,** Perinatal problems, in *The Second Report of the British Perinatal Mortality Survey,* Churchill Livingstone, London, 1969.

28. **Fujikura, T. and Niemann, W. H.,** Birth weight, gestational age, and type of delivery in rhesus monkeys, *Am. J. Obstet. Gynecol.,* 97, 76, 1967.

29. **Brooke, O. G.,** Energy expenditure in the fetus and neonate: sources of variability, in *Perinatal Growth,* Wharton, B. A. and Dunn, P. M., Eds.; *Acta Paediatr. Scand. Suppl.,* 319, 128, 1985.

30. **Brooke, O. G. and McIntosh, N.,** Birthweights of infants born before 30 weeks' gestation, *Arch. Dis. Child.,* 59, 1189, 1984.

31. **Keen, D. V. and Pearse, R. G.,** An analysis of bodyweight by gestation between 14 and 42 weeks, *Arch. Dis. Child.,* 60, 440, 1985.

32. **Falkner, F.,** Some introductory concepts of human growth: an overview, in *Perinatal Growth,* Wharton, B. A. and Dunn, P. M., Eds.; *Acta Paediatr. Scand. Suppl.,* 319, 17, 1985.

33. **Pecorari, D.,** Normal and abnormal development of human embryos and fetuses: embryonic-fetal growth and intrauterine environment, in *Clinical Pharmacology in Pregnancy,* Knemmerle, H. P. and Brendel, K., Eds., Thieme-Stratton, New York, 1984, 34.

34. **Pecorari, D., Costa, L., and Barbone, F.,** Practical application of the Bristol Perinatal Growth Chart to Mediterranean populations, in *Perinatal Growth,* Wharton, B. A. and Dunn, P. M., Eds.; *Acta Paediatr. Scand. Suppl.,* 319, 80, 1985.

35. **Bhargava, S. K., Sachdev, H. P. S., Iyer, P. U., and Ramji, S.,** Current status of infant growth measurements in perinatal period in India, in *Perinatal Growth,* Wharton, B. A. and Dunn, P. M., Eds.; *Acta Paediatr. Scand. Suppl.,* 319, 103, 1985.

36. **Hendrickse, R. G.,** Growth and Development in developing countries, *Bull. Int. Pediatr. Assoc.,* 5, 62, 1984.

37. **Janes, M. D., Macfarlane, B. J., and Moody, J. B.,** Height and weight growth standards for Nigerian children, *Ann. Trop. Paediatr.,* 1, 27, 1981.

Chapter 7

# ULTRASOUND IN DETECTION OF GROWTH RETARDED FETUSES

**Višnja Latin and Jadranka Pavletić**

## TABLE OF CONTENTS

## I. INTRODUCTION

Intrauterine growth retardation (IUGR) continues to represent one of the most significant problems in modern perinatology. Although there is still no specific treatment, early and accurate diagnosis can reduce the hazards of impaired fetal growth by optimal timing delivery.[1,2] Clinical evaluation of fetal growth retardation is difficult and rather inaccurate.[3] In studies evaluating routine antenatal care fewer than 50% of growth-retarded infants were clinically suspected.[4] Biochemical methods are also rather unreliable.[5] With sophisticated ultrasonic techniques, the diagnosis of IUGR is now more accurate than ever before. Nevertheless, detection is associated with many problems, and that is reflected with large number of ultrasonic methods devised for IUGR detection.

Ultrasound screening for IUGR has not been proved to be substantially better than simple serial fundal height measurements.[6,7] However, in selected high-risk groups, ultrasound is the best diagnostic tool for following fetal growth deviation and establishing a diagnosis. It is the only method which safely can provide longitudinal data on fetal growth with reasonable accuracy.

An accurate knowledge of gestational age is essential in order to reliably evaluate ultrasonic measurements in late pregnancy, and thereby diagnose IUGR. The optimal method for detecting IUGR is early ultrasonic assessment of gestational age combined with late assessment of fetal size or, preferably, growth rate. Ultrasound also plays an important role in evaluating fetal activities and functions. Its role in the detection of fetal anatomical abnormalities is irreplaceable.[8]

## II. ASSESSMENT OF FETAL AGE

Clinical assessment of fetal age, based on menstrual history, is rather unreliable. A questionable menstrual history has been found in 20 to 40% of pregnancies.[9,10] The combination of uncertain menstrual dates and any high-risk obstetric situation can result in a fourfold increase in perinatal mortality because it is difficult to assess the appropriate time for delivery.[9] Even when the menstrual history seems reliable, ultrasound dating in early pregnancy more accurately predicts the date of delivery.[10,11] Ovulation can be delayed more than 2 weeks in patients with oligomenorrhoea. Conception may occur early after birthcontrol medication.[12,13] Bleeding during the time of the first missed period may also cause error in dating the pregnancy.

The first trimester of pregnancy is the best period for ultrasonically estimating gestational age for at that stage biological variations are minimal and there is the best growth rate of the embryo. Measurement of the crown-rump length, originally described by Robinson, is the most accurate method for determining gestational age,[14] i.e., $\pm 4.7$ d (2 SD of the mean).[15] The CRL measurement which is obtainable by the 8th week of gestation,[16] is the longest length of embryo, defined as the distance between the outer edge of the crown to the outer edge of the rump. Limbs and yolk sac are not included (Figure 1).

In an earlier study[11] we confirmed that during the first trimester of pregnancy, it is possible to predict gestational age within a confidence limit of $\pm 6$ d in more than 90% of patients. It is observed that the mean CRL increases from 10 mm, at 7 weeks to 84 mm at 14 weeks, i.e., about 10 mm weekly. The original study was performed with a static scanner, but similar accuracy can be obtained by real-time equipment.[17] After the 12th week of gestation the flexion of the fetal spine significantly reduces measurement accuracy.

BPD (biparietal diameter) measurement is a standard and most widely used ultrasonic parameter for the estimation of gestational age in the second trimester of pregnancy.[18,19] From 14 to 16 weeks of pregnancy it has a predictive value of $\pm 7$ d in 90% of cases. During the third trimester its accuracy for estimating gestational age decreases to $\pm 21$ d in 90% of cases.

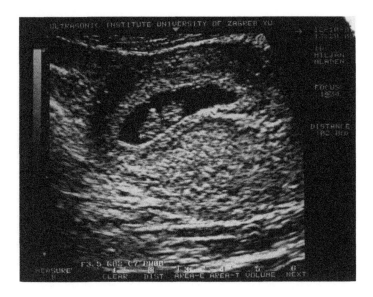

FIGURE 1. The measurement of the crown-rump length. Calipers mark outer edge of the crown and outer edge of the rump.

Accuracy obtained with a static scanner is similar to that obtained by real-time equipment.[20] To obtain reproducibility with the method, the standard plane of measurement is essential.[21] This includes the thalamus and cavum septi pellucidi. The occipito-frontal diameter and head circumference should be measured in the same section. The shape of the skull should be ovoid, and the midline echo, which is generated by the interhemispheric fissure, should be exactly in the middle. After obtaining the proper section, ultrasonic gain should be reduced to avoid apparently "thickening" of the skull. Calipers should be placed at the outer edge of the image of the proximal skull to the inner edge of the distal skull (Figures 2A and 2B).

After 24 weeks of pregnancy, accuracy of BPD measurement is affected by biological variations, pathological growth (mostly IUGR), head abnormalities (microcephaly, hydrocephaly), and head molding. Excessive flattening of the head, dolicocephaly, is frequently present in breech presentation, and can be quantified by the "cephalic index", i.e., the ratio of the BPD to the OFD (occipito-frontal diameter).[22] If the cephalic index is smaller than 0.75, dolicocephaly is present, and the BPD is not a reliable predictor of gestational age. In such circumstances, a complementary method, i.e., fetal limb bones measurement should be performed.[23-28]

Fetal limb bones measurements were originally introduced for the detection of skeletal abnormalities.[29-31] Subsequently those measurements also proved useful in the evaluation of gestational age. Fetal femur length (because it is most easy obtainable) has become the most used parameter. It has been found to be at least as accurate as BPD in the estimation of gestational age.[27-32] Several authors have found it superior.[33,34]

The measurement of fetal femur length is obtained from the greater trochanter to the lateral condyle. The head of the femur is not included. When a clear image of the femur is obtained, the freeze frame is employed and the calcified portion of the bone is measured. In the longitudinal section the entire length of the bone is visualized with characteristic background shadowing (Figure 3).

Many charts have now been developed depicting the growth of various ultrasonic parameters. Sabbagha and Hugney showed that, with BPD measurements using standard techniques and equipment, statistically there is no significant difference between the many available charts.[35]

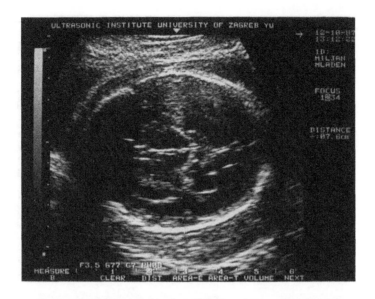

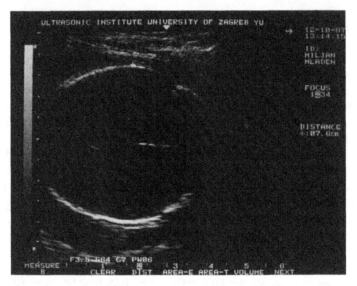

FIGURE 2.    (A) The measurement of biparietal-diameter (BPD). Standard section
includes midline echo, thalamus, and cavum septi pellucidi on the same level.
(B) Same ultrasound picture with reduced gain. Calipers are placed at the outer
edge of the proximal skull and inner edge of the distal skull.

Later experience with ultrasonic measurement has shown that some variation occurs among
different populations when the same ultrasound parameters are measured using the same
methods. Haines et al.[28] reported a difference of more than 5 mm at term in the measurement
of fetal femur length, when compared to the study of O'Brien and Queenan.[36] Such a
discrepancy could cause a significant error in assessment of gestational age if different
normograms are used. Hence, there is a need to establish the normal values for each
population being evaluated.

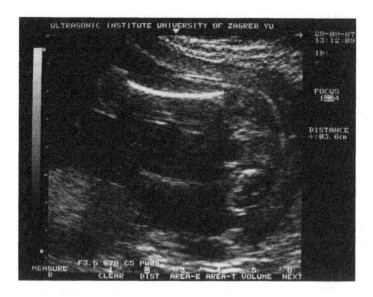

FIGURE 3.   The measurement of femur length. Calipers are placed on trochanter and lateral condyle.

## III. ASSESSMENT OF FETAL GROWTH

The diagnosis of IUGR is associated with difficulties which are partly due to the use of imprecise definitions and inconstant diagnostic criteria. The widely accepted definition of IUGR is based on birthweight. Newborns whose birthweight is below the tenth percentile for gestational age is classified as SGA (small for gestational age). This is the most frequently used criterion, but birthweight below the 25th, 5th, and 3rd percentile, or 2 SD below the mean, are also reported.[37] Another source of discrepancy is the use of various birthweight standards, and this leads to great differences among newborns classified as SGA. For example, the 10th percentile values, given by Thomson et al.,[38] are nearly equal to the 25th percentile values of Lubchenco et al.[39] Moreover, all those birthweight curves, often wrongly called growth curves, are rather inaccurate since they have been obtained cross-sectionally and have not been based on a normal population.[40] A recent study from Secher et al. has confirmed that preterm infants, viewed as a group, are smaller than unborn fetuses of the same age.[41] In order to overcome that problem, several authors have established intrauterine weight curves based on estimated fetal weights.[41-43] It is obvious that such growth curves are more representative of fetal growth since the measurements have been obtained longitudinally and are based on a normal healthy population. However, possible errors in weight estimation limit the usefulness of the method. Also different boundaries between normal and abnormal values of ultrasonic parameters have been reported.

It is clear that the birthweight criterion alone can lead to an underestimation of the number of infants who (due to fast growth potential) are actually growth retarded at birth. Conversely, there are some normal, but constitutionally small infants without any other pathology, who are wrongly diagnosed as being growth retarded.

The term IUGR implies the abnormal restriction of growth of an infant with greater development potential.[44] Hence, IUGR should not to be used as a synonym for SGA. The diagnosis of IUGR requires additional information, such as the pattern of the fetal growth, and particularly, the rate of the fetal growth.

The ultrasound diagnosis of impaired fetal growth has been made by comparing the measurements from individual fetuses to population standards. The limitations of this method have already been mentioned. To overcome this problem, Deter et al. have used Rossavik's growth model[45] to establish individual growth curve standards for various ultrasonic parameters.[46] They reported that individual growth curve models, derived from data obtained before the 28th week of pregnancy, were capable of predicting growth beyond 28 weeks. (It is presumed that comparing a measurement of its expected value provides a sensitive indicator of impaired fetal growth.) Theoretically, a method of individualized assessment of fetal growth seems to be convenient, but the technique needs further investigation. Another, relatively new method, i.e., umbilical artery flow velocity waveforms[47] also is promising, but awaits further assessment.

## A. The Biparietal Diameter

A wide variety of ultrasonic parameters have been used, alone and in different combinations, to diagnose IUGR. At first, cephalometry was probably the most commonly used method of assessing fetal growth.[18,48] Serial cephalometry identified two patterns of impaired fetal growth.[10] In symmetrical IUGR (type I), the BPD growth pattern was steady, but indicated an abnormally low growth rate ("low profile") which began early in the second trimester. In this variety there is high incidence of congenital malformation and the prognosis is poor. In asymmetrical growth retardation (type II), there is a lengthy period of normal BPD growth which is followed by an abrupt flattening of the BPD growth curve ("late flattening") in the third trimester.[10] This type of growth retardation is commonly associated with maternal and placental factors leading to faulty growth support. As there is no strict boundary between types I and II, mixed patterns are also found to occur, and it is not always easy to distinguish one type of growth retardation from another.

Disadvantages of this method include: (1) the need for serial measurements, (2) BPD measurements will detect only the symmetrical type of IUGR which probably includes many healthy genetically small infants,[49] (3) true, symmetrically retarded infants, constitute only about 20% of all growth-retarded infants,[1,8] (4) there are intrinsic limitations to the use of ultrasonic cephalometry for the estimation of fetal weight, and (5) the BPD reflects only one dimension of the head and is frequently not truly representative of the total fetal head and brain size. There is also a biological variation in cranial morphology. Crane and Kopta reported that BPD measurements can be of value even in detecting asymmetrically retarded infants.[50]

The accuracy of antenatal diagnosis of IUGR based upon BPD data by several investigators ranges from 35 to 70%.[42,51,52] We found that both single and serial BPD measurements showed a diagnostic accuracy of approximately 50%.[53] Thus, although the method is simple and reproducible, ultrasonic measurement of the fetal head alone is not a reliable predictor of IUGR.

## B. Abdominal Circumference (AC)

Another relatively old, but much more sensitive method of diagnosis for IUGR, is the abdominal circumference measurement first described by Campbell and Wilkin.[54] The measurement should be performed at the level of the fetal liver. As the fetal liver is the most severely affected organ in infants with type II growth retardation,[55] this ultrasound section is of great importance in the assessment of fetal nutrition. There is also a good correlation with fetal weight.[54,56]

The most important criterion in obtaining a proper abdominal section for measurement is that the section should be as circular as possible. The level of the section is also precisely defined as the bifurcation of the main portal vein into its right and left branches.[57] The portal vein should not reach the anterior abdominal wall. The abdominal circumference can be measured by a map reader, by an electronic digitizer passed along the external circumference, or by multiplying the sum of the two diameters by 1.57 (Figure 4).

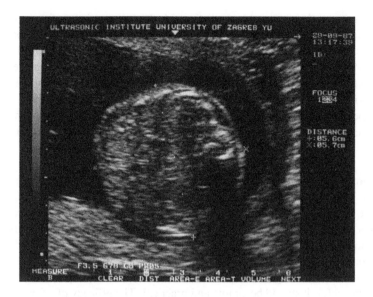

FIGURE 4. The measurement of abdominal circumference on the level of bifurcation of the main portal vein into its right and left branches.

Lateral resolution is very important for perimetrical measurements. It might be expected, therefore, that perimetrical measurements are less accurate when obtained from linear array images than with compound scanning. In practice, the difference between static and real time measurements has been reported to be very small.[58]

We found the AC to be the best single predictor of IUGR.[1,59] In conjunction with other biometric parameters its predictive value is greatly enhanced and capable of accurately predicting IUGR in more than 96% of patients.[1,59]

Recently, Pearce and Campbell reported 83% sensitivity of AC measurements in screening for IUGR.[7] The false-positive rate was rather high — up to 61%. However, in selected patients, detailed ultrasonic biometry with repeated examination will reduce this figure to about 15%.[7] Better results (93% sensitivity) were obtained by Nielson et al.[60] They performed complex measurement involving the product of the CRL and the trunk area in third trimester, which is not suitable for real-time equipment.

Recently, two new ultrasonic parameters have been reported to be of possible value in IUGR detection. Vintzileos et al. described fetal liver measurements and determined fetal liver size for each week of pregnancy from 20 weeks.[61] A linear relationship between fetal liver and abdominal circumference measurements was also described. The fetal liver is the most severely affected organ in deprivational IUGR. However, it has a fast growth rate during the critical third trimester, and this is of great importance for the accurate detection of growth abnormalities. In a preliminary study of ten IUGR infants the authors reported excellent correlation (100%) between IUGR and fetal liver measurements, which decreased by more than 2 SD below the mean.[61]

Several authors have reported on fetal thigh circumference, which reflects the fetal soft tissue mass as a potentially valid parameter for identifying fetuses with IUGR.[62,63]

### C. The Head to Abdomen Ratio

Head to abdomen circumference ratio is reported to be valuable not only in detection of IUGR but also in the distinction of the symmetrical and asymmetrical type.[64] Campbell and Thoms first introduced the ratio in the diagnosis of IUGR[64] and established normal values during the pregnancy. These decline from 1.18 at 17 weeks to 0.96 at 40 weeks of pregnancy.

Using this parameter they were able to distinguish the symmetrical and asymmetrical type of growth retardation in a group of 33 SFD infants, which may be of importance in the long-term assessment of growth retarded infants.[64] A good correlation of elevated head/abdomen ratios and IUGR was reported by Crane and Kopta.[65] In all of the seven growth-retarded fetuses the ratio was 2 SD above the mean. Others found this method less successful in diagnosis of IUGR.[66]

In our experience the accuracy of the head/abdomen ratio is inferior to the abdominal circumference in the diagnosis of IUGR. We use the head/abdomen ratio to demonstrate the pattern of growth (i.e., perinatal risk), rather than the diagnosis of IUGR.

### D. The Estimated Fetal Weight

Estimation of fetal weight is the most practical step in the diagnosis of IUGR. It is also an important factor in management of high-risk pregnancies. A recent survey of over 2 million births concluded that perinatal mortality rates are much more sensitive to birthweight than to gestational age.[67] Based on ultrasonic measurements of various fetal dimensions, a number of formula have been devised for the purpose of estimating fetal weight.[68]

Any method for fetal weight estimation should be as accurate as possible. Also, in order to be clinically useful, it should be simple and practical. The efficacy of a formula for weight estimation depends upon how successful the formula describes the relationship between measured parameters and fetal weight, the accuracy of the measurement, and how the formula deals with altered fetal body proportions, often present in IUGR.

As a single dimension, the BPD is a poor predictor of fetal weight, especially in cases of type II growth retardation. Better results have been obtained using abdominal circumference measurements.[54,56] Campbell and Wilkin estimated fetal weight from abdominal circumference and reported that 95% of actual weights were within 160 g/kg of the estimated weight.[54] Kurjak and Breyer measured two abdominal diameters (the longest and the smallest) and calculated the abdominal circumference using the equation for the circumference of an ellipse.[56] In 83% of the cases the difference between the actual and expected weight was within 150 g. The mean error was 105 g.[56]

Because the fetal mass is contained mostly in the head and trunk, an accurate assessment of fetal weight has to involve measurements of both. A number of formula have been devised which use measurements of both the fetal head and fetal abdomen. Warsof et al. reported that a combination of the BPD and AC predicted fetal weight with an accuracy of 106 g/kg.[69] Using Shepard's formula, which also utilized the BPD and AC,[70] Ott and Doyle calculated fetal weight in 595 patients, both low and high risk, who had undergone ultrasound examination within 72 h before birth.[71] The estimated fetal weight was then plotted on a normal ultrasound fetal weight curve.[42] They found this technique to be 89.9% sensitive and 79.8% specific for the diagnosis of SGA infants.[71] Moreover, all of the 39 severely growth-retarded infants (birthweight below the third percentile) were accurately predicted.[71]

The formula mentioned above does not take into account fetal length, which could have great influence on fetal weight, particularly in extraordinary long or short fetuses. There is, however, no accurate method for fetal length estimation, but good correlation between crown-heel length and femur length has been shown.[72]

Therefore, it has been suggested that femur length (FL) should be added to the formula for estimating fetal weight.[73] Weiner et al. were the first to report a fetal weight estimation using head circumference, abdominal circumference, and femur length in low birthweight infants.[74] FL was used only to adjust the weight estimate if the FL was greater than 2 SD from the mean for gestational age.[74] By using head circumference instead of BPD the problem of dolicocephaly has been resolved. On the other hand, Seeds et al. have suggested the use of a femur equivalent in cases where the BPD is unavailable or distorted.[75] The correlation between femur length and BPD has been reported to be linear with only small variability throughout gestation.[76] Using the formula of Warsof et al.,[69] fetal weight was estimated within 10% of actual birthweight[75] in 77.1% of low birthweight infants (birth weight between 520 and 1500 g). Using femur-equivalent BPD substitution the estimation was only slightly less accurate.

Evaluating three equations,[54,69,70] Deter et al. reported that Campbell and Wilkin's formula[54] overestimated fetal weight, whereas Warsof et al.'s formula[69] underestimated fetal weight.[77] They concluded that the best estimates were provided by Shepard et al.'s method. Data from Hill et al. also confirmed underestimation of fetal weight using Warsof et al.'s formula.[78] They also found Campbell and Wilkin's equation most reliable in estimation fetal weight greater than 2000 g, whereas Shepard et al.'s method was more accurate at the ends of the weight scale (<2000 g and >4000 g).[78] Recently, Dudley and co-workers devised a method for estimating fetal weight by calculating an approximate fetal volume from abdominal area, head area, and femur length.[79] The new method was then compared to those of Campbell and Wilkin and Warsof et al. in estimating birthweights in 434 cases. It was reported that in the middle range of birthweights all three methods performed equally, while the new method had greater accuracy in the important low and high birthweight group.[79] Several authors have studied a group of low birthweight infants and derived their own formulas for weight estimation.[80-82]

### E. Fetal Urinary Production Rate

Oligohydramnios is often associated with severe IUGR.[83] This association probably relates to the diminished fetal urine output seen in IUGR.[1] Campbell and co-workers were the first to describe fetal urine production rates.[84] This is estimated by taking serial bladder volume measurements and calculating the hourly rate of increase. A strong correlation between reduced fetal urine production rate and IUGR was reported.[84] However, this method is rather time consuming, less accurate than others, and therefore, is not suitable for widespread use.

### F. The Total Intrauterine Volume (TIUV)

A measurement of TIUV is theoretically useful to detect IUGR, since in IUGR pregnancies not only the fetal mass, but also placental volume and amniotic fluid volume are often diminished. Normal growth curves for TIUV have been reported[85] and a significantly increased risk of IUGR has been found when the TIUV is below the 2.5% confidence limit.[86] In a nonselected antenatal clinic population of 362 women Geirsson reported this method to be more sensitive in predicting IUGR than abdominal area and BPD measurements.[87] However, a large number of false-positive tests resulted in a lower predictive value for positive tests (mean 34%), than for the abdominal area measurements (mean 54%).[87] Several other authors have also reported high false-positive rates with TIUV.[85,88]

Since the measurement of the TIUV is rather indirect in relation to fetal size, and can be obtained only by static scanner, it is not convenient for the detection of IUGR and has been supplanted by more accurate and easily obtainable parameters.

### G. Quantitative Amniotic Fluid Volume Determination (QAFV)

Similar to TIUV, a QAFV determination has been reported to be useful for predicting IUGR.[89] QAFV is defined as abnormal if the examiner cannot find one pocket of AF at least 1 cm wide.[89] In their study of 120 pregnant women Manning et al. correctly predicted 85 out of 91 (93.4% accurate) infants to be non-IUGR, while 26 out of 29 patients with decreased QAFV were accurately predicted to have growth-retarded infants (89.9% accurate).[89] Other investigators have not confirmed the same level of correlation.[83,90] Although it is a valuable method of diagnosis oligohydramnios, which frequently indicates a severe level of fetal deprivation, QAFV is not a useful method for IUGR detection.

## H. Placental Maturation Grading

Kazzi et al. found that ultrasonic placental maturity (grade III placenta), associated with a small fetus, successfully detects IUGR in 62% of patients.[91] As a single method, it is not sensitive enough for IUGR detection, but it may be useful in connection with other methods.

In conclusion, IUGR should be detected as early as possible because of the fact that intensive surveillance and optimal timing of delivery could save many affected infants. Undoubtedly, ultrasound is the most powerful diagnostic tool for the IUGR detection although there is a tendency to "over" diagnose. To improve diagnostic accuracy of IUGR by ultrasound we need the following: (1) a precise definition of IUGR based not only on birth weight, (2) an optimal and consistent boundary between normal and abnormal values for various ultrasonic parameters, and (3) normograms of each parameter measured and these should be obtained by longitudinal studies of the same population.

## REFERENCES

1. **Kurjak, A., Kirkinen, P., and Latin, V.,** Biometric and dynamic ultrasound assessment of small-for-dates infants: report of 260 cases, *Obstet. Gynecol.,* 56, 281, 1980.
2. **Pearce, J. M. and Campbell, S.,** Ultrasonic monitoring of normal and abnormal fetal growth, in *Modern Management of High Risk Pregnancy,* Laurensen, N. H., Ed., Plenum Press, New York, 1983.
3. **Beazley, J. M. and Kurjak, A.,** Prediction of fetal maturity and birth weight by abdominal palpation, *Nurs. Times,* 69, 14, 1973.
4. **Hall, M. H. and Ching, P. K.,** Is routine antenatal care worthwhile, *Lancet,* 278, 1980.
5. **Campbell, S. and Kurjak, A.,** Comparison between urinary aestrogen assay and serial ultrasonic cephalometry in assessment of fetal growth retardation, *Br. Med. J.,* 4, 336, 1972.
6. **Warsof, S. L., Pearce, J. M., and Campbell, S.,** The present place of routine ultrasound screening, *Clin. Obstet. Gynaecol.,* 10, 445, 1983.
7. **Pearce, J. M. and Campbell, S.,** A comparison of symphysis-fundal height and ultrasound as screening tests for light-for-gestational age infants, *Br. J. Obstet. Gynaecol.,* 94, 100, 1987.
8. **Linn, C. C.,** Intrauterine growth retardation, in *Obstetrics and Gynecology Annual,* Vol. 14, Wynn, R. M., Ed., 1985, 127.
9. **Dewhurrst, C. J., Beazley, J. M., and Campbell, S.,** Assessment of fetal maturity and dysmaturity, *Am. J. Obstet. Gynecol.,* 113, 141, 1972.
10. **Campbell, S.,** The assessment of fetal development by diagnostic ultrasound, *Clin. Perinat.,* 1, 507, 1974.
11. **Kurjak, A., Čečuk, S., and Breyer, B.,** Prediction of maturity in first trimester of pregnancy by ultrasonic measurement of fetal crown-rump length, *J. Clin. Ultrasound,* 4, 83, 1976.
12. **Boyce, A., Mayaux, M., and Schwartz, J.,** Classical and "true" gestational postmaturity, *Am. J. Obstet. Gynecol.,* 125, 911, 1976.
13. **Kurjak-Funduk, B. and Kurjak, A.,** Ultrasound monitoring of follicular maturation and ovulation in normal menstrual cycle and in ovulation induction, in Weinstein Peds. Recent Advances in EPH Gestosis, Schenker, I. R. and Rippmann, E. T., Eds., Excerpta Medica, Amsterdam, 1984.
14. **Robinson, H. P.,** Sonar measurement of fetal crown-rump length as means of assessing maturity in first trimester pregnancy, *Br. Med. J.,* 4, 28, 1973.
15. **Robinson, H. P. and Fleming, J. E. E.,** A critical evaluation of sonar "crown-rump-length" measurements, *Br. J. Obstet. Gynaecol.,* 82, 705, 1975.
16. **Sabbagha, R. E. and Kipper, I.,** The first trimester pregnancy, in Sabbagha, R. E., Ed., *Diagnostic Ultrasound Applied to Obstetrics and Gynecology,* Harper & Row, Hagerstown, MD, 1980.
17. **Adam, A. H., Robinson, H. P., and Dunlop, C.,** A comparison of crown-rump length measurement using a real-time scanner in an antenatal clinic and a conventional B-scanner, *Br. J. Obstet. Gynaecol.,* 86, 521, 1979.
18. **Campbell, S.,** An improved method of fetal cephalometry by ultrasound, *J. Obstet. Gynecol. Br. Commonw.,* 75, 568, 1968.
19. **Campbell, S.,** The prediction of fetal maturity by ultrasonic measurement of the biparietal diameter, *J. Obstet. Gynaecol. Br. Commonw.,* 76, 603, 1969.
20. **Docker, M. F. and Settatree, R. S.,** Comparison between linear array real time ultrasonic scanning and conventional compound scanning in the measurement of fetal biparietal diameter, *Br. J. Obstet. Gynaecol.,* 84, 924, 1977.

21. **Shepard, M. and Filly, R. A.,** A standard plane for biparietal diameter measurement, *J. Ultrasound Med.,* 1, 145, 1982.
22. **Hadlock, F. P., Deter, R. L., Carpenter, R. J., and Park, R. S.,** Estimating fetal age: effect of head shape on BPD, *Am. J. Radiol.,* 137, 83, 1981.
23. **Queenan, J. T., O'Brien, G. D., and Campbell, S.,** Ultrasound measurement of fetal limb bones, *Am. J. Obstet. Gynecol.,* 138, 277, 1980.
24. **O'Brien, G. D., Queenan, J. T., and Campbell, S.,** Assessment of gestational age in the second trimester by real-time ultrasound measurement of the femur length, *Am. J. Obstet. Gynecol.,* 139, 540, 1981.
25. **Seeds, J. W. and Cefalo, R. C.,** Relationship of fetal limb lengths to both biparietal diameter and gestational age, *Obstet. Gynecol.,* 60, 680, 1982.
26. **Hadlock, F. P., Harrist, R. B., Deter, R. L. et al.,** Fetal femur length as a predictor of menstrual age: Sonographically measured, *Am. J. Roentgenol.,* 138, 875, 1982.
27. **Jeanty, P., Rodesch, F., Delbeke, D. et al.,** Estimation of gestational age from measurement of fetal long bones, *J. Ultrasound Med.,* 3, 75, 1984.
28. **Haines, C. J., Langlois, S. L., and Jones, W. R.,** Ultrasonic measurement of fetal femoral length in singleton and twin pregnancies, *Am. J. Obstet. Gynecol.,* 155, 838, 1986.
29. **Filly, R. A., Golbus, M. S., Carey, J. C. et al.,** Short-limbed dwarfism: ultrasonographic diagnosis by mensuration of fetal femoral length, *Radiology,* 138, 653, 1981.
30. **Filly, R. A. and Golbus, M. S.,** Ultrasonography of the normal and the pathologic fetal skeleton, *Radiol. Clin. North Am.,* 20, 311, 1982.
31. **Hobbins, J. C., Bracken, M. B., and Mahoney, M. J.,** Diagnosis of fetal skeleton dysplasias with ultrasound, *Am. J. Obstet. Gynecol.,* 142, 306, 1982.
32. **Hadlock, F. P., Harrist, R. B., Deter, R. L., et al.,** A prospective evaluation of fetal femoral length as a predictor of gestational age, *J. Ultrasound Med.,* 2, 111, 1983.
33. **Yeh, M. N., Bracero, L., Reilly, K. B., et al.,** Ultrasonic measurement of the femur length as an index of fetal gestational age, *Am. J. Obstet. Gynecol.,* 144, 519, 1982.
34. **Tse, C. H. and Lee, K. W.,** A comparison of the fetal femur length and biparietal diameter in predicting gestational age in the third trimester, *Aust. N.Z. J. Obstet. Gynecol.,* 24, 186, 1984.
35. **Sabbagha, R. and Hugney, M.,** Standardization of sonar cephalometry and gestational age, *Obstet. Gynecol.,* 52, 402, 1978.
36. **O'Brien, P. C. and Queenan, J. T.,** Growth of the ultrasound fetal femur length during normal pregnancy, *Am. J. Obstet. Gynecol.,* 141, 833, 1981.
37. **Deter, R. L., Harrist, R. B., Hadlock, F. P., and Carpenter, R. J.,** The use of ultrasound in the detection of intrauterine growth retardation: a review, *J. Clin. Ultrasound,* 10, 9, 1982.
38. **Thomson, A. M., Billewicz, W. Z., and Hytten, F. E.,** The assessment of fetal growth, *J. Obstet. Gynaecol. Br. Commonw.,* 75, 903, 1968.
39. **Lubchenco, L. O., Hansman, C., Dressler, M., and Boyd, E.,** Intrauterine growth as estimated from liveborn birthweight data at 24 to 42 weeks of gestation, *Pediatrics,* 32, 793, 1963.
40. **Miller, H. C.,** Intrauterine growth retardation, An unmet challenge, *Am. J. Dis. Child.,* 135, 944, 1981.
41. **Secher, N. J., Hansen, P. K., Thompsen, B. L., and Keiding, N.,** Growth retardation in preterm infants, *Br. J. Obstet. Gynaecol.,* 94, 115, 1987.
42. **Ott, W. J. and Doyle, S.,** Normal ultrasonic fetal weight curve, *Obstet. Gynecol.,* 59, 603, 1982.
43. **Persson, P. H. and Weldner, B. M.,** Intra-uterine weight curves obtained by ultrasound, *Acta Obstet. Gynecol. Scand.,* 65, 169, 1986.
44. **Seeds, J. W.,** Impaired fetal growth: ultrasonic evaluation and clinical management, *Obstet. Gynecol.,* 64, 577, 1984.
45. **Rossavik, J. K. and Deter, R. L.,** Mathematical modeling of fetal growth. I. Basic principles, *J. Clin. Ultrasound,* 12, 529, 1984.
46. **Deter, R. L., Rossavik, I. K., Harrist, R. B., and Hadlock, F. P.,** Mathematic modeling of fetal growth: development of individual growth curve standards, *Obstet. Gynecol.,* 68, 156, 1986.
47. **Trudinger, B. J., Warwick, B. G., Cook, C. M., Bombardieri, J., and Collins, L.,** Fetal umbilicae artery flow velocity wave forms and placental resistance: clinical significance, *Br. J. Obstet. Gynaecol.,* 92, 23, 1985.
48. **Campbell, S. and Dewhurst, C. J.,** Diagnosis of the small-for-dates fetus by serial ultrasound cephalometry, *Lancet,* 6, 1002, 1971.
49. **Kierse, M. J. N. C.,** Aetiology of intrauterine growth retardation, in *Fetal Growth Retardation,* Van Assche, F. A. and Robertson, W. B., Eds., Churchill Livingstone, Edinburgh, 1981.
50. **Crane, J. P. and Kopta, M. M.,** Comparative newborn anthropometric data in symmetric versus asymmetric intrauterine growth retardation, *Am. J. Obstet. Gynecol.,* 138, 518, 1980.
51. **Arias, F.,** The diagnosis and management of intrauterine growth retardation, *Obstet. Gynecol.,* 49, 293, 1977.

52. **Sabbagha, R. E.,** Intrauterine growth retardation, antenatal diagnosis by ultrasound, *Obstet. Gynecol.,* 52, 252, 1978.

53. **Kurjak, A., Latin, V., and Polak, J.,** Ultrasonic recognition of two types of growth retardation by measurement of four fetal dimensions, *J. Perinat. Med.,* 6, 102, 1978.

54. **Campbell, S. and Wilkin, D.,** Ultrasonic measurement of fetal abdomen circumference in the estimation of fetal weight, *Br. J. Obstet. Gynaecol.,* 82, 689, 1975.

55. **Rosso, P. and Winick, M.,** Intrauterine growth retardation: A new systematic approach based on the clinical and biochemical characteristics of this condition, *J. Perinat. Med.,* 2, 147, 1974.

56. **Kurjak, A. and Breyer, B.,** Estimation of fetal weight by ultrasonic abdominometry, *Am. J. Obstet. Gynecol.,* 1, 962, 1976.

57. **Chinn, D. H., Filly, R. A., and Callen, P. V.,** Ultrasonic evaluation of fetal umbilical and hepatic vascular anatomy, *Radiology,* 144, 153, 1982.

58. **Weiner, C. P., Sabbagha, R. E., Tamura, R., and DalCompo, S.,** Sonographic abdominal circumference: dynamic versus static imaging, *Am. J. Obstet. Gynecol.,* 139, 953, 1981.

59. **Kurjak, A., Breyer, B., and Olajoš, J.,** Ultrasonic assessment of fetal growth and gestational age by measurement of three fetal dimensions, in *Ultrasound in Medicine,* White, D. and Brown, R. E., Eds., Plenum Press, New York, 3A, 681, 1977.

60. **Neilson, J. P., Munjanja, S. P., and Whitfield, C. R.,** Screening for small for dates fetuses: a controlled trial, *Br. Med. J.,* 289, 1179, 1984.

61. **Vintzileos, A. M., Neckles, S., Campbell, W. A., Andreoli, J. W., Jr., Kaplan, B. M., and Nochimson, D. J.,** Fetal liver ultrasound measurements during normal pregnancy, *Obstet. Gynecol.,* 66, 477, 1985.

62. **Deter, R. L., Warda, A., Rossavik, I., Duncan, G., and Hadlock, F. P.,** Fetal thigh circumference: a critical evaluation of its relationship to menstrual age, *J. Clin. Ultrasound,* 14, 105, 1986.

63. **Warda, A. H., Deter, R. L., Duncan, G., and Hadlock, F. P.,** Evaluation of thigh circumference measurements: a comparative ultrasound and anatomical study, *J. Clin. Ultrasound,* 14, 99, 1986.

64. **Campbell, B. and Thoms, A.,** Ultrasound measurement of the fetal head to abdomen circumference ratio in the assessment of growth retardation, *Br. J. Obstet. Gynaecol.,* 84, 165, 1977.

65. **Crane, J. P. and Kopta, M. M.,** Prediction of IUGR via ultrasonically measured head abdominal circumference ratios, *Obstet. Gynecol.,* 54, 497, 1979.

66. **Ellis, C. and Berrnet, M. J.,** Detection of intrauterine growth retardation by ultrasound: preliminary communication, *Journal of the Royal Society of Medicine,* 74, 739, 1981.

67. **Williams, R. L., Creasy, R. K., Cunningham, G. C., Hawes, W. E., Norris, F. D., and Tashiro, M.,** Fetal growth and perinatal viability in California, *Obstet. Gynecol.,* 50, 624, 1982.

68. **Morgenstern, J., Burzik, C., Soffke, U., and Bokelmann, J.,** Estimation of birth weight, *J. Perinat. Med.,* 14, 147, 1986.

69. **Warsof, S. L., Gohari, P., Berkowitz, R. L., and Hobbins, J. C.,** The estimation of fetal weight by computer-assisted analysis, *Am. J. Obstet. Gynecol.,* 128, 881, 1977.

70. **Shepard, M. T., Richards, V. M., Berkowitz, R. T. et al.,** An evaluation of two equations for the prediction of fetal weight by ultrasound, *Am. J. Obstet. Gynecol.,* 142, 47, 1984.

71. **Ott, W. J. and Doyle, S.,** Ultrasonic diagnosis of altered fetal growth by use of a normal ultrasonic fetal weight curve, *Obstet. Gynecol.,* 63, 201, 1984.

72. **Fazekas, I. and Kosa, F.,** *Forensic Fetal Osteology,* Ileyden, Philadelphia, 1978.

73. **Hadlock, F. P., Harrist, R. B., Carpenter, R. J. et al.,** Sonographic estimation of fetal weight: the value of femur length in addition to head and abdomen measurements, *Radiology,* 150, 535, 1984.

74. **Weiner, C. P., Sabbagha, R. E., Vasirub, N. et al.,** Sonographic weight prediction of the low birthweight infants, SGI Meeting Abstract, Washington, D.C., 1983, 67.

75. **Seeds, J. W., Cefalo, L. C., and Bowes, W. A.,** Femur length in the estimation of fetal weight less than 1500 grams, *Am. J. Obstet. Gynecol.,* 149, 232, 1984.

76. **Seeds, J. W. and Cefalo, R. C.,** Relationship of fetal limb lengths to both biparietal diameter and gestational age, *Obstet. Gynecol.,* 60, 680, 1982.

77. **Deter, R. L., Hadlock, F. P., Harrist, R. B. et al.,** Evaluation of three methods for obtaining fetal weight estimates using dynamic image ultrasound, *J. Clin. Ultrasound,* 9, 421, 1981.

78. **Hill, L. M., Breckle, R., Wolfram, K. R., and O'Brien, P. C.,** Evaluation of three methods for estimating fetal weight, *J. Clin. Ultrasound,* 14, 121, 1986.

79. **Dudley, N. J., Lomb, M. P., and Copping, C.,** A new method for fetal weight estimation using real-time ultrasound, *Br. J. Obstet. Gynecol.,* 94, 110, 1987.

80. **Eden, R. R., Jelovsek, F. R., Kodack, L. D. et al.,** Accuracy of ultrasonic fetal weight prediction in preterm infants, *Am. J. Obstet. Gynecol.,* 147, 43, 1983.

81. **Thurnau, G. R., Tamura, R. K., Sabbagha, R. et al.,** A simple estimated fetal weight equation based on real-time ultrasound measurements of fetuses less than thirty-four weeks gestation, *Am. J. Obstet. Gynecol.,* 145, 557, 1983.

82. **Weinberger, E., Cyr, D. R., Hirsch, J. H. et al.,** Estimating fetal weights less than 2000 g, an accurate and simple method, *Am. J. Roentgenol.,* 142, 973, 1984.
83. **Philipson, E. H., Sokol, R. J., and Williams, T.,** Oligohydramnios-clinical association and predictive value for intrauterine growth retardation, *Am. J. Obstet. Gynecol.,* 146, 271, 1983.
84. **Campbell, S., Wladimiroff, J., and Dewhurst, C. J.,** The antenatal measurement of fetal urine production, *Br. J. Obstet. Gynecol.,* 80, 680, 1973.
85. **Chinn, D. H., Filly, R. A., and Callen, P. W.,** Prediction of intrauterine growth retardation by sonographic estimation of total intrauterine volume, *J. Clin. Ultrasound,* 9, 175, 1981.
86. **Levine, S. C., Filly, R. A., and Creasy, R. K.,** Identification of fetal growth retardation by ultrasonographic estimation of total intrauterine volume, *J. Clin. Ultrasound,* 7, 21, 1979.
87. **Geirsson, R. T.,** Intrauterine volume in pregnancy, *Acta Obstet. Gynecol. Scand. Suppl.,* 136, 1986.
88. **Grossman, M., Flynn, J. J., Aufrichtig, D., and Handler, R. C.,** Pitfalls in ultrasonic determination of total intrauterine volume, *J. Clin. Ultrasound,* 10, 17, 1982.
89. **Manning, F. A., Hill, L. M., and Platt, L. D.,** Qualitative amniotic fluid volume determination by ultrasound — antepartum detection of intrauterine growth retardation, *Am. J. Obstet. Gynecol.,* 139, 254, 1981.
90. **Hill, L. M., Breckle, R., Wolfgram, K. R. et al.,** Oligohydramnios: Ultrasonically detected incidence and subsequent outcome, *Am. J. Obstet. Gynecol.,* 147, 407, 1983.
91. **Kazzi, G. M., Gross, T. L., Sokol, R. J. et al.,** Detection of intrauterine growth retardation — a new use for sonographic placental grading, *Am. J. Obstet. Gynecol.,* 145, 733, 1983.

Chapter 8

# ULTRASOUND GUIDED PROCEDURES IN SMALL-FOR-GESTATION FETUSES

**R. J. Bradley and K. H. Nicolaides**

## TABLE OF CONTENTS

# I. INTRODUCTION

Small-for-gestational-age (SGA) fetuses are a heterogeneous group that can be broadly classified into: (1) constitutionally small because of familial or racial factors (the majority of SGA fetuses can be regarded as "normal small" babies that are not at increased risk of intrauterine death or perinatal asphyxia) and (2) growth retarded, due to uteroplacental insufficiency, genetic disease, intrauterine infection, or toxic damage. (These fetuses are at increased risk of intrauterine, intrapartum, or neonatal death and chronic handicap.)

Distinguishing between "normal small" and "growth-retarded" fetuses remains one of the major challenges of antenatal management. This chapter reviews how ultrasound-guided invasive techniques can be used in this context.

# II. ANTENATAL DETECTION OF SGA FETUSES

## A. Clinical

The prenatal detection of SGA fetuses by abdominal palpation is poor,[1] with up to 50% of cases being undiagnosed prior to delivery.[2] Measurement of the symphysis-fundal height, may improve the detection rate to 75%.[3,4]

## B. Ultrasound

The ultrasound diagnosis of SGA is usually made when the fetal abdominal circumference falls below the fifth centile of the normal range for gestational age. Other ultrasonic features which help establish the nature and severity of the underlying pathology include:

1.  Fetal malformation — many of which are associated with SGA fetuses.
2.  Fetal morphometry — ultrasound will distinguish between asymmetrical SGA (ratio of head circumference to abdomen circumference above the 95th centile for gestation), which is thought to be the result of uteroplacental insufficiency, and symmetrical SGA which includes normal small babies and those whose growth is stunted by chromosomal or structural abnormalities or intrauterine infection.[5]
3.  Amniotic fluid volume — oligohydramnios markedly worsens the prognosis for the growth retarded fetus, especially when noted in the second trimester,[6,7] reflecting the severity of uteroplacental insufficiency.
4.  Fetal activity — a decrease in fetal movements being associated with fetal compromise as a result of uteroplacental insufficiency and fetal hypoxia.

### 1. Oligohydramnios

The finding of severe oligo- or anhydramnios in the mid-trimester presents a difficult diagnostic problem. This may be due to three causes: (1) ruptured membranes, (2) fetal renal agenesis or urinary tract malformation, or (3) uteroplacental insufficiency. It is usually possible to exclude leakage of liquor by taking a careful history. An obstructive uropathy can be reliably diagnosed by ultrasound examination. The main difficulty lies in differentiating renal agenesis from intrauterine growth retardation (IUGR), as fetuses with renal agenesis are often small for gestational age[8] and the absence of liquor makes the identification of fetal kidneys difficult. Doppler ultrasound is proving to be a useful tool in this situation, as in renal agenesis the uteroplacental and fetal blood flow velocity waveforms are usually normal, in contrast to the findings in uteroplacental insufficiency.[9] Alternatively, the ultrasonographic image can be improved by the instillation of normal saline either into the amniotic cavity or the fetal peritoneal cavity.

## III. FETAL KARYOTYPING

The finding of an SGA fetus, especially when severely affected and of early onset, in the second trimester, raises the possibility of the fetus being chromosomally abnormal.[10,11] Fetal structural malformations, detected by ultrasound, increase the likelihood of an underlying abnormal karyotype,[12] as do some more subtle morphological markers.[13] The finding of an abnormal chromosomal complement in the second trimester will allow the option of abortion, but we feel that this investigation should be performed even in the third trimester, as the knowledge of a serious chromosomal defect may alter the management of labor and delivery. For example, at present, up to 53% of fetuses with trisomy 18 are delivered by caesarean section, being undiagnosed before delivery.[14] Fetal karyotype can be determined by cytogenetic analysis of amniotic fluid, placental biopsy material, or fetal blood.

### A. Amniocentesis

Under continuous ultrasound visualization[15] a needle (20 gauge) is introduced transabdominally into the amniotic cavity. This can be done by either employing the free-hand technique or by use of a special guide attached to the ultrasound transducer.

Amniotic fluid culture and cytogenetic analysis requires 3 to 4 weeks. This delay may mean that, if the fetus is abnormal, the result is available too late for the option of abortion to be available. Furthermore, in the third trimester, fast results are necessary for planning the time and mode of delivery. In cases of SGA associated with oligohydramnios, the lack of amniotic fluid may make amniocentesis technically difficult.

### B. Placental Biopsy (Chorionic Villus Sampling)

It is possible to obtain samples of placental tissue by transabdominal needle aspiration under ultrasound guidance at any stage of pregnancy.[16] The technique we employ involves the use of a 17/19 gauge double-needle system. The outer needle, with its stylet in place, is inserted into the placenta under local anaesthesia and with continuous ultrasound guidance. The stylet is then withdrawn and replaced by the sampling needle and placental tissue obtained by aspiration with a 10-ml syringe. Using this technique the inner needle may be atraumatically reinserted if the first aspiration does not yield an adequate sample. Alternatively we have successfully obtained satisfactory quantities of tissue from a single aspiration through a 20-gauge needle.

The advantage over amniocentesis is that chromosomal analysis can be performed directly without the need for prolonged culture and therefore the diagnosis of aneuploidy can be made within 24 h of sampling. However, for more detailed cytogenetic studies it is still necessary to culture the tissue, and this requires 2 to 3 weeks.

### C. Cordocentesis

The first method of obtaining pure fetal blood samples was by fetoscopy.[17] However, the disadvantages of heavy sedation, a 2- to 3-d stay in the hospital, and the relatively high incidence of amniotic fluid leakage, led to the development of cordocentesis. The technique of cordocentesis[18,19] has allowed the sampling of pure fetal blood as a single operator outpatient procedure. The site and direction of the umbilical cord at its insertion into the placenta are identified by real-time ultrasound scanning. With the transducer in one hand, held parallel to the intended course of the needle, the chosen site of entry is cleaned with an antiseptic solution and infiltrated with a 1% lignocaine solution to achieve local anaesthesia down to the myometrium. In cases where the placenta is anterior or lateral, a 20-gauge needle is introduced transplacentally into the umbilical cord. When the placenta is posterior, the needle is introduced transamniotically and the cord punctured close to its placental insertion (Figure 1). The umbilical artery and vein are differentiated by the turbulence seen

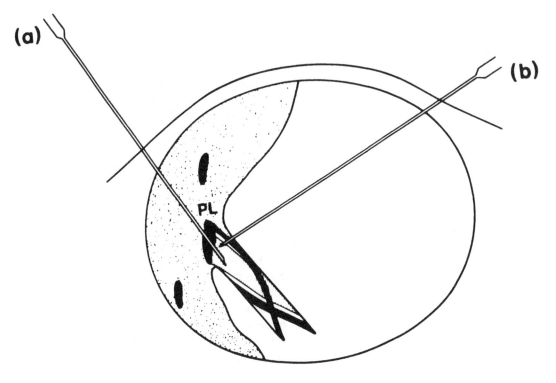

FIGURE 1.    Transplacental (a) and transamniotic (b) approaches for fetal blood sampling by cordocentesis.

ultrasonically when sterile saline (0.2 ml) is injected via the sampling needle. In addition, when the needle is inserted transplacentally, as in 60% of cases, intervillous maternal blood can be aspirated as the needle is withdrawn, thus enabling the study of placental transfer. The technique is safe, with the risk of fetal loss as a result of the procedure being less than 1% in our unit, which is in agreement with published studies,[20] and comparable with the loss rates from amniocentesis or placental biopsy.

The ability to obtain fetal blood safely by an outpatient technique now enables not only rapid karyotyping of the growth retarded fetus, but also an assessment of the fetal condition, which may be of vital importance in planning the timing and mode of delivery.

## IV. FETAL BLOOD GASES AND ACID-BASE STUDIES

### A. Normal Fetuses

A reference range for fetal blood gases and acid-base status has been constructed from analysis of blood obtained for prenatal diagnosis from fetuses that were subsequently shown to be unaffected by the condition under investigation.[21] This data has shown that the fetal $pO_2$ falls with increasing gestation (Figure 2), while the $pCO_2$, lactate and base excess all increase. The umbilical venous pH does not change with gestation (7.38; SD 0.04). The fetal hemoglobin concentration, perhaps as a compensatory mechanism for the falling $pO_2$, increases with increasing gestation, resulting in the calculated oxygen content of the blood remaining surprisingly constant throughout pregnancy.

### B. Small-for-Gestation Fetuses

In our study of 38 fetuses with SGA, where venous blood was obtained by cordocentesis, it was found that 36% were hypoxic (Figure 3).[22] In addition there was a significant correlation

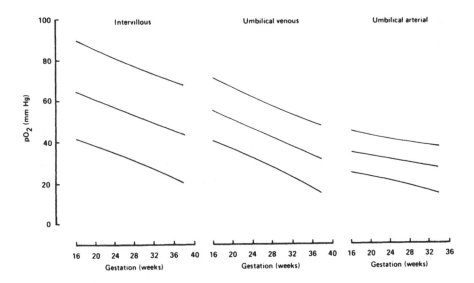

FIGURE 2. Effect of gestation on intervillous, umbilical venous, and umbilical arterial pO₂ (mean and 95% confidence interval). (From Soothill, P. W., Nicolaides, K. H., Rodeck, C. H., and Campbell, S., *Fetal Ther.*, 1, 168, 1986. With permission.)

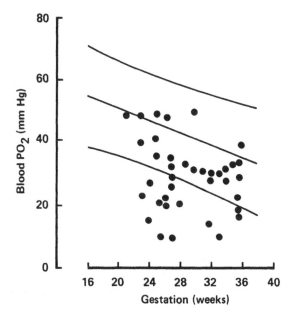

FIGURE 3. Umbilical venous pO₂ in 38 growth-retarded fetuses plotted against mean and 95% confidence interval for normal fetuses. (From Soothill, P. W., Nicolaides, K. H., and Campbell, S., *Br. Med. J.*, 294, 1051, 1987. With permission.)

between the severity of fetal hypoxia and the degree of hypercapnia, acidosis, hyperlacti-caemia, hypoglycemia, and erythroblastosis. This group of hypoxic growth-retarded fetuses are presumably those most at risk of intrauterine death or birth asphyxia. However, the traditional noninvasive methods of assessing fetal well-being, such as ultrasound measurement of fetal growth or cardiotocography, were unable to differentiate those small fetuses that were shown by cordocentesis to be hypoxic, from those with normal pO₂ values.

## C. Doppler Blood Flow Studies

The use of Doppler ultrasound to analyze blood flow velocity waveforms[23] has provided a noninvasive means of assessing the fetal condition. The development of cordocentesis has allowed an evaluation of the correlation between fetal hypoxia and abnormal Doppler blood-velocity waveforms.

### 1. Uteroplacental Blood Flow Velocity Waveforms

The maternal blood flow to the utero-placental interface may be assessed by Doppler studies of the "uteroplacental" vessels.[23] It is not possible to visualize these vessels with real-time ultrasound and, as a result, the velocity of blood within these vessels cannot be calculated. However, it is possible to make an analysis of the resistance to flow by studying the nature of the blood flow velocity waveform. A high resistance index (RI) suggests that there is failure of trophoblastic invasion of the maternal spiral arteries and their conversion into low resistance vessels. By performing Doppler blood flow studies, along with cordo-centesis for blood gas and acid-base status in pregnancies complicated by SGA, we have shown significant correlations between a high resistance pattern in the uteroplacental vessels and fetal hypoxia, acidosis, hypercapnia, and hyperlacticaemia.[24] These findings support the concept that one of the causes of IUGR is poor maternal blood supply to the placental bed, leading to fetal undernutrition.

### 2. Fetal Blood Flow Velocity Waveforms
### a. Mean Aortic Velocity

The use of a combined linear array and pulsed doppler ultrasound system allows calculation of the mean velocity of blood in the fetal descending thoracic aorta. Hackett et al. (1986)[25] have shown an association between abnormal fetal blood-velocity waveforms and poor perinatal outcome. In a recent study[26] we compared doppler blood flow studies in SGA fetuses with blood gas and acid-base status of fetal blood samples obtained by cordocentesis. There were significant negative correlations between the mean velocity of blood in the fetal aorta and the severity of fetal hypoxia (Figure 4), hypercapnia, acidosis, and hyperlacti-caemia, and a significant positive correlation between the mean velocity and pH. Thus, in SGA fetuses, the slower the velocity of blood in the fetal aorta, the more likely the fetus is to be hypoxic or acidotic.

### b. End Diastolic Frequencies in the Umbilical Artery

Umbilical venous blood $pO_2$ and pH were measured in samples obtained by cordocentesis, and the umbilical artery blood velocity waveforms were recorded, using Doppler ultrasound, in 38 small-for-gestational-age fetuses. In 22 fetuses Doppler frequencies were not detected at the end of diastole (EDF negative); of these, 21 (95%) were hypoxic and/or acidotic. In contrast, of the 17 fetuses with Doppler frequencies at the end of diastole (EDF positive), only two were hypoxic and none were acidotic (Figure 5). The equipment required for detection of umbilical arterial EDF is relatively cheap, and this screening test of fetal condition relatively easy to learn. Since it has been demonstrated that "birth asphyxia" is not necessarily due to the process of birth,[22] the responsibility for hypoxic fetal damage is moving from the labor ward to the antenatal clinic. Should the study of umbilical artery FVWs in apparently well-grown fetuses prove to be as reliable in predicting prenatal asphyxia as has been demonstrated for the SGA fetuses, it may provide an explanation for hitherto "unexplained" macerated stillbirths.

### c. Carotid Artery Blood Flow

The so-called "brain sparing effect" in asymmetrical IUGR has long been recognized and has been suggested to be due to diversion of blood from the fetal splanchnic circulation

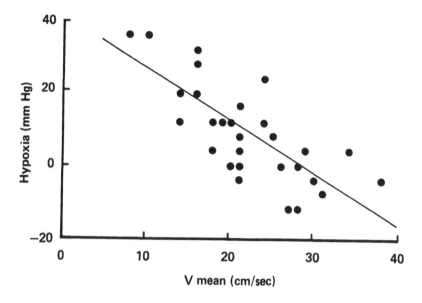

FIGURE 4. Relation between mean velocity of blood in the fetal aorta (V mean) and umbilical venous hypoxia in cases of intrauterine growth retardation. (Hypoxia is expressed as the normal mean for gestational age minus the observed value). (From Soothill, P. W., Nicolaides, K. H., Bilardo, C. M., and Campbell, S., *Lancet,* 1, 1118, 1986. With permission.)

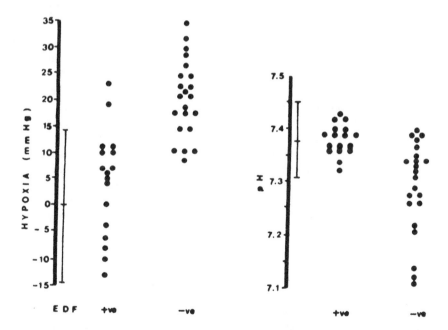

FIGURE 5. Relation between the fetal aortic doppler velocity waveform and fetal hypoxia (deviation from the mean for gestation) and acidosis in 39 cases of intrauterine growth retardation. EDF positive = end diastolic frequencies present; EDF negative = end diastolic frequencies absent. Normal ranges shown as mean and 95% confidence intervals.

to the brain. Doppler blood flow can now study this redistribution and has shown that in cases of placental insufficiency the velocity of blood in the fetal carotid circulation increases as the fetal aortic velocity decreases. Thus, in fetal hypoxia this mechanism may maintain adequate oxygen delivery to the fetal head and allow normal growth and development of the fetal brain. It is of interest that "placental insufficiency" of early onset results in symmetrical growth retardation in the second trimester. This may be because the autonomic nervous system is not sufficiently developed in early pregnancy to achieve the cardiovascular readjustments necessary to maintain preferential brain growth.

## V. MATERNAL HYPEROXYGENATION

It is estimated that severe IUGR and oligohydramnios in the second trimester complicates approximately 1% of pregnancies. In two reports on second-trimester oligohydramnios, only 8 of 34 (19%)[6] and 1 out 28 (4%),[7] pregnancies resulted in live births. These studies, however, included pregnancies with fetal abnormalities and also elective abortions. When only normal fetuses are considered the survival rates were 8 out of 24 (32%) and 1 out of 7 (14%), respectively. In a more recent study reporting on 14 cases of second-trimester oligohydramnios associated with fetal growth retardation and abnormal Doppler blood velocity waveforms, only two fetuses survived (14%) with the rest dying *in utero*.[9] The present management of such cases is simply to wait, in the hope that the fetus reaches the stage of viability so that it can be delivered before intrauterine death occurs. Maternal administration of oxygen immediately before delivery results in an increase in fetal $pO_2$ and is used widely in the management of fetal distress in labor.[27,28] In an investigation of the effect of long-term maternal hyperoxygenation on the hypoxic, growth-retarded fetus,[29] humidified oxygen (55%) was administered continuously through a face mask to five patients whose pregnancies (four singleton and one twin) were complicated by the following features: severe IUGR, oligohydramnios, high blood flow impedance in the fetal aorta and umbilical artery, and low mean blood velocity in the fetal thoracic aorta. All the fetuses sampled were hypoxic and two (cases A and C) were acidotic. Maternal hyperoxygenation raised the fetal $pO_2$ to within or near the normal range (Figure 6), and resulted in a sustained rise in the mean blood velocity in the fetal thoracic aorta, though fetal growth did not improve (Figure 7). In case C, the most hypoxic and acidotic fetus, maternal hyperoxygenation failed to completely correct the hypoxia and acidosis, and the fetus died *in utero* 5 d after starting oxygen therapy. The other five fetuses survived and after delivery experienced minimal neonatal morbidity. These preliminary observations suggest that, if a hypoxic or acidotic fetus is too immature for delivery, maternal hyperoxygenation may prevent intrauterine death and allow the pregnancy to continue long enough for the fetus to be viable after delivery.

## VI. CONCLUSION

Only the minority of SGA fetuses are at risk of intrauterine death or asphyxia at birth. Some will be small because of a low growth potential due to structural or chromosomal malformation; ultrasound examination and tissue sampling will identify this group. Others achieve their full growth potential, but are small because of familial or racial factors. Some fetuses however, that are structurally and chromosomally normal, are small because, due to adverse conditions *in utero* ("uteroplacental insufficiency"), they fail to achieve their full growth potential. It is this latter group that are at risk of intrauterine death or asphyxial damage in labor, as a proportion will be chronically hypoxic *in utero*. The use of cordocentesis in cases of IUGR enables the identification of those fetuses that are hypoxic and has allowed validation of Doppler blood flow measurement as a noninvasive means of monitoring the condition of SGA fetuses.

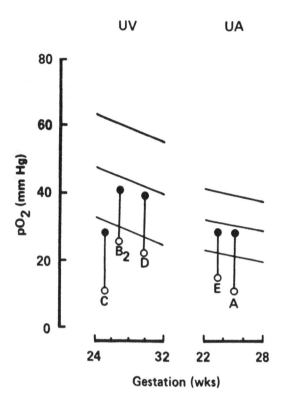

FIGURE 6. Fetal blood pO$_2$ in five growth-retarded fetuses before (○) and at the end of (●) 10 min of maternal hyperoxygenation. Normal range for gestation shown as mean and 95% confidence interval. UV = umbilical vein; UA = umbilical artery. (From Nicolaides, K. H., Soothill, P. W., Rodeck, C. H., and Campbell, S., *Lancet,* 1, 942, 1987. With permission.)

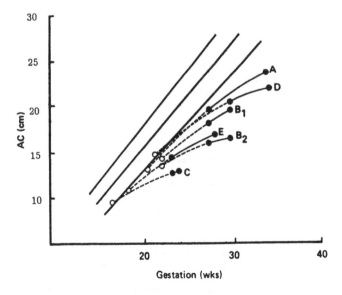

FIGURE 7. Fetal abdominal circumference (AC) growth measured by two weekly ultrasound scans before (○) and after (●) maternal hyperoxygenation. Reference range shows mean with 5th and 95th percentiles. (From Nicolaides, K. H., Soothill, P. W., Rodeck, C. H., and Campbell, S., *Lancet,* 1, 942, 1987. With permission.)

# REFERENCES

1. **Beazley, J. M. and Underhill, R. A.,** Fallacy of the fundal height, *Br. Med. J.,* 4, 404, 1970.
2. **Rosenberg, K., Grant, J. M., and Hepburn, M.,** Antenatal detection of growth retardation: actual practice in a large maternity hospital, *Br. J. Obstet. Gynaecol.,* 89, 12, 1982.
3. **Quaranta, P., Currell, R., Redman, C. W. G., and Robinson, J. S.,** Prediction of small for dates infants by measurement of the symphysis-fundal height, *Br. J. Obstet. Gynaecol.,* 88, 115, 1981.
4. **Calvert, J., Crean, E. E., Newcombe, R. G., and Pearson, J. F.,** Antenatal screening by measurement of symphysis-fundus height, *Br. Med. J.,* 285, 846, 1982.
5. **Campbell, S. and Thoms, A.,** Ultrasound measurement of the fetal head to abdominal circumference ratio in the assessment of growth retardation, *Br. J. Obstet. Gynaecol.,* 84, 165, 1977.
6. **Mercer, L. J. and Brown, L. G.,** Fetal outcome with oligohydramnios in the second trimester, *Obstet. Gynecol.,* 67, 840, 1986.
7. **Barss, V. A., Benacerraf, B. R., and Frigoletto, F. D.,** Second trimester oligohydramnios, a predictor of poor fetal outcome, *Obstet. Gynecol.,* 64, 608, 1984.
8. **Hansmann, M.,** in *Ultrasound Diagnosis in Obstetrics and Gynaecology,* Hansmann, M., Hackeloer, B.-J., and Staudach, A., Eds., Springer-Verlag, New York, 1985, 223.
9. **Hackett, G. A., Nicolaides, K. H., and Campbell, S.,** The value of Doppler ultrasound assessment of fetal and uteroplacental circulations when severe oligohydramnios complicates the second trimester of pregnancy, *Br. J. Obstet. Gynaecol.,* 94, 1074, 1987.
10. **Chen, A. T. and Falek, A.,** Chromosome aberrations in full-term low birthweight neonates, *Hum. Genet.,* 21, 13, 1974.
11. **Anderson, N. G.,** A five year survey of small for dates infants for chromosome abnormalities, *Aust. Paediatr. J.,* 12, 19, 1976.
12. **Nicolaides, K. H., Rodeck, C. H., and Gosden, C. M.,** Rapid karyotyping in non-lethal malformations, *Lancet,* 1, 283, 1986.
13. **Benacerraf, B. R., Frigoletto, F. D., and Laboda, L. A.,** Sonographic diagnosis of Down syndrome in the second trimester, *Am. J. Obstet. Gynecol.,* 153, 49, 1985.
14. **Schneider, A. S., Mennuti, M. T., and Zackai, E. J.,** High caesarean section rate in trisomy 18 births: a potential indication for late prenatal diagnosis, *Am. J. Obstet. Gynecol.,* 140, 367, 1981.
15. Medical Research Council Working Party, An assessment of the hazards of amniocentesis, *Br. J. Obstet. Gynaecol.,* Suppl. 2, 85, 1978.
16. **Nicolaides, K. H., Soothill, P. W., Rodeck, C. H., and Warren, R. C.,** Why confine chorionic villus (placental) biopsy to the first trimester? *Lancet,* 1, 543, 1986.
17. **Rodeck, C. H. and Campbell, S.,** Sampling pure fetal blood by fetoscopy in the second trimester of pregnancy, *Br. Med. J.,* 2, 728, 1978.
18. **Daffos, F., Cappella-Pavlovsky, M., and Forestier, F.,** Fetal blood sampling via the umbilical cord using a needle guided by ultrasound. Report of 66 cases, *Prenatal Diagn.,* 3, 271, 1983.
19. **Nicolaides, K. H., Soothill, P. W., Rodeck, C. H., and Campbell, S.,** Ultrasound-guided sampling of umbilical cord and placental blood to assess fetal wellbeing, *Lancet,* 1, 1065, 1986.
20. **Daffos, F., Cappella-Pavlovsky, M., and Forestier, F.,** Fetal blood sampling during pregnancy with use of a needle guided by ultrasound: a study of 606 consecutive cases, *Am. J. Obstet. Gynecol.,* 153, 655, 1985.
21. **Soothill, P. W., Nicolaides, K. H., Rodeck, C. H., and Campbell, S.,** The effect of gestational age on blood gas and acid-base values in human pregnancy, *Fetal Ther.,* 1, 166, 1986.
22. **Soothill, P. W., Nicolaides, K. H., and Campbell, S.,** Prenatal asphyxia, hyperlacticaemia, and erythroblastosis in growth retarded fetuses, *Br. Med. J.,* 294, 1051, 1987.
23. **Cohen-Overbeek, T., Pearce, J. M., and Campbell, S.,** The assessment of uteroplacental and fetoplacental blood flow using Doppler ultrasound, *Ultrasound Med. Biol.,* 11, 329, 1985.
24. **Soothill, P. W., Nicolaides, K. H., Bilardo, C., Hackett, G., and Campbell, S.,** Uteroplacental blood velocity resistance index and umbilical venous $pO_2$, $pCO_2$, pH , lactate and erythroblast count in growth retarded fetuses, *Fetal Ther.,* 1, 174, 1986.
25. **Hackett, G. A., Campbell, S., Gamsu, H., Cohen-Overbeek, T., and Pearce, J. M. F.,** Doppler studies in the growth retarded fetus and prediction of necrotising enterocolitis, haemorrhage and neonatal morbidity, *Br. Med. J.,* 294, 13, 1986.
26. **Soothill, P. W., Nicolaides, K. H., Bilardo, C. M., and Campbell, S.,** Relation of fetal hypoxia in growth retardation to mean blood velocity in the fetal aorta, *Lancet,* 1, 1065, 1986.
27. **McClure, J. H. and James, B. S.,** Oxygen administration to the mother and its relation to blood oxygen in the newborn infant, *Am. J. Obstet. Gynecol.,* 80, 554, 1960.
28. **Willcourt, R. J., King, J. C., and Queenan, J. T.,** Maternal oxygen administration and the fetal transcutaneous $pO_2$, *Am. J. Obstet. Gynecol.,* 146, 714, 1983.
29. **Nicolaides, K. H., Campbell, S., Bradley, R. J., Bilardo, C., Soothill, P. W., and Gibb, D.,** Maternal oxygen therapy for intrauterine growth retardation, *Lancet,* 1, 942, 1987.

Chapter 9

# UTERO-PLACENTAL AND FETAL CIRCULATION IN INTRAUTERINE GROWTH RETARDATION

**Asim Kurjak, Žarko Alfirević, Giuseppe Rizzo, and Domenico Arduini**

## TABLE OF CONTENTS

## I. MEASUREMENT OF UTERO-PLACENTAL AND FETAL BLOOD FLOW

The interest for the fetal cardiovascular system was expressed as early as the 5th century B.C. when pre-Hippocrates philosophers Diogenes of Appolonia and later Diokles of Canisto spoke about the so-called cotyledons or acetabula of the uterine inner surface from which the fetus feeds sucking, preparing itself for postnatal breast feeding.[1] The continuing research can be followed through writings of Da Vinci, Harwey, Sabatier, and others[1,2] but systematic measurements of the fetal blood flow began to emerge from the 1950s onwards. Although those experimental studies and measurements using the Fick principle with nitrousoxide, or 4-aminoantipyrine, or using radioactive tracers[1-3] have given fundamental information about the fetal physiology, they cannot be used for studies and clinical purposes in human fetuses due to their invasivity, low reproducibility, and potential hazards for the mother and fetus.

Newly developed direct measurement of both fetal and utero-placental blood flow by means of ultrasonic Doppler techniques seems to allow accurate, noninvasive, and clinically valuable investigations of circulatory changes in normal and pathologic pregnancies.

## II. TECHNICAL PRINCIPLES OF DOPPLER MEASUREMENT

The measurement of blood flow velocity, using ultrasound, is based on the effect which is named after Christian Johan Doppler (1803—1853), a professor of physics at the University of Vienna. The principle that now bears his name implies that the frequency of sound or light waves depends on the motion of the wave source and the observer. The wave emitted from a stationary source and reflected from a moving interface changes according to the velocity and the direction of the moving interface. Movements towards the wave source will increase the frequency and the movement away from it will decrease the frequency of the emitted signal. The change of the frequency is directly proportional to the velocity of the moving interface. This change of frequency is called the Doppler shift. During the measurements of blood flow the ultrasound wave is sent towards a blood vessel in which moving erythrocytes act as reflectors causing a change of the reflected sound frequency.

That change of Doppler shift is proportional to the velocity of a blood stream and the angle of insonation and could be calculated from the following equation:

$$F_d = \frac{2 \times F \times v \times \cos\Theta}{c}$$

where $F_d$ is the Doppler shift, F the frequency of the emitted ultrasound, v the velocity of the blood, $\Theta$ the angle between the sound wave and direction of the blood stream, and c the velocity of ultrasound in tissue (1540 cm s$^{-1}$). Once the standard form of the Doppler equation is used for quantification of blood volume (v) the total rate of blood flow in the vessel can be easily calculated by multiplying the average velocity by the cross-sectional area of the vessel:

$$\text{Flow} = \frac{v \times r^2 \times \Pi}{\cos\Theta}$$

where v is the mean blood velocity over the vessel cross-sectional area, r is the vessel radius ($r^2\pi$ = vessel area), and $\Theta$ is the angle of approach of the Doppler beam to the vessel.

### A. Potential Problems in Doppler Measurement

The vast majority of Doppler ultrasound units for obstetrical purposes use pulsed-wave Doppler. Although it is far more complicated and more expensive than continuous wave

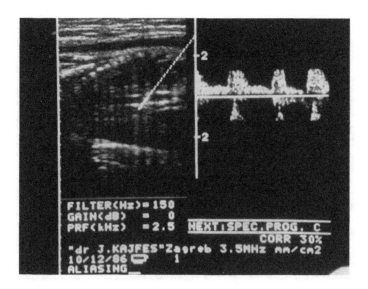

FIGURE 1. The aliasing phenomenon during FVW analysis of the fetal aorta. Peak velocities in each systole are shifted on the opposite side of the zero line.

Doppler the pulsed-wave Doppler is range selective, which means that last short pulse of ultrasound has to travel to the vessel and back before next one is emitted. Thus, signals from a certain depth can be sampled and analyzed separately.

A potential problem could be the depth limitation of measurement determined by pulsed repetition frequency (PRF). If the vessel of interest lies deep and has high velocities, the highest Doppler frequency can be picked up with ambiguity.

According to Nyquist's theorem, the aliasing occurs when Doppler shift exceeds half the value of the pulse repetition frequency. With the insonation angle of 40 to 60° the pulse repetition frequency should be at least 5 kHz for accurate recording of a peak maximum velocities in investigated vessels, especially arcuate arteries and fetal aorta. Fortunately, aliasing can be easily detected during measurements. In the currently used Doppler ultrasound machines, the peak maximum velocities that exceeds the half value of pulse repetition frequency are shifted on the other side of the zero line (Figure 1).

Another limitation factor of a pulsed-wave Doppler is the length of the sample volume along the beam axis. It must be long enough to cover entire diameter of the insonated vessel (more than 10 mm).

In the cheap and highly portable continuous wave Doppler unit, the transmitting and receiving of ultrasound beam is done continuously. Consequently, it has no depth resolution and there are no limitations regarding high velocity measurements (no PRF limitations). Continuous wave Doppler has been widely used in detection of peripheral vascular disease and has been also successfully used in recording signals from the umbilical cord.[4] Unfortunately, it seems that for comprehensive assessment of utero-placental and fetal blood flow localization of vessel is indispensable. The potential value of clinical application of the continuous wave Doppler ultrasound in obstetrics is a screening program for detection of end diastolic flow in umbilical artery.

## B. High Pass Filters

Before spectral analysis, the Doppler audio signal must go through a high pass filter to remove low frequency signals produced by slowly moving tissue, namely the vessel wall. The filters of 600 Hz, used some years ago,[3] caused underestimation of flow calculations.

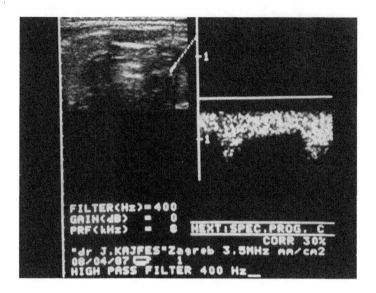

FIGURE 2.    Doppler sonogram of the arcuate artery obtained with the high pass filter set on 400 Hz. All frequencies lower than 400 Hz are not displayed on the screen.

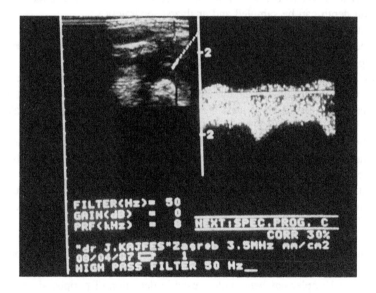

FIGURE 3.    Same signal recorded with the high pass filter setted on 50 Hz.

The 150 Hz, as a cutoff frequency of the high pass filter, is generally accepted in the recent studies although it should be as low as possible, especially in the angle independent (qualitative) studies (Figures 2 and 3).

## III. VOLUME FLOW DOPPLER MEASUREMENTS

It has been already mentioned that for quantitative information of the total rate of blood flow *in utero*, several problems should have been solved. The method should allow visualization of the vessel and vessel diameter measurement, estimation of the angle between the vessel and the Doppler beam, and finally accurate Doppler calculation of blood flow velocity in ml/min.

In 1979 Gill and Kossoff[5] described a method which made possible such noninvasive quantification of blood flow in umbilical vein. The method involves a combination of B-mode ultrasonic imaging (VI Octoson) and pulsed 2 MHz Doppler ultrasound. The intraabdominal part of the umbilical vein was located by the real-time scanner. Calipers were placed on the inner edges of the vessel to determine both the lumen diameter and the spatial orientation of the vessel. The pulsed Doppler unit was then activated with known information of the angle between the beam and the vessel, and the Doppler shift electronically measured. Due to limitations of the range velocity, the system did not allow recording of the high velocities, such as in arteries.

A more sophisticated system was described by Eik-Nes et al.,[6] which could quantify blood flow in fetal veins as well as arteries. The duplex scanner which can be handled easily on the abdomen of pregnant woman consist of real-time B-mode transducer and a pulsed Doppler transducer firmly attached to each other at an angle of 45°. Current machines offer a choice of a fixed angle Doppler transducer or Doppler transducer attached to the B-mode by a jointed arm.[3] The direction of the Doppler beam with the position of the time gate is displayed on the screen. In order to avoid artifacts, the obtained Doppler shift frequencies are analyzed before displaying by means of a real-time, on-line spectrum analyzer.

The distribution and intensities (represented by the gray scaling) of the Doppler shifts are displayed against the time (the Doppler sonogram). The analyzer also has the ability to separate forward and reverse flow into opposite channels. The sonogram is displayed by means of a television monitor, its audio signal is fed to a loudspeaker, and it could be stored by means of a tape recorder for an off-line spectral analysis.

## A. Possible Source of Errors

Before any judgment can be made about the clinical value of volume flow measurement in obstetrics, some error sources should be described. Some of them could be easily overcome, but a few of them are constant, nonsystematic errors often causing unacceptable low reproducibility of the measurement.

The error in vessel diameter measurement seems to be the most significant, since the error will be squared when calculating volume blood flow (see the Doppler equation). Therefore, those measurements should be done, if possible, in a zoomed two-dimensional real-time image. For example, the error of 0.4 mm will cause a 10% error in a vessel with diameter between 6 and 8 mm, and up to 25% if the vessel diameter is below 5 mm[7,8] (Figure 4). Another problem during the vessel diameter measuring is the pulsatility of the arterial vessel wall. The calculated errors, if the measurement is carried out from one frozen two-dimensional image, vary between +9 and −19%, and if the M-mode recordings are used, the error can be decreased to 5%.[2]

The correct angle measurement is also important for the flow velocity calculation. Fortunately, for measurements around 50°, the velocity measurement with a ±4° angle, error would still be within ±5% accuracy range.[8]

However, if the angle between investigated vessel and Doppler beam exceeds 60°, the errors become unacceptably high.[2,8] That is the major reason for which the sector scanners with combined real-time and Doppler facilities should not be used for variable volume flow measurements.

Volume flow is usually expressed in ml/min/kg because it is essential to know whether the flow is simply reduced in proportion to the reduced size of the fetus or if the reduction is even more severe. Although the calculation of volume flow per kg provides an answer to that question, antenatal estimation of fetal weight by ultrasound compounds significant errors in estimation of volume flow.

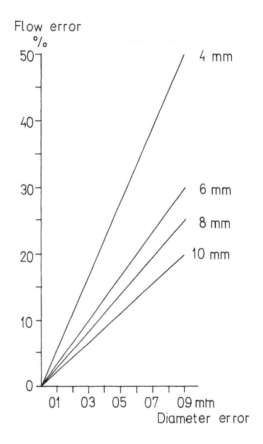

FIGURE 4. Flow measurement error at four different vessel diameters. (From *Measurements of Fetal Blood Flow*, Kurjak, A., Ed., CIC, Rome, 1983, 81. With permission.)

Two other possible sources of errors are incorrect positioning of sample gate and incorrect high pass filters. It should be kept in mind that the sample gate should cover the entire lumen of the vessel in order to detect all moving structures inside the vessel. The sample volume should not be too large since it might include signals from other moving structures in the surrounding tissue. It has been already emphasized, that high pass filters should be set to at most 150 Hz in order to eliminate low frequency signals, originating mainly from the vessel wall.

## B. Clinical Application of Volume Flow Measurement in Detection of IUGR

Although the volume flow measurement (quantitative, angle dependent) has various limitations, it has been widely used in the early 80s in order to detect impaired circulation in some pathological states in pregnancy, such as intrauterine growth retardation (IUGR), EPH gestosis, Rh incompatibility, etc.[9-13]

The rate of umbilical blood flow was first calculated in normal pregnancies. Our team[9] examined 200 normal pregnant patients from 30 to 41 weeks gestation. An almost constant flow per kg of fetal body weight of 120 ml/min/kg was found with a gradual decrease towards the end of the pregnancy (Figures 5 and 6). Similar results were obtained in studies performed by Gill and Warren[13] and Joupilla and Kirkinen.[14]

The investigations of those authors, in high-risk group patients for IUGR, showed that volume flow measurements may have diagnostic value. In our study, 155 measurements of blood flow were carried out in 45 patients with ultrasonic and clinical signs of IUGR by means of Kranzbühler 8130 Doppler Duplex equipment. The average umbilical blood flow

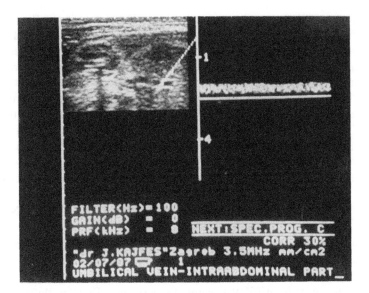

FIGURE 5. Doppler signal from the intrahepatic part of the umbilical vein. The vessel diameter could be easily measured on the left side on the screen.

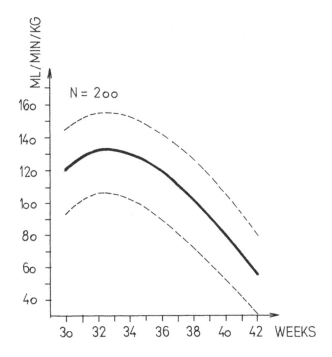

FIGURE 6. Values of umbilical vein flow measured in 200 healthy pregnant women.

was 73.4 ml/min/kg, significantly lower when compared with the control group (106 ml/min/kg).

Joupilla and Kirkinen[14] measured the blood flow in the umbilical vein and descending aorta in 74 fetuses in which the weight at birth was under the tenth weight percentile. From the 101 single values from the umbilical vein, 34% were below the normal range.

In the recent study performed by the Australian group,[15] a total number of 29 small-for-date fetuses (below fifth percentile) were examined. The sensitivity of flow measurement for the identification of small-for-dates was 69%, while the specificity was 90%. It is evident from the above-mentioned data that reduced umbilical flow is strongly associated with growth retardation, but we still do not have the answer whether that kind of measurement can be clinically valuable, both for the diagnosis of IUGR and for its exclusion. It must be emphasized that satisfactory high sensitivity, specificity, positive, and negative predicted value, were obtained only in group of experts from Australia who introduced the technique.[13,15] Although the value of volume flow measurement in obstetrics should not be underestimated, it is hard to believe that that technique will be widely accepted for the clinical purposes, especially now, when relatively simple and reproducible flow velocity wave-form analysis for the assessment of utero-placental and fetal circulation have been introduced.

## IV. FLOW VELOCITY WAVEFORM ANALYSIS IN DETECTION OF IUGR

Since it has been obvious that errors in measurement of volume flow in routine clinical practice are unacceptably high, the attention has been turned to the flow velocity waveforms, their quantification, and possibility to predict impaired utero-placental and fetal circulation. The flow velocity waveform (FVW) represents maximum Doppler shifts throughout the cardiac cycle, reflecting the pulsatile nature of blood flow in arterial vessels. The advantage of that alternative new method, is that FVW quantification is angle independent and there is no need for simultaneous vessel visualization and diameter measurement.

More than ten various FVW indices have been used for assessment of vascular bed resistance in pregnancy,[3,16] but the A/B ratio,[17] resistance index (RI),[18] and pulsatility index (PI)[19] are predominantly used (Figure 7). According to recently published data,[20] no arguments were found to prefer one index to the other.

### A. Potential Problems in FVW Analysis

Aliasing and high pass filters as a potential source of errors have already been described, and using present machines, should be easily overcome.

It is necessary to stress again that fetal movements, breathing, and behavioral states significantly alter the shape of waveforms (Figure 8). Therefore, the recording of signals should be performed during the fetal apnea and quiescence.

Probably the most frequent source of error is the calculation of chosen index. To obtain relevant, reproducible data about vascular resistance, it is essential to calculate the chosen index for each of at least five consecutive cardiac cycles. The average value should be calculated and used for further analysis. Unfortunately, such on-line analysis is not possible in currently used machines because softwares are incomplete and often unable to detect noise.

### B. Arcuate Arteries Waveforms Analysis in Prediction of IUGR

Several studies have shown that physiological changes in the placental bed known as "trophoblast invasion" normally extend from the decidua into the inner myometrium.[21,22] That process which converts spiral arteries into low resistance vessels is well established by 18 weeks' gestation. However, it seems that in preeclampsia and in a proportion of pregnancies with IUGR infants, the physiological vascular changes are restricted to the decidual segments of utero-placental arteries.[23] It has been speculated that that could reduce perfusion of intervillous space because the myometrial spiral arteries retain their musculoelastic coat.

Indeed, Campbell et al.[24] demonstrated that in pregnancies complicated by hypertension and IUGR, decreased end-diastolic flow reflect increased peripheral vascular resistance (Figure 9).

To obtain the Doppler sonogram of arcuate artery, the transducer should be directed to

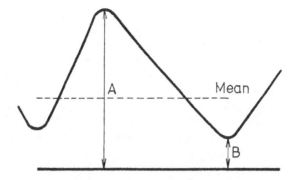

$$\frac{A}{B} = A/B \ \text{ratio}$$

$$\frac{A-B}{A} = \text{Resistance index}$$

$$\frac{A-B}{\text{Mean}} = \text{Pulsatility index}$$

FIGURE 7. The indices used in flow velocity waveforms analysis enabling calculation independent of the angle of insonation.

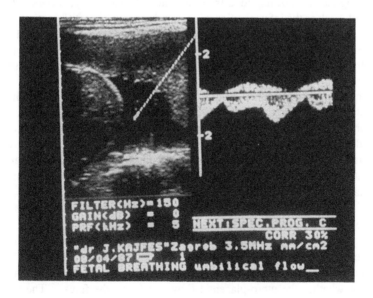

FIGURE 8. Obvious difference in shape of two subsequent waveforms from the umbilical artery caused by fetal breathing movements.

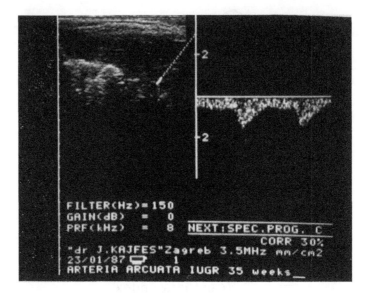

FIGURE 9.   Low-end diastolic flow in the arcuate artery in IUGR at 35 weeks'
gestation.

the lateral pelvic wall to identify external or internal iliac artery. The typical signal of arcuate
artery (which is only seldom seen in two-dimensional real-time image), showing a pattern
of low pulsatility with high velocities in diastole, is than recorded from the lateral wall.

Since the abnormally high pulsatile waveform would imply pathologic findings, care must
be taken that signals are not recorded from the internal iliac artery, uterine artery, or even
abdominal wall, such as the inferior epigastric artery branches. The differentiation of channels
in which the vessels are recorded is quite helpful and should decrease "quid pro quo" to
the minimum. The arcuate artery should therefore be recorded in the opposite channel from
that in which the characteristic signal of external iliac artery is obtained (Figures 10 a and
b).

Using that technique, Campbell et al.[25] have studied 126 singleton pregnancies at 18
weeks' gestation in order to assess the value of arcuate artery FVW analysis in predicting
the risk of pregnancy-induced hypertension, IUGR, and fetal asphyxia. Since 66% of the
growth-retarded fetuses were predicted correctly, it was concluded "that measurement of
utero-placental blood flow in the second trimester appears promising as an early screening
tool to indicate those pregnancies at risk from pregnancy-induced hypertension, IUGR, and
fetal asphyxia".

The usage of inexpensive and portable continuous wave Doppler apparatus, as an alternative tool for that purpose, has been also investigated.[26]

According to our opinion, the cost effectiveness of such a screening program has not been
fully evaluated, neither in normal nor in high-risk populations of pregnant women. There
is still much speculation as to whether the fetus determines its placenta and utero-placental
blood flow, or whether the utero-placental flow constrains the fetus.[27] The recent investigations suggest that in some cases of growth retardation a change in uterine perfusion is a
primary event.[25,26] However, the proportion of such events in overall population of IUGR
(determined as infants whose birthweight is below the tenth centile) seems to be relatively
small, and therefore the belief that screening for only one possible factor of impaired fetal
growth would be justifiable is, at the moment, too enthusiastic.

According to our opinion, the FVW of arcuate arteries should be an important part of the
comprehensive assessment of utero-placental and fetal circulation in the high-risk pregnan-

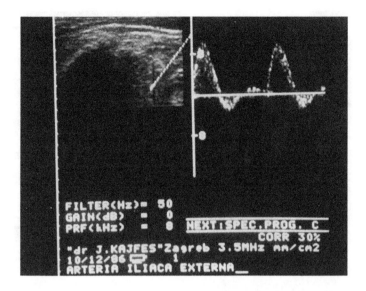

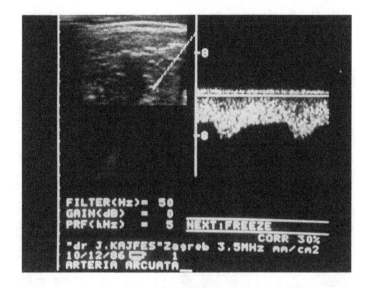

FIGURE 10.    (a) Characteristic signal from the external iliac artery and (b) normal arcuate artery waveform obtained from the same patient without changes in the transducer position. Note the opposite direction of flow.

cies. Only then could the Doppler measurement have a major impact on the diagnosis of the third trimester pathology.

## C. Flow Velocity Waveforms in the Fetal Aorta and IUGR

The fetal aorta is studied by orienting the transducer longitudinally along the fetus. In normal pregnancies there is more or less constant pulsatility with the evident end-diastolic flow in fetal aorta during the third trimester[2,28] (Figure 11).

Several studies have shown that in the majority of asymmetrical IUGR the pulsatility of FVW express, either by resistance index or by pulsatility index, is significantly elevated.[2,29] Those findings suggest increased peripheral vascular resistance and selective redistribution

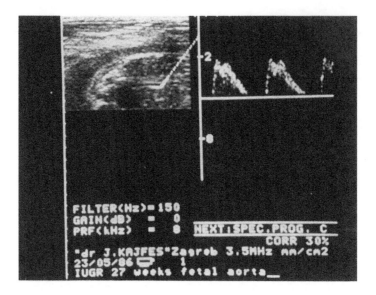

FIGURE 11. Waveform from the fetal aorta in normal pregnancy with clearly visible end-diastolic flow.

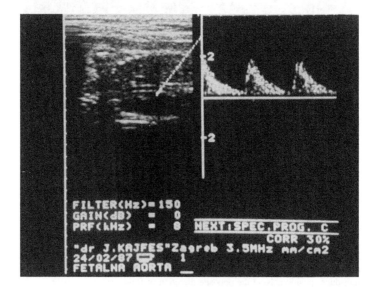

FIGURE 12. Lack of end-diastolic flow in the aorta of growth-retarded fetus at 27 weeks' gestation.

of the cardiac output to the upper part of the body (brain-sparing effect), resulting in diminished flow through the descending aorta (Figures 12 and 13).

Hackett et al.[29] compared 26 fetuses with absence of end diastolic frequencies in the fetal aorta with 20 fetuses with discernible aortic and diastolic flow. Although all of them were growth retarded, the former group were more likely to suffer perinatal death ($p < 0.05$), necrotising enterocolitis ($p < 0.01$) and hemorrhage ($p < 0.05$).

All those above-mentioned data suggest that Doppler ultrasound visualization of circulatory changes in fetal aorta of IUGR fetuses (especially the lack of forward end diastolic flow)

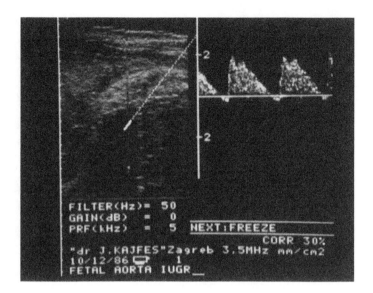

FIGURE 13.   Severe growth retardation with reverse flow during diastole in fetal aorta.

could provide a more sensitive measure of the critical fetal compromise than current techniques.

## D. Flow Velocity Waveforms in the Umbilical Artery and IUGR

The signals from the umbilical artery are so characteristic, and their recording is so simple, that the continuous wave equipment can be used for that purpose.[29,30] The signal from the umbilical artery should be analyzed only if it could be displayed simultaneously with the characteristic low frequency signal from the umbilical vein (Figure 14). We have already suggested combined B imaging and the pulsed Doppler system for clinical purposes in order to evaluate complete utero-placental and fetal circulation. If so, the technique is the same as previously described. The real-time scanner is used to locate a loop of umbilical cord in the amniotic fluid, then sample volume is placed in the luminal center of the artery and the characteristic signal obtained. Recordings are made during the period of fetal rest without breathing movements on patients lying in a comfortable semirecumbent position. The pulsatility of the obtained signals decrease over the last trimester of pregnancy indicates a decrease in peripheral vascular resistance in the normal placenta.

Recently, several groups have published data in relation to the clinical relevance of predicting growth retardation.[3,9,15,20,29,31]

There is general agreement that in the majority of IUGR fetuses an increase in pulsatility, due to decreasing diastolic flow velocity, can be observed. The increase in the pulsatility index, A/B ratio, or RI, decrease or even reverse-end diastolic flow indicate a rise in the peripheral impedance (Figures 15 and 16).

The most probable explanation for the observed changes would be the adrenergic vasoconstriction in the fetal limbs combined with increased placental resistance.

As a diagnostic test the FVW analysis of umbilical artery seems to have an unacceptable low sensitivity of 78.3% as reported by Fleisher et al.[31] or 53.3% in the study of Mulders et al.[20] It can be partially explained with our present definition of IUGR (birthweight below tenth percentile) in which the constitutionally small fetuses are also included. Therefore, it is not surprising that the FVW analysis in the umbilical artery seems to be more valuable in predicting fetal distress than in predicting growth retardation.

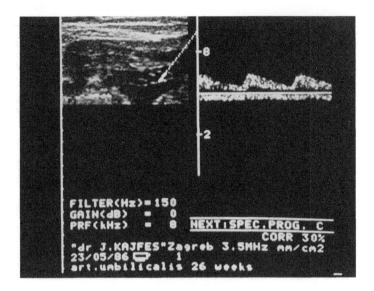

FIGURE 14.   Doppler signal from the umbilical cord with the pulsatile flow in the umbilical artery and consonant flow in umbilical vein (below).

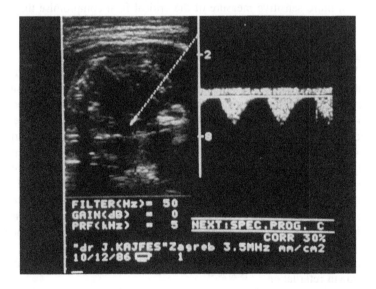

FIGURE 15.   Marked reduction of flow during diastole in the umbilical artery of the severely growth-retarded fetus.

## V. CEREBRAL CIRCULATION IN IUGR

Recently, the combined use of high-resolution real-time equipments and the pulsed Doppler system has also allowed the recording of cerebral blood flow in the human fetus. To date, the analysis of fetal cerebral blood FVW is considered a very useful tool in the management of IUGR fetuses, as it provides valuable information concerning cerebral resistances and the ''brain sparing effect''.

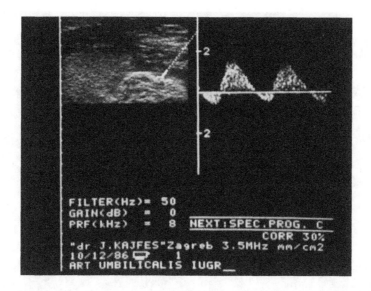

FIGURE 16. "Reverse flow" in the umbilical artery. Ominous sign indicating fetal jeopardy.

Furthermore, cerebral resistance may also be analyzed after birth in order to identify newborns at risk of neurological sequelae.

## A. Methods of Recording

Studies of human fetal cerebral circulation using Doppler ultrasound equipment were first reported in 1984 by Marŝal and co-workers[32] who recorded velocity waveforms from common carotid artery. Recordings of velocity waveforms from common carotid artery are obtained by performing a longitudinal scan of the fetal head and neck. In that section, the common carotid artery appears in its longitudinal axis from the aortic arch origin (Figure 17). However, in our experience, the common carotid artery is difficult to visualize, due to the usually curved position of fetal neck. Furthermore, the common carotid artery divides into the internal and external carotid arteries, and is therefore only partially representative of cerebral blood flow. For the above-mentioned reasons the analysis of fetal blood flow at this level has not been extensively applied.

Wladimiroff et al.[33] reported a technique for recording velocity waveforms from fetal internal carotid artery (ICA) at the level of its bifurcation into anterior and middle cerebral artery. To visualize the intracerebral portion of this vessel, it is necessary to first obtain a transverse scan of the fetal head at the same plane normally used for the measurement of biparietal diameter. The operator will then direct the ultrasound transducer, in a parallel fashion, towards the base of the skull in order to visualize, on either side of the midline, two pulsing structures representing the terminal parts of ICA. The sample volume will then be placed on one of those pulsing areas for the recordings of velocity waveforms. Velocity waveforms from ICA are characterized in physiological conditions by low diastolic velocity and exhibit a shape similar to that of descending aorta waveforms (Figure 18). The reproducibility of that technique is excellent in our experience. The coefficient of variation in repeated measurements is <0.03. Reliable recordings have been easily obtained in about 90% of the cases investigated in our laboratory from 26 weeks' gestation onwards.

We have also recently started to record velocity waveforms from fetal middle cerebral artery (MCA). The MCA could be easily visualized in a transverse section intermediate, between that previously described for visualizing ICA and that used for biparietal diameter

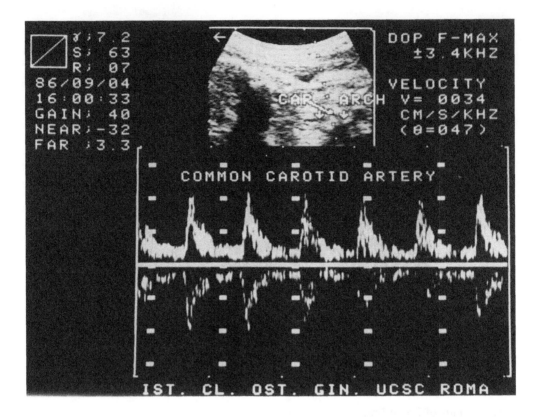

FIGURE 17.    Flow velocity waveforms from common carotid artery during normal pregnancy.

measurements. At that level (Figure 19), MCA appears in its longitudinal axis as a pulsing structure.

In that position the angle of insonation of Doppler beam is usually reduced, thus allowing the recording of maximum velocities (Figure 20). Two of the most evident advantages of recording cerebral velocity waveforms from MCA must be pointed out. First, the reduced angle of insonation allows a high level of reproducibility (coefficient of variation (0.01); on the other side, as MCA is one of the vessels usually investigated in the newborn, its prenatal analysis allows direct comparison with postnatal events.

A potential limitation of that technique is represented by the reduced dimension of the vessel diameter. In our experience, however, from 30 weeks' gestation onwards, recordings from MCA are as reliable as those from ICA.

Arbeille[34] suggested a technique to record velocity waveforms at the level of anterior cerebral artery (ACA) by performing a parasagittal view of the fetal face and directing the transducer towards the base of the skull (Figure 21).

In newborns, cerebral velocity waveforms, are usually investigated at the level of ACA and MCA.

ACA velocity waveforms are recorded (Figure 22) by placing the probe in a sagittal plane on the anterior fontanelle and directing the transducer towards the base of the skull.[35] Velocity waveforms can also be easily obtained with continuous wave Doppler equipments. Moreover, the use of pulsed Doppler equipment allows us to distinguish signals from two different points on the ACA: the first site is situated at the initial straight portion of the vessel, as it ascends towards the corpus callosum, whereas the second site represents the anterior bend of corpus callosum, as the vessel turns with its direction of blood flow toward the anterior fontanelle. A better reproducibility is usually achieved when the inferior position (first site) is selected.[36]

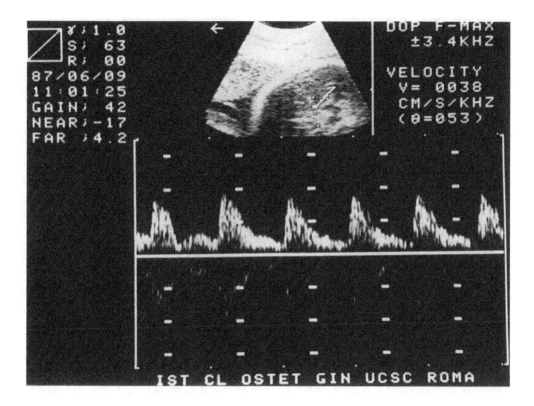

FIGURE 18.   Flow velocity waveforms from internal carotid artery in a healthy fetus (PI = 1.62).

Velocity waveforms can be easily obtained in the newborn from MCA (Figure 23) by placing the pulsed Doppler transducer in a coronal plane, over the temporal bone, just above and anterior to the elix of the ear.[37] A clear localization of the vessel under examination, in addition to a Doppler signal with quality (signal/noise ratio), permitting adequate analysis, is obtained in about 95% of the cases of MCA analysis.[38]

The PI in ICA remains almost constant throughout pregnancy in healthy fetuses. Wladimiroff[33] reported a mean value ranging between 1.5 and 1.6 with a standard deviation of 0.2 from 26 to 41 weeks' gestation. Figure 24 provides our ranges of normality of PI from ICA calculated on the basis of more than 400 fetuses.

Our experience concerning MCA is limited. However, the results obtained in a longitudinal study in ten healthy fetuses analyzed at 2 weeks interval from 30 weeks' gestation onward are reported in Figure 25. The PI values obtained from MCA are similar to those obtained from ICA. Moreover, we noticed a nonsignificant, slight reduction of PI values near term.

The correlation between RI from ACA and MCA is also high (r = 0.75) in the newborn.[36] Thus, comparison of resistance indices of those two vessels is usually performed.

RI has been shown to fall with postnatal age over the first 48 h in both ACA and MCA.[38] Moreover, RI values are usually considered abnormal when equal or below 0.55.[39]

## B. Applications

Several applications of the cerebral Doppler ultrasonography have been suggested for the management of growth retardation.

The results of experimental animal models demonstrated that during chronic hypoxia the preferential perfusion of the brain and myocardium, i.e., the so-called "brain-sparing effect", precedes the advent of the growth defect.[40] The human fetus with already evident clinical or ultrasonographic signs of asymmetrical growth retardation shows a marked al-

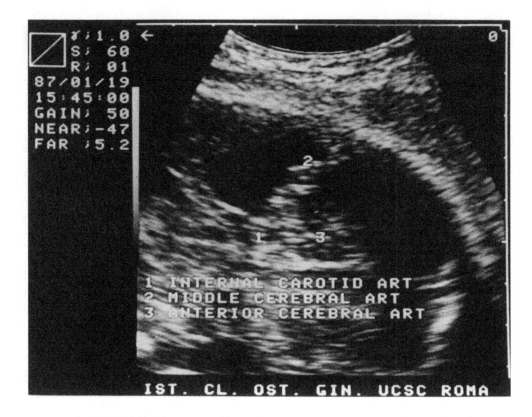

FIGURE 19.   Cross-section through the fetal head showing the middle cerebral artery in its longitudinal axis. (1 = internal carotid artery, 2 = middle cerebral artery, 3 = anterior cerebral artery).

teration of velocity waveform profile from ICA. Those alterations are predominantly due to the increased diastolic velocity (Figure 26), which suggests a decrease in cerebral vascular resistance in IUGR fetuses.

However, the isolated analysis of cerebral blood flow in fetuses at risk or suspected of asymmetrical IUGR resulted, according to our experience, in limited usefulness in the prediction of growth defects. On the other side, the combined analysis of fetal peripheral vessels and ICA provides an improved accuracy in the prediction of IUGR fetuses. The best results for IUGR screening are achieved using the ratio between the PI of umbilical and internal carotid artery (UA/ICA ratio). That ratio probably reflects more accurately than others the "brain-sparing effect" which is characterized by an increase of vascular resistance associated with cerebral vasodilation.

In order to establish the clinical value of the fetal blood flow assessment in the prediction of IUGR, we carried out a prospective study on high-risk pregnancies.

To date, we have investigated 140 pregnancies at risk of asymmetrical IUGR (hypertensive disease, heavy smokers, previous asymmetrical IUGR infants). All those pregnancies had a reliable gestational age and no ultrasonographic signs (BPD, AC, femur) of impaired growth at the time of blood flow measurements. Doppler blood flow assessments were performed at the level of umbilical artery, descending aorta, and ICA between 26 and 28 weeks' gestation.

Table 1 reports the results obtained in the prediction of IUGR fetuses (below the tenth centile) using either the isolated analysis of different fetal vessels or their combined analysis.

The UA/ICA ratio was confirmed to be the best predictor of IUGR and reached an adequate level of accuracy. In conclusion, that technique seems to represent an improvement in the

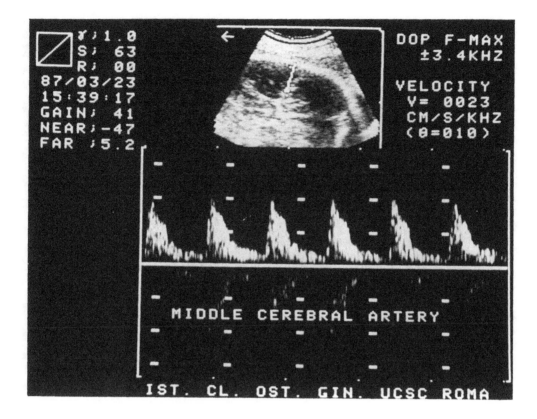

FIGURE 20. Flow velocity waveforms from fetal middle cerebral artery during normal pregnancy.

prediction of IUGR. The combined analysis of PI in umbilical artery and ICA proves to be a useful tool for an early screening of pregnancies at risk of IUGR.

## C. Differential Diagnosis of IUGR Fetuses

Recently, Wladimiroff et al.[41] suggested employment of the analysis of the fetal blood flow in the differential diagnosis of IUGR fetuses in the presence of severe growth retardation and marked oligohydramnios. In his experience, with ten selected cases, the PI from ICA resulted useful to differentiate IUGR fetuses with "placental insufficiency" (characterized by cerebral vasodilation due to chronic hypoxia) from IUGR fetuses with structural defects (characterized by normal cerebral resistance).

It must be pointed out that the assessment of fetal peripheral resistance is not always helpful in the differential diagnosis of IUGR[42] as oligohydramnios may influence the resistance in umbilical artery.

## D. Monitoring of Fetal Oxygenation

Asymmetrical IUGR fetuses are characterized by a chronic deprivation of nutrients, including oxygen, derived from an impaired transport from mother to fetus. The recent application of cordocentesis[43] has confirmed the presence of a chronic hypoxia in human IUGR fetuses. Great potential of the new technique is described in the chapter "Ultrasound-Guided procedures in SGA fetuses".

Soothill et al.[44] correlated measurements of fetal blood flow with fetal blood-gas and acid-base parameters obtained by cordocentesis. They found relationships between the mean velocity in fetal descending aorta, and pH values, plasma lactate concentrations, $pCO_2$, and $pO_2$ levels in the umbilical vein. However, significant correlations, with fetal aortic mean

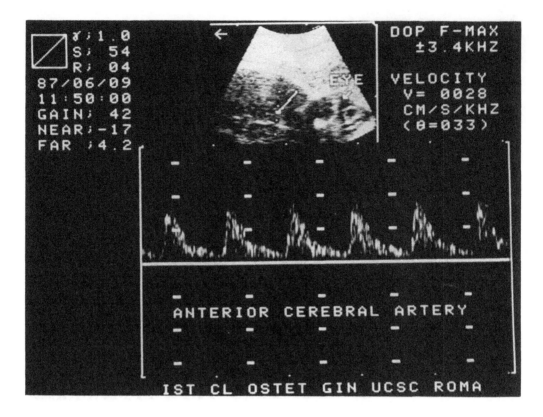

FIGURE 21.   Flow velocity waveforms from anterior cerebral artery in a healthy fetus. Recording was obtained by performing a sagittal scan of the fetal face.

velocity, were found only after adjusting for gestational age all those biochemical measurements except pH.

Pardi (personal communication) similarly correlated the acid-base balance in umbilical vein to the PI in umbilical artery. No correlation was found with oxygen levels, but a very significant correlation with fetal acidosis, as expressed by the level of lactate, bicarbonate, and basis excess, was evidenced.

We recently analyzed fetal blood flow at the level of ICA, descending aorta, and umbilical artery in 30 high-risk pregnancies immediately before elective cesarian section. The acid-base balance at the level of the umbilical artery and vein was evaluated immediately after clamping the cord. A significant positive correlation was found between the Pulsatility Index (PI) in ICA and umbilical venous $pO_2$ ($r = 0.001$) as shown in Figure 27. Moreover, significant correlations were evident between the severity of fetal hypercapnea and acidosis (i.e., basis excess and bicarbonate) in the umbilical artery and the PI evaluated in the descending aorta (Figure 27).

Therefore, our data confirm the results obtained in animal models, and suggest a direct relationship between oxygen content in the umbilical vein and cerebral vascular impedance. On the other side, the degree of peripheral vascular resistance is strictly related to the level of fetal acidosis measured in the umbilical artery.

Cerebral Doppler ultrasonography seems to be a helpful, noninvasive method for monitoring fetal oxygenation. However, further studies are required to establish the clinical significance of application in the early diagnosis of the fetal jeopardy.

### E. Intrauterine Prediction of Neonatal Neurological Sequelae
The newborn brain is particularly vulnerable to a variety of pathological conditions, and

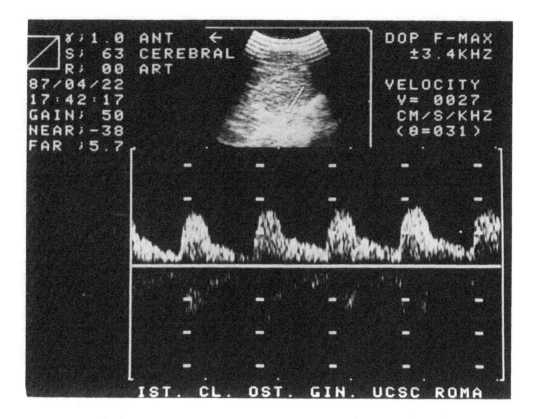

FIGURE 22.  Flow velocity waveforms from anterior cerebral artery in a healthy newborn.

those lesions may cause death or serious neurodevelopmental handicaps. Cerebral hemorrhage and postasphyxial encephalopathy (PAE) are frequently present in asymmetrical IUGR and are due to modifications in cerebral haemodynamics. Those changes secondary to hypoxia are generally established before birth, as recently demonstrated by fetal cerebral Doppler ultrasonography. Therefore, neurological sequelae may be predicted already in the fetus with a technique similar to that, employed in the newborn.

In order to assess whether there is a continuity in cerebral resistance in the perinatal period, we compared RI values obtained from MCA at the onset of delivery with RI measured from the same vessel in the first day of life in 30 infants. The correlation between the prenatal and postnatal RI was adequate ($r = 0.81$), suggesting that a comparison of cerebral resistance during the perinatal period is practicable.

We therefore analyzed short-term neurological sequelae (i.e., cerebral hemorrhage and PAE) in 87 fetuses at high risk of hypoxia by cerebral Doppler ultrasonographic examinations performed within 3 d from delivery.In fetuses with normal growth and birthweight above 2500 g, the prediction of neurological abnormalities was good with a specificity of 93.7%, a sensitivity of 71.4%, and an accuracy of 89.7%. Unfortunately, the predictive value was lower in IUGR fetuses and this difference was particularly evident in fetuses with birthweight below 1500 g as shown in Table 2.

Our data suggest that a prediction of eventual neurological sequelae may be performed near term in fetuses with normal growth with an accuracy similar to that reported in newborns.[39]

The imperfect predictive value found in IUGR fetuses can be due to various multiple factors, influencing exclusively the postnatal period such as the presence of patent ductus arteriosus, respiratory distress syndrome, fluctuations in arterial pressure, and therapeutic

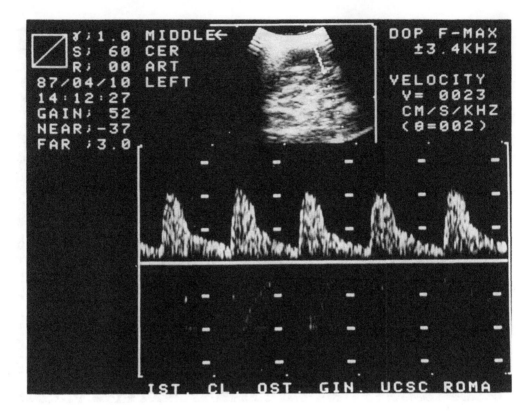

FIGURE 23.   Flow velocity waveforms from middle cerebral artery in a healthy newborn.

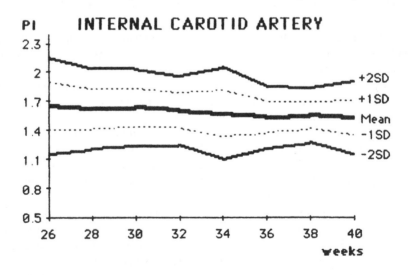

FIGURE 24.   Mean values ($\pm 2$ SD) of PI in fetal internal carotid from 26 weeks' gestation onwards. Data are obtained from 404 fetuses.

measures. Those factors cannot be predicted before birth and predispose IUGR fetuses to neurological sequelae. However, we feel that also in the presence of IUGR the assessment of cerebral resistance should provide valuable additional information concerning the risk of neurological complications.

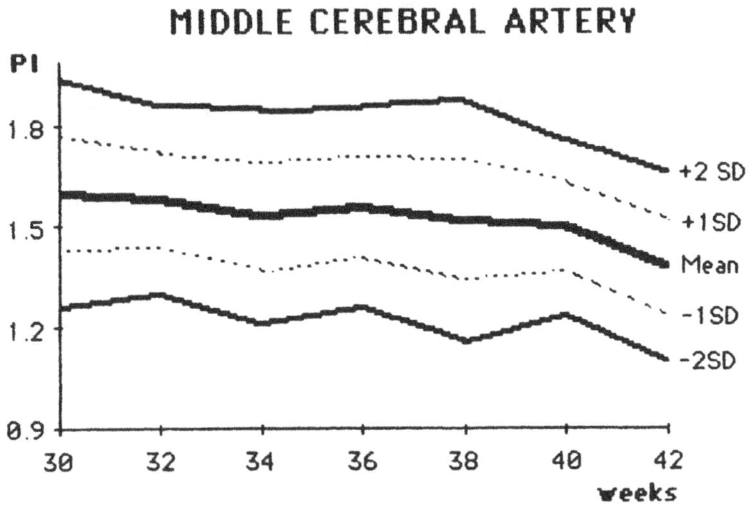

## MIDDLE CEREBRAL ARTERY

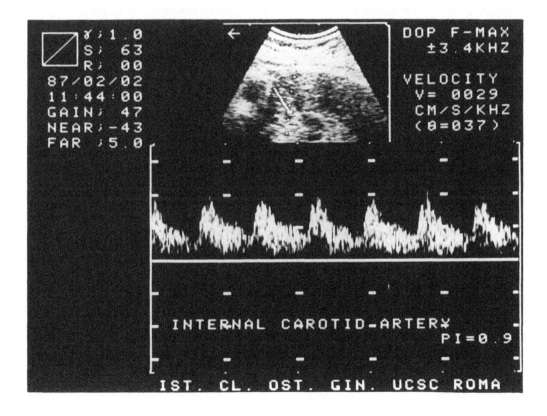

FIGURE 25. Mean values (±2 SD) of PI in fetal middle cerebral artery from 30 weeks' gestation onwards. Data are obtained from a longitudinal study in 10 healthy fetuses recorded at 2 weeks' interval.

FIGURE 26. Flow velocity waveforms from internal carotid artery in an asymmetrical growth-retarded fetus. Waveforms are characterized by increased diastolic velocity. (PI = 0.9.)

**Table 1**

## COMPARISON OF STANDARD DIAGNOSTIC TEST PARAMETERS IN THE DIFFERENT VESSELS INVESTIGATED AS PREDICTORS OF IUGR IN 140 HIGH-RISK FETUSES

|                          | UA   | DA   | ICA  | DA/ICA | UA/ICA |
|--------------------------|------|------|------|--------|--------|
| Specificity              | 68.4 | 57.2 | 71.3 | 73.9   | 91.4   |
| Sensitivity              | 59.3 | 54.3 | 67.4 | 68.2   | 78.5   |
| Positive predictive value | 46.2 | 43.2 | 74.7 | 75.8   | 81.4   |
| Negative predictive value | 72.3 | 60.3 | 73.3 | 69.3   | 87.9   |
| Accuracy                 | 57.6 | 54.2 | 71.4 | 74.8   | 87.6   |

## VI. CONCLUSION

In the last decade ultrasound has helped us tremendously to solve a lot of intrauterine life mysteries. However, the recognition of the fetal compromise in the third trimester still poses many challenges. It seems that with Doppler ultrasound we finally have the tool which can help us solve the majority of obstetrics puzzles providing comprehensive, noninvasive assessment of the utero-placental and fetal circulation, which complements the morphological and biometric data, obtained by two-dimensional ultrasound.

In the last few years Doppler ultrasound was mainly used in obstetrics to document altered blood flow in IUGR and to enable a better understanding of its nature and pathophysiology.

Despite many improvements, the observed changes in volume blood flow measurement in IUGR could only be guidelines for the investigation and should not be used for clinical purposes because of major limitations and pitfalls.

On the other hand, the analysis of the FVW recordings from uterine circulation, umbilical artery, fetal aorta, and fetal intracranial circulation seems to be a sensitive agent in assessing and monitoring the well being of a growth-retarded fetus. The FVW analysis has proved to be simple and reproducible even in less-experienced hands. The encouraging preliminary results are behind use, and it is time for the wide prospective controlled trials. With enough information on specificity and sensitivity of FVW analysis in detection of growth-retarded fetuses in jeopardy, it will be possible to draw the final conclusions about screening programs and extended clinical application.

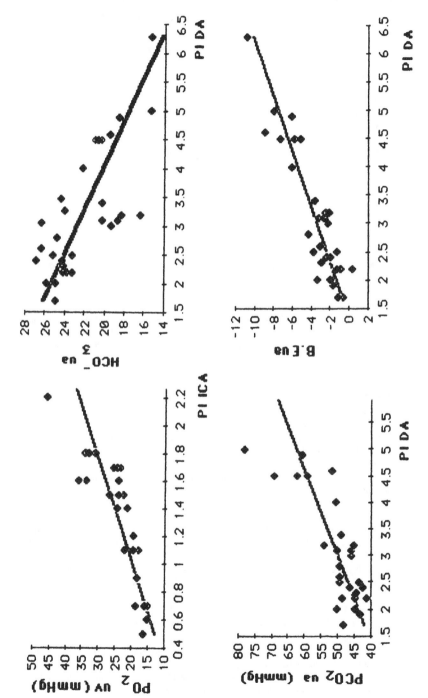

FIGURE 27. Correlations between PI from fetal internal carotid artery and pO₂ levels in umbilical vein and between PI in fetal descending aorta and pCO₂, HCO₃, and base excess levels in umbilical artery.

**Table 2**

**VALUES OF THE PRENATAL ASSESSMENT OF PI FROM INTERNAL
CAROTID ARTERY IN PREDICTING NEUROLOGICAL SEQUELAE
(CEREBRAL HEMORRHAGE AND POSTASPHYXIAL ENCEPHALOPATHY)
OF IUGR FETUSES DIVIDED ACCORDING TO THEIR BIRTHWEIGHT**

| Birthweight | <1500 g | 1500—2500 g |
|---|---|---|
| Specificity | 68.6 | 74.6 |
| Sensitivity | 74.6 | 76.6 |
| Positive predictive value | 68.4 | 58.3 |
| Negative predictive value | 83.3 | 75.1 |
| Accuracy | 63.6 | 75.9 |

# REFERENCES

1. **Salvadori, B. A.,** History of the measurement of fetal blood flow, in *Measurements of Fetal Blood Flow,* Kurjak, A., Ed., CIC, Rome, 1984, 1.
2. **Tonge, H. M.,** A Doppler ultrasound study of human fetal vascular dynamics, Thesis, Drukkerij, J. H., Ed., Pasmans, Gravenhage, 1987, chap. 1.
3. **Cohen-Overbeek, T., Pearce, J. M., and Campbell, S.,** The antenatal assessment of utero-placental and feto-placental blood flow using Doppler ultrasound, *Ultrasound Med. Biol.,* 11, 329, 1985.
4. **Fitzgerald, D. E. and Drumm, J. E.,** Non-invasive measurement of the fetal circulation using ultrasound: a new method, *Br. J. Obstet. Gynecol.,* 2, 1450, 1977.
5. **Gill, R. W. and Kossoff, G.,** Pulsed Doppler combined with B mode imaging for blood flow measurement, *Contrib. Gynecol. Obstet.* 6, 139, 1979.
6. **Eik-Nes, S. H., Maršal, K., Brubakk, A. O., and Ulstein, M.,** Ultrasonic measurement of human fetal blood flow, *J. Biomed. Eng.,* 4, 28, 1982.
7. **Eik-Nes, S. H., Maršal, K., and Kristoffersen, K.,** Non-invasive measurement of human fetal blood flow, in *Measurement of Fetal Blood Flow,* Kurjak, A., Ed., CIC, Rome, 1984, 73.
8. **Warnking, K.,** Errors in Quantitative Doppler Measurements, in *Doppler Techniques in Obstetrics,* Jung, H. and Fendel, H., Eds., Georg Thieme Verlag, Stuttgart, 1986, 2.
9. **Kurjak, A., Rajhvajn, B., and Aradi, M.,** Clinical application of ultrasonically measured umbilical blood flow, in *Measurement of Fetal Blood Flow,* Kurjak, A., Ed., CIC, Rome, 1984, 103.
10. **Kurjak, A. and Rajhvajn, B.,** Ultrasonic measurements of umbilical blood flow in normal and complicated pregnancies, *J. Perinat. Med.,* 10, 3, 1982.
11. **Kurjak, A., Latin, V., Klobučar, A., and Rajhvajn, G.,** *Clinical Applications of Blood Flow Measurements, Doppler Techniques in Obstetrics,* Jung, H. and Fendel, H., Eds., Georg Thieme Verlag, Stuttgart, 1986, 68.
12. **Kirkinen, P., Joupilla, P., and Eik-Nes, S.,** Fetal blood flow in Rh-incompatibility, in *Recent Advances in Ultrasound Diagnosis 3,* Kurjak, A. and Kratochwil, A., Eds., Excerpta Medica, Amsterdam, 1981, 243.
13. **Gill, R. W. and Warren, P. S.,** Doppler measurement of umbilical blood flow, in *The Principles and Practise of Ultrasonography in Obstetrics and Gynecology,* Appelton-Century-Crofts, New York, Sanders, R. C. and James, A. E., Eds., 1985, 87.
14. **Joupilla, P. and Kirkinen, P.,** The role of fetal blood flow measurements in obstetrics, in *Measurements of Fetal Blood Flow,* Kurjak, A., Ed., CIC, Rome, 1983, 139.
15. **Gill, R. W., Kossoff, G., Warren, P. S., Stewart, A., and Garrett, W. J.,** Umbilical artery velocity waveform and umbilical vein volume flow in the assessment of high risk pregnancies in the third trimester, Anali Dr. J. Kajfeš, 1987, in press.
16. **Thompson, R. S., Trudinger, B. J., and Cook, C. M.,** A comparison of doppler ultrasound waveform indices in the umbilical artery. I. Indices derived from the maximum velocity waveform, *Ultrasound Med. Biol.,* 12, 835, 1986.

17. **Gosling, R. C.,** Extraction of physiological information from spectrum analysed Doppler-shifted continuous wave ultrasound signal obtained non-invasively from the arterial tree, in *IEE Medical Monographis*, Hill, D. M. and Watson, B. W., Eds., Peter Peregrinus, London, 1976, 73.

18. **Pourcelot, L.,** Applications cliniques de l'examen Doppler transcutane, in *Velocimetric Ultrasonor Doppler*, Peronnean, P., Ed., INSERM, Paris, 1974, 625.

19. **Gosling, R. C. and Kong, D. H.,** Continuous wave ultrasound as an alternative and complement to X-rays in vascular examinations, in *Cardio-Vascular Applications of Ultrasound*, Reneman, R. S., Ed., North-Holland, New York, 1974, 266.

20. **Mulders, L. G. M., Wijn, P. F. F., Jonsma, H. W., and Heni, R. R.,** A comparative study of three indices of umbilical blood flow in relation to prediction of growth retardation, *J. Perinat. Med.*, 15, 3, 1987.

21. **Brosens, I., Robertson, W. B., and Dixon, H. G.,** The physiological response of the vessels of the placental bed to normal pregnancy, *J. Pathol. Bacteriol.*, 93, 569, 1967.

22. **Pijneborg, R., Bland, J. M., Robertson, W. B., and Brosens, I.,** Uteroplacental arterial changes related to intersitial thropoblast migration in early human pregnancy, *Placenta*, 4, 387, 1983.

23. **Khtong, T. Y., De Wolf, F., Robertson, W. B., and Brosens, I.,** Inadequate maternal vascular response to placentation in pregnancies complicated by pre-eclampsia and by small-for-gestational age infants, *Br. J. Obstet. Gynecol.*, 93, 19049, 1986.

24. **Campbell, S., Diaz-Recasens, J., Griffin, D. et al.,** New doppler technique for assessing uteroplacental blood flow, *Lancet*, 1, 675, 1983.

25. **Campbell, S., Pearce, J. M. F., Hackett, G., Cohen-Overbeek, T., and Hernandez, C.,** Qualitative assessment of utero-placental blood flow: early screening test for high-risk pregnancies, *Obstet. Gynecol.*, 68, 649, 1986.

26. **Trudinger, B. J., Giles, W. B., and Cook, C. M.,** Uteroplacental blood flow velocity-time waveforms in normal and complicated pregnancies, *Br. J. Obstet. Gynecol.*, 92, 39, 1985.

27. **Rankin, J. H. G. and Mc Laughlin, M. K.,** The regulations of placental blood flows, *J. Dev. Physiol.*, 1, 3, 1979.

28. **Lingman, G. and Marŝal, K.,** Fetal central blood circulation in the third trimester of normal pregnancy — a longitudinal study. II. Aortic blood velocity waveform, *Early Hum. Dev.*, 13, 151, 1986.

29. **Hackett, G. A., Campbell, S., Gamsu, H., Cohen-Overbeek, T., and Pearce, J. M. F.,** Doppler studies in the growth retarded fetus and prediction of neonatal necrotising enterocolitis, haemorrhage and neonatal morbidity, *Br. Med. J.*, 294, 13, 1987.

30. **Trudinger, B. J., Giles, B. W., Cook, C. M., Bombardieri, J., and Collins, L.,** Fetal umbilical artery flow velocity waveforms and placental resistance: clinical significance, *Br. J. Obstet. Gynecol.*, 92, 23, 1985.

31. **Fleisher, A., Schulman, H., Farmakides, G. et al.,** Umbilical artery velocity waveforms and intrauterine growth, *Am. J. Obstet. Gynecol.*, 151, 502, 1985.

32. **Marŝal, K., Lingman, G., and Giles, W.,** Evaluation of the carotid, aortic and umbilical blood velocity, in *Proc. Soc. Study of Fetal Physiology*, 11th Annual Conference, Oxford, 1984, chap. 33.

33. **Wladimiroff, J. W., Tonge, H. M., and Stewart, P. A.,** Doppler ultrasound assessment of cerebral blood flow in the human fetus, *Br. J. Obstet. Gynecol.*, 93, 471, 1986.

34. **Arbeille, Ph., Patat, F., Body, G., Berson, M., Roncin, A., Berger, C. H., Saliba, E., Magnin, G., Berger, Ch., and Pourcelot, L.,** Exploration Doppler des circulations arterielles ombelicale et cerebrale du foetus, *J. Gynecol. Obstet. Biol. Reprod.*, 16, 45, 1987.

35. **Bada, H. S., Hajjar, W., Chua, C., and Summer, D. S.,** Non-invasive diagnosis of neonatal asphyxia and intraventricular haemorrhage by Doppler ultrasound, *J. Pediatr.*, 95, 775, 1979.

36. **Levine, M.,** Doppler assessment of cerebral haemodinamics: what can it tell us, in *Obstetrical and Neonatal Blood Flow*, Vol. 2, Sheldon, C. D., Evans, D. H., and Salvage, J. R., Eds., Biological Engineering Society, London, 1987, 91.

37. **Aaslid, R., Markwalder, T. M., and Nornes, H.,** Non-invasive transcranial Doppler recording of flow velocity in basal cerebral arteries, *J. Neurosurg.*, 57, 763, 1982.

38. **Archer, L. N. J., Evans, D. H., and Levene, M. I.,** Doppler examination of the anterior cerebral arteries of normal infants: the effect of postnatal age, *Early Hum. Dev.*, 10, 255, 1985.

39. **Archer, L. N. J., Levene, M. I., and Evans, D. H.,** Cerebral artery doppler ultrasonography for prediction of outcome after perinatal asphyxia, *Lancet*, 2, 1116, 1986.

40. **Bernham, R. E., Lees, M. H., Peterson, E. N., De Lamncy, C. W., and Seeds, A. E.,** Distribution of the circulation in the normal and asphyxiated fetal primate, *Am. J. Obstet. Gynecol.*, 108, 956, 1970.

41. **Wladimiroff, J. W., Tonge, H. M., Stewart, P. A., and Reuss, A.,** Severe intrauterine growth retardation; assessment of its origin from fetal arterial flow velocity waveforms, *Eur. J. Obstet. Gynecol. Reprod. Biol.*, 22, 23, 1986.

42. **Trudinger, B. J. and Cook, C. M.,** Umbilical and blood flow velocity waveforms in pregnancy associated with major fetal abnormalities, *Br. J. Obstet. Gynecol.,* 32, 1985.
43. **Nicolaides, K. H., Soothill, P. W., Rodeck, C. H., and Campbell, S.,** Ultrasound-guided sampling of umbilical cord and placental blood to assess fetal wellbeing, *Lancet,* 1, 1065, 1986.
44. **Soothill, P. W., Nicolaides, K. H., Rodeck, C. H., and Campbell, S.,** Relation of fetal hypoxia in growth retardation to mean blood velocity in the fetal aorta, *Lancet,* 2, 1118, 1986.

Chapter 10

# THE USE OF MAGNETIC RESONANCE IMAGING IN INTRAUTERINE GROWTH RETARDATION

**A. S. Garden**

## TABLE OF CONTENTS

## I. HISTORY AND DEVELOPMENT

The clinical use of magnetic resonance imaging (MRI) today has its roots in atomic physics in the first part of this century. In 1924, the Austrian physicist Wolfgang Pauli first suggested the concept of "nuclear spin", the intrinsic spinning motion demonstrated by the nuclei of some atoms. Since these nuclei bear positive or negative charges the spin produces a magnetic field. The independent discovery in 1946 by two American scientists, Felix Bloch from Stanford University and Edward Purcell from Harvard University, of a means of measuring the strength of the nuclear magnet, was the foundation of the clinical use of nuclear magnetic resonance (Bloch and Purcell were awarded the 1952 Nobel Prize for Physics).

A detailed study of the physics and chemistry of nuclear magnetic resonance (NMR) is beyond the scope of this book and would be of limited interest to most obstetricians. For those who would like more information, the articles by Pykett[1] and Pykett et al.[2] are recommended. For clinical purposes, it is sufficient to say that the resonance of nuclei can be measured within a magnetic field using pulses of radiowaves. The strength of the signal is in part proportional to the number of freely mobile nuclei present, with tissue contrast further dependent on how the signal relaxes after each pulse of radiowaves. The proton nucleus is useful in NMR imaging as it has a large magnetic moment and is present in water and fat in the human body. Different resonance will be obtained from a proton in the chemical configuration $CH_2$ from that in the configuration $CH_3$. Unfortunately, the large numbers of proton nuclei occurring in many different chemical environments limit its use in spectroscopy that is the measurement of the spectrum of resonances used in biochemical measurements. Phosphorous- and carbon-13, however, present in much smaller quantities in the body, have great potential in this situation. It is this application of NMR which makes it a powerful, noninvasive method of biochemical investigation.

Although the term "nuclear magnetic resonance" is the more correct, clinicians tend to refer to its as "magnetic resonance imaging" (MRI), due to the implications of "nuclear" in the minds of most lay people.

MRI was first used to obtain signals from a live animal by Jasper Jackson in 1967. In 1971, Damadian used MRI in the diagnosis of cancer. It was first used for the examination of the fetus *in utero* by Smith et al. in 1983.[3]

## II. SAFETY OF MAGNETIC RESONANCE IMAGING

Magnetic resonance imaging has no known significant adverse biological effects. Biomedical investigation using bacteria, cell culture, *in vivo* studies, as well as the clinical follow-up of patients, has identified no adverse effects from MRI.[4-8] Three specific potential adverse areas have been considered by the National Radiation Protection Board (NRPB):

1. The potential biological effects of the static magnetic field
2. The time varying magnetic fields which may induce electric currents of sufficient magnitude to cause depolarization in nerve muscle cells, thus causing cardiac arrhythmias or epilepsy
3. Heat production in tissues from radio frequency magnetic fields, which may cause damage to avascular tissues; heat production has also been reported to be teratogenic in rats and mice

Guidelines laid down by the NRPB[9] in Britain are aimed at avoiding these potential hazards. Similar guidelines are published in the U.S., Germany, and Japan. McRobbie and Foster[10] in a study of pregnant mice showed no significant difference between the litter numbers and growth rates of the exposed litters compared with controls. Despite this, the

NRPB has prudently advised against imaging the fetus during the first trimester, i.e., during the period of rapid organogenesis, unless the patient is having a termination of pregnancy.

There are some very practical hazards in the use of MRI. People (either patients or staff) with ferromagnetic aneurysm clips should not be placed in the magnetic field as there is a risk of the clips being displaced with fatal consequences. (Clips used by gynecologists for tubal occlusion are not usually ferromagnetic and so are not susceptible to this hazard!) Also, some cardiac pacemakers may be affected by the magnetic field, causing a malfunction. No one with a pacemaker *in situ* — particularly those programmed by magnetic fields — should be permitted in the vicinity of the magnet.

## III. OBSTETRIC APPLICATIONS

The major limitation of MRI in obstetrics is the length of time taken to obtain an image; this may be up to 12 min, and distortion is caused by fetal movement in that time. This creates, in addition, further image distortion due to movement of the large amount of nuclei in the amniotic fluid. Nonetheless, several studies are now published describing the applications of MRI in obstetrics. McCarthy et al.,[11] studying nine high-risk obstetric patients at 34 to 36 weeks' gestation, saw the fetal heart (resolved into left- and right-sided chambers), fetal lungs, liver, and brain in all patients examined. They commented that the location and extent of fetal fat was easily documented. In addition, longitudinal studies have shown sequential changes in tissue structure as the pregnancy continues. For example, images of the fetal brain at 22 weeks' gestation showed a uniformly white appearance, but by 39 weeks, the myelination of the basal ganglia was visible as a light grey area.[12] Sequential changes in the appearance of the liver were also noted.

Magnetic resonance imaging has been used to confirm the presence of fetal anomalies. McCarthy et al.[13] found MRI to be a useful complementary tool to ultrasound in the diagnosis and management of patients with fetal abnormalities. They reported five cases. In three, magnetic resonance was equal to, or superior to ultrasonography in the prenatal diagnosis of intracranial lesions. In the fourth case, (a fetus with a large cystic hygroma), MRI was less helpful than ultrasound in making the diagnosis, partly due to the similar relaxation behavior of the fluid in the cystic hygroma and in the amniotic cavity. Magnetic resonance imaging showed the pelvic anatomy more clearly in the fifth patient, who had a partial mole, than did ultrasound. In addition, in this study, MRI was found to be superior to ultrasound in the diagnosis of coincidental maternal anomalies. In one patient, a subseptate uterus was noted with MRI which had been completely missed on ultrasound examination.

Magnetic resonance imaging has some advantages over other existing techniques. Magnetic resonance imaging gives better soft tissue definition than X-rays, (Figures 1 and 2) and does not expose patients to ionizing radiation and the associated risk of childhood cancer. More tissue-specific images than those obtained by computerized tomography are obtained, again without the hazards of ionizing radiation. It has, however, the disadvantages of being more expensive than either of these techniques.

Ultrasound is cheaper and has the advantage of being a bedside mobile unit. Because of the size of the magnet required in magnetic resonance, it is unlikely that a mobile unit could be developed. Magnetic resonance imaging, however, can give much clearer pictures of the fetus in obese patients. It does not suffer from artifacts due to maternal or fetal bone, or from bowel gas. In addition, MRI can provide much clearer images in patients with oligohydramnios. The lack of amniotic fluid works to the detriment of ultrasound scanning, but works to the benefit of MRI. Magnetic resonance imaging also allows visualization of the internal structure of the fetal brain (Figure 3) and has the potential for biochemical and metabolic studies.

Magnetic resonance imaging is well tolerated by pregnant patients, although a few patients

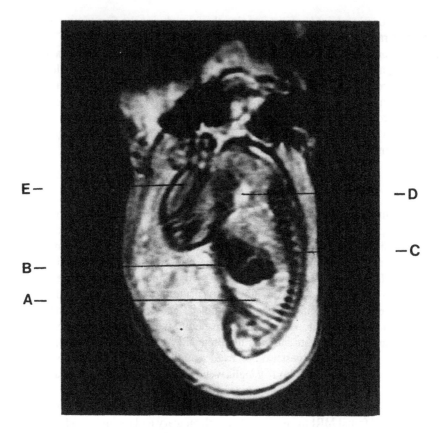

FIGURE 1.    Coronal section through maternal abdomen showing sagittal section of fetal trunk, abdomen and lower limb at 39 weeks gestation. (A) lung; (B) liver with ductus verosus; (C) spinal column; (D) bladder; and (E) soft tissues of lower limb and foot. Field 1.5T; TR — 22; 256 × 128/2 NEX; Thickness 10 mm; P. Seq. GRE/10; TE — 13; FOV — 48 cm.

feel slightly claustrophobic inside the magnet. The lack of the necessity of a full bladder is a much-appreciated advantage.

## IV. MAGNETIC RESONANCE IMAGING IN INTRAUTERINE GROWTH RETARDATION

The diagnosis of intrauterine growth retardation (IUGR) is traditionally made on clinical examination, in combination with ultrasound. However, the detection rate by measurement of symphysis-fundal height (SFH) is only 76%, and screening, with both SFH and ultrasound measurement of fetal abdominal circumference, has a sensitivity of 93%, a specificity of 67%, and a positive predictive value of only 32%.[14] Underdiagnosing the condition results in poor fetal surveillance and is associated with a higher perinatal mortality. Overdiagnosing produces unnecessary intervention, which is costly, and causes increased anxiety for the mother. Good tissue resolution, and the ability to visualize fetal fat clearly, which appears bright with MRI, suggests that MRI is a potentially useful tool in the diagnosis and management of IUGR. In addition, the presence of oligohydramnios may limit fetal movement and thus improve visualization.

Depletion of fetal body fat is known to occur earlier than reduced body size in IUGR. In the fetus, subcutaneous fat storage commences around 27 weeks.[15] Wienreb et al.,[16] in a series of 24 patients, reported only one fetus which had no discernible fat after the 30th

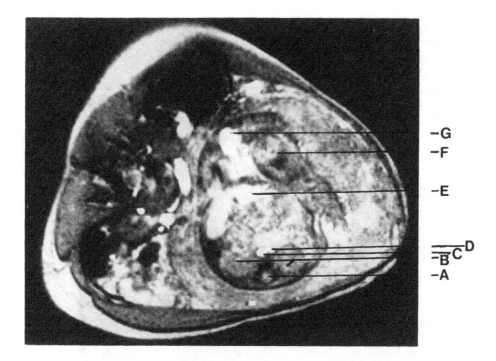

FIGURE 2. Axial section through both maternal and fetal abdomen of same fetus as Figure 1. (A) fetal vertebral body spinal cord; (B) fetal kidneys; (C) fetal aorta; (D) fetal inferior vera cava; (E) fetal transverse colon; (F) lower limb; and (G) umbilical cord. Field 1.5T; TR — 22; 256 × 256/1 NEX; Thickness 10 mm; P. Seq. GRE/30; TE — 13; FOV — 40 cm.

week. Ultrasound examination was not helpful in confirming a diagnosis of IUGR. At delivery at 39 weeks, the infant weighed 2420 g (i.e., below the tenth percentile). These investigators suggested that the absence of subcutaneous fat after 30 weeks may be a good indicator of IUGR.

Stark et al.[17] studied 11 fetuses, 9 of whom had suspected IUGR, by ultrasound examination and by magnetic resonance. Two fetuses, with little or no subcutaneous fat detectable MRI, had moderate to severe IUGR by birthweight criteria, low Apgar scores, perinatal complications, and neonatal morbidity. Nine fetuses, with subcutaneous fat noted on MRI, had normal deliveries, with normal neonatal examinations in infant development. The presence of fetal fat, however, did not correlate directly with birthweight. Two fetuses who, by ultrasound and birthweight criteria, had IUGR, had normal amounts of subcutaneous fat on magnetic resonance examination. These two fetuses were normal on clinical examination and outcome. The authors concluded that magnetic resonance may be able to separate well-nourished small fetuses from malnourished ones.

A study of 62 women undergoing a total of 92 examinations measured fetal dimensions such as head, chest, and abdominal circumference as a means of estimating fetal size. The researchers also assessed fetal growth by measuring uterine size, which they found an easy procedure with MRI, as all uterine dimensions were available on a single sagittal image. In seven patients, who they were able to follow sequentially, they found that the "take-off" points for uterine size in early pregnancy were fairly uniform. However, the lines diverged with advancing pregnancy and different growth rates. The individual growth slopes correlated closely with birthweight.[6]

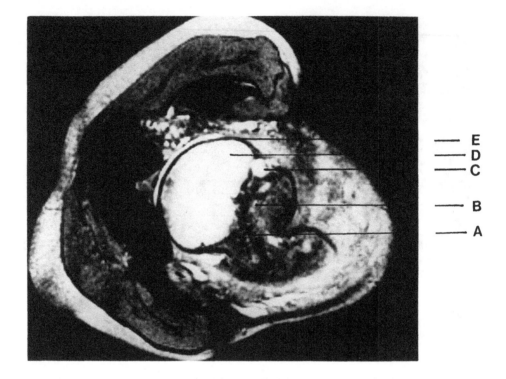

FIGURE 3.    Axial section through maternal abdomen and sagittal section through same fetus as Figures 1 and 2. (A) cervical spine; (B) nasopharynx; (C) orbit and lens; (D) brain; and (E) skull. Field 1.5T; TR — 22; 256 × 256/1 NEX; Thickness 10 mm; P. Seq. GRE/30; FE — 13; FOV — 40 cm.

## V. POTENTIAL DEVELOPMENT OF MAGNETIC RESONANCE IMAGING IN INTRAUTERINE GROWTH RETARDATION

Further work is required to be done in the measurement of fetal subcutaneous fat as a predictor of IUGR. Studies of the placenta may also be helpful, both in measuring the volume of the placenta, and in assessing placental architecture. Placental perfusion studies to detect areas of ischemia, infarction, or retroplacental hemorrhage, may give helpful pointers in the detection of an at-risk fetus.

It is not in areas where its function is complementary to traditional imaging techniques that MRI is likely to make the greatest impact. The availability, mobility, and relative inexpensiveness of ultrasound scanning will probably cause it to remain the mainstay of fetal imaging, despite the imminent development of real-time MRI.

The greatest diagnostic use in IUGR will be in the development of phosphorous spectroscopy. The development of spectroscopy should enable investigators to study, *in vivo,* the pH of fetal tissue such as the brain, and allow *in vivo* monitoring. A noninvasive technique of this type would be of great benefit in the management of high-risk pregnancy.

*In vivo* analysis of amniotic fluid would also be helpful, particularly in the measurement of meconium concentration. This can, at present, be done *in vitro* by magnetic resonance, and an *in vivo* application would be of benefit.

Blood flow studies using MRI have already been reported,[18] and development of this to provide a reliable noninvasive technique of assessing fetoplacental circulation, without the use of radio isotopes would be of inestimable value.

Initial research with MRI suggests many advances in noninvasive monitoring for the fetomaternal medicine specialist. Future developments in spectroscopy, and increased magnetic strength, may provide more answers.

## REFERENCES

1. **Pykett, I. L.,** N.M.R. imaging in medicine, *Sci. Am.,* 246, 78, 1982.
2. **Pykett, I. L., Newhouse, J. H., Buoanno, F. S., Brady, T. J., Goldman, M. R., Kistler, J. P., and Pohost, G. M.,** Principles of nuclear magnetic resonance imaging, *Radiology,* 143, 157, 1982.
3. **Smith, F. W., Adam, A. M., and Phillips, W. D. P.,** NMR Imaging in pregnancy, *Lancet,* 1, 61, 1983.
4. **Thomas, A. and Morris, P. G.,** The effects of NMR exposure on living organisms, a microbial assay, *Br. J. Radiol.,* 54, 615, 1981.
5. **Budinger, T. F.,** Nuclear magnetic resonance (NMR) *in vivo* studies: known threshold for health effects, *J. Comput. Assisted Tomography,* 5, 800, 1981.
6. **Reid, A., Smith, H. W., and Hutchison, J. M. S.,** Nuclear magnetic resonance imaging and its safety implications: follow-up of 181 patients, *Br. J. Radiol.,* 55, 784, 1982.
7. **Schwartz, J. L. and Crooks, L. E.,** NMR imaging produces no observable mutations or cytotoxity in mammalian cells, *Am. J. Radiol.,* 139, 583, 1982.
8. **Johnson, I. R., Symonds, E. M., Kean, D. M. et al.,** Imaging the pregnant human uterus with nuclear magnetic resonance, *Am. J. Obstet. Gynecol.,* 148, 1136, 1984.
9. NRPB ad hoc Advisory Group on NMR clinical imaging, Revised guidelines on acceptable limits of exposure during nuclear magnetic resonance clinical imaging, *Br. J. Radiol.,* 56, 974, 1983.
10. **McRobbie, D. and Foster, M. A.,** Pulsed magnetic field exposure during pregnancy and implications for NMR foetal imaging: a study with mice, *Magn. Reson. Imaging,* 3, 231, 1985.
11. **McCarthy, S. M., Filly, R. A., Stark, D. D., Hricak, H., Brant-Zawadzki, M. N., Callen, P. W., and Higgins, C. B.,** Obstetrical magnetic resonance imaging: fetal anatomy, *Radiology,* 154, 427, 1985.
12. **Smith, F. W., Kent, C., Abramovich, D. R., and Sutherland, H. W.,** Nuclear magnetic resonance imaging — a new look at the fetus, *Br. J. Obstet. Gynaecol.,* 92, 1024, 1985.
13. **McCarthy, P. W., Filly, R. A., Stark, D. D., Callen, P. W., Golbus, M. S., and Hricak, H.,** Magnetic resonance imaging of fetal anamolies in utero: early experience, *Am. J. Radiol.,* 145, 677, 1985.
14. **Pearce, J. M. and Campbell, S.,** A comparison of symphysis-fundal height and ultrasound as screening tests for light-for-gestational age infants, *Br. J. Obstet. Gynaecol.,* 94, 100, 1987.
15. **England, M. A.,** *Color Atlas of Life Before Birth: Normal Fetal Development,* Year Book Medical Publishers, Chicago, 1983.
16. **Weinreb, J. C., Lowe, T. W., Cohen, J. M., and Kutler, M.,** Human fetal anatomy: magnetic resonance imaging, *Radiology,* 157, 715, 1985.
17. **Stark, D. D., McCarthy, S. M., Filly, R. A., Callen, P. W., Hricak, H., and Parer, J. T.,** Intrauterine growth retardation: evaluation by magnetic resonance, *Radiology,* 155, 425, 1985.
18. **Bradley, W. G. and Waluch, V.,** Blood flow: magnetic resonance imaging, *Radiology,* 154, 443, 1985.

Chapter 11

# LOW BIRTHWEIGHT AND FETAL GROWTH RETARDATION: SOME PREVENTABLE ASPECTS

**Peter M. Dunn**

## TABLE OF CONTENTS

# I. INTRODUCTION

Low birthweight (LBW) is defined by WHO as "less than 2500 g" (up to and including 2499 g). Although no lower limit is included in this definition, most workers take 500 g as a cut-off point. LBW infants have either been born early or have failed to grow *in utero*. In fact we now appreciate that a fetus that is chronically distressed due to hypoxia or malnutrition may make hormonal signals to the mother that early delivery would be to his or her advantage. Indeed, the obstetrician also contemplates elective premature delivery when he detects evidence of fetal distress. Thus, many LBW infants are both preterm and growth retarded.

Low birthweight constitutes the most important challenge for maternal and child health today. Throughout the world some 21 million LBW babies are born each year, more than 90% of them in developing countries. The significance and importance of LBW lies in the fact that such infants, whether preterm or small-for-dates or both, attract far more, perhaps ten times their share of perinatal and infant mortality and also short- and long-term morbidity. Quite apart from the tragedy and suffering involved, the immediate and subsequent care of such infants, especially those with handicaps, presents an enormous burden to both family and the community and, by consuming scarce resources, may seriously frustrate efforts to improve other necessary health services, especially those of preventative and primary care.

In developed countries the incidence of LBW ranges from 3 to 12% of all births. On average, 60% of babies are preterm, while 40% are small-for-date infants born after the 37th week of gestation. In developing countries such figures as are available suggest that the incidence of LBW ranges from 12 to 40%; in contrast to developed countries, the great majority of such babies, perhaps 80% of them, are small-for-dates term infants.[1] Many factors probably contribute to this fetal growth retardation but probably a central role is played by the synergistic efforts of maternal malnutrition, anemia, and infection, exacerbated by over-frequent pregnancies.[2,3] The influence of these factors is not confined to pregnancy. By operating after delivery and retarding growth throughout childhood they may have a profound effect on ultimate maternal stature, and hence on the size at birth of the following generation. Therefore, any strategy to reduce the incidence of LBW in developing countries should include vigorous efforts to improve hygiene and the general health and nutrition of children and expectant mothers. Such problems are likely to remain as long as world population escalates, especially in the developing countries, with its exacerbating effect on poverty, pollution, and exhaustion of natural resources leading to malnutrition and disease.

# II. ANTENATAL FACTORS

The cumulative energy cost of pregnancy to a mother has been estimated at nearly 70,000 kcal.[4,5] While the fetus is recognized as being an efficient "parasite", it would seem inevitable that maternal malnutrition would to some extent lead to fetal malnutrition. Yet this view has been challenged on the evidence of the failure of some maternal supplementation studies to significantly influence birthweight. Perhaps this should not surprise us, as such studies are notoriously difficult to control. If instead we turn to similar studies conducted on domestic animals there can be no doubt as to the importance of maternal nutrition especially in the second half of pregnancy. Arthur[6] has reviewed some of the evidence. To cite him, for example: "Stillbirths are numerous among the offspring of underfed ewes. In ordinary farming conditions supplementation of the ewe's diet during the last quarter of pregnancy increases lamb weights by 25% and leads to a fourfold increase in survival of twin lambs." And again he writes: "In varying the diets of pregnant sows, Pike and Boaz[7] have shown that variable feeding from conception to 70 d gestation (gestation period 114 d) exerted no effect. Only in the last 45 d did maternal nutrition influence birthweight. Of course, this should be expected because normally there is a tenfold increase in porcine fetal weight during this later period.''

There is increasing evidence that nutritional deficiency is not confined to the developing world but may also be a major cause of LBW in industrialized countries. Perhaps too frequently in the past, the emphasis in some of our antenatal clinics has been on dieting and the restriction of weight gain during pregnancy. The time has come to recognize that the expectant mother is eating for two and that a good weight gain during pregnancy (11 kg) is a very healthy sign.

Multiple pregnancy throws an extra burden on the mother's ability to adequately nourish her fetuses and on the uterus' ability to retain them until term. As a result, intrauterine growth retardation and preterm delivery are commonplace and at least half of all twins are of low birthweight.[8] In a developed country such as the U.K. where multiple pregnancy occurs 1 in 80 times, twins account for about 15% of all LBW infants. Optimal management depends on early diagnosis and in this ultrasound examination has proved most valuable. But over and above this we have a responsibility not to *cause* multiple pregnancy by the overenthusiastic use of drugs that stimulate ovulation in the treatment of subfertility or by the insertion of too many ova with *in vitro* fertilization.[9]

Malnutrition is not confined to lack of protein or calories. Deficiency of other factors such as vitamins or trace elements may also play a part. Recent work has focused on the importance of zinc deficiency in association with fetal growth retardation. In a recent study by Simmer and Thompson,[10] 55% of the mothers of small-for-dates infants were zinc deficient, a state that appears to be related to and exacerbated by maternal smoking. Zinc is an essential element in many important enzymes concerned not only with growth but also with immunity. Therefore, when zinc deficient, both mother and baby may be prone to infection, another significant cause of both fetal growth retardation and preterm delivery.

After malnutrition, infection is likely to be the second most important cause of both fetal growth retardation and preterm delivery throughout the world.[11] The infection may just involve the mother with a knock-on effect on the fetus through her illness (e.g., malnutrition, pyrexia, drugs, etc.). Alternatively the infection may involve the fetus and/or placenta as with blood-born organisms such as syphilis, rubella, and malaria. Or infection, usually bacterial, may pass up the birth canal to cause chorion-amnionitis, a condition being increasingly recognized in association with both premature labor and fetal growth retardation, especially in developing countries.[12,13] It has been suggested that coitus may on occasion precipitate such infection by dislodging the cervical plug of mucus and permitting organisms to reach the amniotic mambranes. Most vaginal organisms will metabolize prostaglandin precursors in the amnion into prostaglandins. Chorion-amnionitis, rupture of the membranes, placental infection, and premature labor are among the complications which may ensue.[14] A similar train of events may be precipitated by the examining finger of the obstetrician or midwife. Indeed the ''membrane sweep'' used to be a popular method of inducing labor. Trainee obstetricians are now usually taught not to insert a finger into the cervix before the time for delivery has arrived.

Another maternal factor recognized in association with LBW and raised perinatal mortality is anemia. In many instances this may be related to malnutrition or a deficiency of iron or folic acid. In other cases it is related to infections such as malaria or hookworm, or to genetic disease such as sickle cell anemia and thalassemia. Often in the background is the draining impact of repeated pregnancies. Often the primary cause of the anemia as well as the anemia itself, is both preventable and treatable.[15]

The strategy occupying most obstetric attention in developed countries, with respect to reducing the incidence of preterm delivery, has been the inhibition of premature labor using a variety of drugs. Yet such a strategy has only limited value. In one U.K. study, half the 6% of preterm deliveries were either electively induced or were of malformed infants, while another 2% had already reached the comparative safety of 35 to 37 weeks gestation. In addition, a proportion of the remaining 1% were already too far advanced in labor by the time they presented in hospital.[16]

Another major obstetrical strategy in some developed countries has been the elective induction of labor. This makes sound sense in the case of pregnancies in which the fetus is small-for-date and/or is exhibiting signs of distress. However, while the proportion of such pregnancies is unlikely to exceed 10%, the incidence of reported elective induction has been as high as 25 to 50%. Such excessive use of this technique has its dangers, among them unexpected and iatrogenic prematurity. In some studies, 10 to 20% of all LBW infants fall into this category.[17]

Surely we should turn our energy towards more productive lines of action. Ranking high in priority must be the prevention of smoking during pregnancy. It has now been established in studies in a number of developed countries that maternal smoking is associated both with a significant degree of fetal growth retardation at term and a 30% higher perinatal mortality. More recently, Meyer and Tonascia[18] have shown from the Ontario data that maternal smoking is also associated with a significant increase in both premature rupture of the membranes and antepartum hemorrhage, especially between 20 and 32 weeks' gestation. Here then is a major challenge. So far medical propaganda directed at the smoking mother has proved ineffective. Probably we should be aiming much more at children during their formative years (5 to 10 years) in this as well as in many other matters concerning reproductive health.

Another of the major health problems of modern life is "stress", particularly in our overcrowded cities. It is well established that stress can lead to abortion and premature labor in a variety of animals.[19] Whether the same is true for the human has not been definitely established, although there are indications to suggest that it is. Recently Newton and his colleagues[20,21] in Manchester have shown that stressful events occur two or three times more frequently among mothers delivering prematurely than among those delivering at term. This, then, is yet another promising line of enquiry and potential prevention, especially as, if the world population continues to increase at its present rate, stress is likely to dominate all our lives in the future.

One form of stress which may divert blood flow and energy away from the utero-placental circulation is physical work. In developing countries in particular, women may be engaged in physical activity around the home, collecting water and fuel or working in the fields for 18 h/d. For many years obstetricians have recommended "rest" to mothers whose pregnancies were "at risk", either because of maternal hypertension, cervical imcompetance, multiple pregnancy, fetal growth retardation, or threatened premature delivery. Recent experience in France, reported by Papiernik and colleagues,[22] appears to support the value and importance of this approach.

A most important background factor leading to LBW is lack of family planning, especially when combined with the social custom prevalent in many developing countries of marriage in the early "teens". Repeated pregnancies not only take their toll on the mother's nutritional status and health, but of course present her with an ever-increasing workload in the home.[23]

One of the socio-medical strategies for birth control since the war has been therapeutic abortion. Not surprisingly, as the years have passed, we have learned more of the price that has to be paid in the form of a variety of complications, not the least being an increased chance of a subsequent LBW infant due to preterm delivery. National statistics from Hungary, for example, have demonstrated the cumulative effect of repeated abortion. In the years since therapeutic abortion was introduced in Hungary after the war, the incidence of LBW has nearly doubled.[24] It appears that forcible dilatation of the cervix in early pregnancy may lead to tearing of the spiral fibrous strands that play such an important part in maintaining cervical competence. Here too, then, we have another potential method of preventing LBW, even if the lesson is a negative one. In other words, avoidance of abortion, or minimization of preliminary cervical dilatation.

Clearly there are better methods of birth control than therapeutic abortion which is, at the best, an expression of failure in prevention. Cheap contraceptive methods should surely be made readily available and instruction in their use part of the normal education of every child. The value of contraception lies as much in spacing pregnancies as in preventing them. Time and again studies have shown that too short an interval between successive births is associated with a raised incidence of LBW and perinatal mortality. Data from the national British study in 1970[25] dramatically illustrated the importance of spacing births, preferably with intervals of 18 to 36 months. If this matter is important for developed countries, it has even greater significance for those that are still developing. As Ebrahim has shown,[26] the number of children under the age of 5 years which a mother will have after 8 years will be just one or four, depending on whether the birth interval was 34 months or 17 months. The effect that this must have on a mother's health, nutrition, and ability to care for her children is obvious.

The importance of breast feeding in determining a satisfactory birth interval is often insufficiently appreciated. In part, its effect is due to the temporary inhibition or reduction in ovulation and in part to the widespread taboo in developing countries against sexual intercourse with a lactating woman.[23] Sadly there has been a dramatic decline in breast feeding throughout the world. This decline represents an extremely serious threat to health, especially in developing countries. Apart from the reason just given, failure to breast feed in some parts of the world is almost tantamount to a death sentence, usually from gastroenteritis. In Chile the infant mortality of nonbreast-fed infants has been shown to be twice that of those given breast milk.[27] In addition, weight gain during infancy was often found to be very suboptimal. If breast feeding in important for the term infant, it is doubly essential for the LBW baby. Such infants are particularly prone to infection, failure to thrive, and malnutrition. Another important point to be made about this subject is in relation to economics. Human milk costs little or nothing while artificial milk is relatively expensive; and the less developed a country, the greater the financial burden. Thus, while the cost of artificially feeding a 6-month-old infant in the U.K. may represent 3% of the family's income, in many developing countries the figure may be 50% or more.[26] Therefore we must make an all-out effort to educate our mothers and our future mothers to breast feed their children.

## III. OBSTETRIC AND PEDIATRIC FACTORS

The obstetrician's role in the prevention of LBW and fetal growth retardation must include preconception education on family planning and reproduction health. Once a pregnancy has commenced, the doctor must attempt to establish the gestational age, then exclude, or diagnose and treat maternal disease such as infection or anemia, and advise the mother on good nutrition, on the avoidance of smoking, alcohol and drugs, and also untoward stress or physical activity (especially in first and multiple pregnancies or when there is a poor obstetric history). Thereafter, the main duty is to monitor the progress of the pregnancy with a view to the early detection of signs suggesting that all is not well, two of the most important being evidence of pre-eclampsia, or of fetal growth retardation.[28] While ultrasound now provides a more accurate method of measuring fetal growth, much can still be achieved by careful charting of maternal weight and fundal height.[29]

Once the fetus is known to be at risk there is a need to introduce more frequent and careful monitoring and assessment, whether by clinical (kick charts), sonographic, or biochemical means, or by using CTG (with or without stress tests). At the same time there is a need to screen the pregnancy again carefully for preventable or treatable causes of the fetal problem, and to institute appropriate therapy whenever possible.[30] The detection of serious fetal malformation is important as it may greatly influence management.

In due course the obstetrician will need to weigh the risks to the fetus of continued pregnancy against those following elective delivery. When the gestation is preterm, a knowledge of the likely postnatal outcome of neonatal care at any given gestational age is essential, and most obstetricians these days consult closely with their pediatric colleagues. If suitable facilities are not available locally, then mother and fetus should, if possible, be transferred to wherever they are. The uterus is rightly regarded as the ideal transport incubator. Next, a decision must be made on method of delivery — vaginal or caesarean. Many factors need to be taken into account including the age, parity, and past obstetric history of the mother, the gestational age and presentation of the fetus, the presence or absence of malformation, and the likely ability of the compromised bably to withstand labor. If vaginal delivery is sought, then labor must be monitored most carefully and everything done to avoid and treat maternal hypoxia, hypovolemia, hypotension, and acidosis. The dorsal position should be avoided. Oxytocic drugs, when absolutely necessary, should be used with the utmost caution. At the first sign of serious fetal distress, caesarean section should be considered.

Whichever route is chosen, the pediatric staff should be available in the delivery room in order to promptly resuscitate the infant,[31] to protect "him" from chilling, and to deal with any complications of the LBW infant, such as respiratory distress syndrome, meconium aspiration, hypoglycemia, and polycythaemia. The importance of breast feeding has already been discussed.

In conclusion, the best approach to the problem of LBW and fetal malnutrition may be summed up by five words: standards, organization, education, prevention, and therapy.

# REFERENCES

1. WHO Report of the Meeting on Etiology, Prevention and Social Implications of Low Birthweight, Geneva, September 1 to 5, 1975, MCH/LBW/78.
2. **Lechtig, A., Habicht, J.-P., Delgardo, H., Klein, R., Yarborough, C., and Martonelli, R.,** Effect of food supplementation during pregnancy on birthweight, *Pediatrics*, 56, 508, 1975.
3. **Mata, L. J.,** *The Children of Santa Maria Canque: A Prospective Field Study of Health and Growth*, MIT Press, Cambridge, 1978.
4. **Hytten, F. E.,** Nutritional aspects of human pregnancy, in *Maternal Nutrition During Pregnancy and Lactation*, Aebi, H. and Whitehead, R., Eds., Hans Huber, Berne, 1980, 36.
5. **Hytten, F. E.,** Nutrition in relation to fetal growth, in *Fetal Growth Retardation*, Van Assche, F. A. and Robertson, W. B., Eds., Churchill Livingstone, Edinburgh, 1981, 57.
6. **Arthur, G. H.,** Fetal growth in domestic species, in *Fetal Growth Retardation*, Van Assche, F. A. and Robertson, W. B., Eds., Churchill Livingstone, Edinburgh, 1981, 219.
7. **Pike, J. H. and Boaz, T. G.,** The effect of condition at service and plane of nutrition in early pregnancy in the sow, *Anim. Prod.*, 15, 147, 1972.
8. **Dunn, P. M.,** Some perinatal observations on twins, *Develop. Med. Child. Neurol.*, 7, 121, 1965.
9. **Levene, M. I.,** Grand multiple pregnancies and demand for neonatal intensive care, *Lancet*, 2, 347, 1986.
10. **Simmer, K. and Thompson, R. P. H.,** Zinc in the fetus and newborn, in *Perinatal Growth: the Quest for an International Standard for Reference*, Wharton, B. A. and Dunn, P. M., Eds.; *Acta Paediatr. Scand. Suppl.*, 319, 158, 1985.
11. **Peckham, C. S. and Marshall, W. C.,** Infections in pregnancy, in *Obstetrical Epidemiology*, Academic Press, London, 1983, 209.
12. **Higgs, S. C., Malan, A. F., and Heese, H de V.,** The perinatal infective environment and infants of very low birth weight, *S. Afr. Med. J.*, 51, 621, 1977.
13. **Naeye, R. L., Tafari, N., Judge, D., Gilmour, D., and Marboe, C.,** Amniotic fluid infections in an African city, *J. Paediatr.*, 90, 965, 1977.
14. **Naeye, R. L. and Ross, S.,** Coitus and chorioamnionitis, a prospective study, *Early Hum. Dev.*, 6, 91, 1982.

15. **Dunn, P. M.,** Low birthweight—incidence, aetiology and prevention, in *Maternity Services in the Developing World—What the Community Needs, Proc. 7th Study Group of Royal College of Obstetricians and Gynaecologists,* Philpott, R. H., Ed., Royal College of Gynecologists, London, 1980, 233.

16. **Turnbull, A. C.,** Aetiology of pre-term labour, in *Pre-Term Labour, Proc. 5th Study Group of Royal College of Obstetricians and Gynaecologists,* Anderson, A., Beard, R., Brudenell, J. M., and Dunn, P. M., Eds., Royal College of Gynecologists, London, 1978, 56.

17. **Flaksman, R. J., Vollman, J. H., and Benfield, D. G.,** Iatrogenic prematurity due to elective termination of the uncomplicated pregnancy: a major perinatal health care problem, *Am. J. Obstet. Gynecol.,* 132, 885, 1978.

18. **Meyer, M. R. and Tonascia, J. A.,** Maternal smoking, pregnancy complications and perinatal mortality, *Am. J. Obstet. Gynecol.,* 128, 494, 1977.

19. **Naaktgeboren, C. and Bontekoe, E. H. M.,** in *The Family,* 4th Int. Congr. of Psychosomatic Obstetrics and Gynaecology, Tel Aviv, 1974, S. Karger, Basel, 1975, 519.

20. **Newton, R. W., Webster, P. A. C., Binn, P. S., Maskrey, N., and Phillips, A. B.,** Psycho-social stress in pregnancy and its relation to the onset of premature labour, *Br. Mod. J.,* 2, 411, 1979.

21. **Newton, R. W.,** Influence of psychological stress in low birthweight and pre-term labour, in *Pre-term Labour and its Consequences,* Proc. 13th Study Group of Royal College of Obstetricians and Gynaecologists, Beard, R. W. and Sharpe, F., Eds., Royal College of Gynecologists, London, 1985, 225.

22. **Papiernik, E., Bouyer, J., and Dreyfus, J.,** Risk factors for pre-term births and results of a prevention policy—the Haguenau Perinatal Study 1971—1982, in *Pre-term Labour and its Consequences, Proc. 13th Study Group of Royal College of Obstetricians and Gynaecologists,* Beard, R. W., and Sharpe, F., Eds., Royal College of Gynecologists, London, 1985, 15.

23. **Morley, D.,** Birth interval and family planning, in *Paediatric Priorities in the Developing World,* Butterworths, London, 1973, 296.

24. **Makoi, Z.,** The impact of abortion policy on prematurity in Hungary, in *Perinatal Growth: the Quest for an International Standard for Reference,* Wharton, B. A. and Dunn, P. M., Eds.; *Acta Paediatr. Scand. Suppl.,* 319, 84, 1985.

25. **Chamberlain, G., Phillip, E., Howlett, B., and Masters, K., Eds.,** British Births 1970, Vol. 2, William Heinemann, London, 1978.

26. **Ebrahim, G. J.,** *Breast Feeding, the Biological Option,* MacMillan, London, 1978.

27. **Plank, S. J. and Milanesi, M. L.,** Infant feeding and infant mortality in Chile, *Bull.,* WHO 48, 203, 1973.

28. **Keirse, M. J. N. C.,** Aetiology of intrauterine growth retardation, in *Fetal Growth Retardation,* Van Assche, F. A. and Robertson, W. B., Eds., Churchill Livingstone, Edinburgh, 1981, 37.

29. **Pearce, J. M. and Campbell, S.,** A comparison of synthesis-fundal height and ultrasound as screening tests for light-for-gestational age infants, *Br. J. Obstet. Gynaecol.,* 94, 100, 1987.

30. **Hibbard, B.,** The aetiology of pre-term labour (editorial), *Br. Med. J.,* 294, 594, 1987.

31. **Dunn, P. M.,** In the delivery room, in *A Neonatal Vade-Mecum,* Fleming, P. J., Speidel, B. D., and Dunn, P. M., Eds., Lloyd-Luke Limited, London, 1986, 15.

Chapter 12

# PREVENTION OF INTRAUTERINE GROWTH RETARDATION BY MAGNESIUM SUBSTITUTION IN PREGNANCY

**L. Kovács**

## TABLE OF CONTENTS

# I. INTRODUCTION

Recent reports have emphasized the important role of magnesium in the physiology of pregnancy, including the development of the fetus. Although magnesium sulphate has long been used in the treatment of preeclamptic toxemia, the widening of the indications of its use seems to be causing a therapeutic renaissance of this almost forgotten cation.

Magnesium is now used as a tocolytic agent,[1,2] or as an adjuvant to betamimetic tocolysis,[3] and in the treatment of EPH gestosis.[4] Several retrospective evaluations have indicated its usefulness in the prevention of gestosis,[5] premature birth, and intrauterine growth retardation.[6,7] Two prospective controlled clinical studies have been published on the use of magnesium substitution during pregnancy. The first was a preliminary report on our own study in 1985,[8] while the second paper was published by Vetter and Spaetling[9] from Zürich in 1986. The beneficial effect of magnesium prophylaxis as regards the outcome of pregnancy was convincing in both studies. A detailed report on our study will be given in the second part of this paper.

# II. MAGNESIUM METABOLISM

Magnesium is one of the most abundant intracellular cations. Only 1% of the total body magnesium is present in the extracellular fluid, and 30% of this is protein bound. Sixty percent of the total body magnesium is found in the bones, incorporated in the crystal mineral lattice, or in the surface-limited exchangeable pool. Twenty percent is located in the skeletal muscle, and the remainder in other body tissues, especially the heart and the liver. It is clear that, while determination of the serum magnesium concentration remains the best readily available test for magnesium deficiency, it provides only a rough index of the total body magnesium stores.

Magnesium is required for the activation of about 300 enzyme systems, including those that involve adenosine triphosphate (ATP). This element is also essential for the transfer, storage, and utilization of intracellular energy, for the metabolism of protein, carbohydrate, fat, and nucleic acids, for the maintenance of the normal cell membrane function, and for neuromuscular transmission.

The magnesium balance is achieved through intestinal absorption and renal excretion. The mechanisms leading to hypomagnesemia (serum levels <0.7 mmol/l) can include a decreased intake or absorption, an internal redistribution, and an increased renal or nonrenal loss.

The normal range of the serum magnesium level is between 0.7 and 1.05 mmol/1.

Various daily intakes have been estimated by the different authors; on average the daily intake is about 12 to 15 mmol (300 to 400 mg). The daily need for adults is assessed as about 12 to 18 mmol (300 to 450 mg). It is the general opinion of the investigators that the daily need is usually not covered by the daily intake in the industrialized countries. This causes a latent hypomagnesemia in the population.

Several factors are responsible for this condition. The use of chemical fertilizers in agriculture causes a calcination of the soil and as a consequence, a decreasing magnesium level in drinking water and in agricultural products; the situation is worsened by the refining of cereals. Further, modern dietary habits tend to lead to hypomagnesemia. The intake of magnesium is reduced by the decreasing proportion of vegetable to animal food. The high protein and calcium intake (milk, cheese, and other dairy products) increases the magnesium need, whereas the restriction of fats reduces the magnesium resoprtion. Alcohol consumption is also disadvantageous, because it increases the renal magnesium excretion.

Foodstuffs rich in magnesium include fruits, vegetables, nuts, and bran.

**Table 1**
**STUDY POPULATION**

| Admitted<br>subjects | Total<br>997 | Magnesium<br>490 | Placebo<br>507 |
|---|---|---|---|
| Excluded | 12 | 5 | 7 |
| Nonpregnant | 4 | | |
| Multiple pregnancy | 7 | | |
| Anencephalus | 1 | | |
| Evaluated | 985 | 485 | 500 |

## III. MAGNESIUM METABOLISM IN PREGNANCY

In pregnancy, the danger of hypomagnesemia is greater. The magnesium need is higher throughout pregnancy than in a nonpregnant condition; the need increases as pregnancy progresses, and in the third trimester hypomagnesemia is commonplace. The minimum necessary magnesium intake in pregnancy and lactation is 450 mg or 18.5 mmol daily. The usual alimentation cannot cover this need, and magnesium substitution throughout pregnancy, therefore, seems to be an important task in modern antenatal care. The recommended substitution is 10 to 20 mmol/d.

## IV. THE "SZEGED MAGNESIUM STUDY"

The above ideas led us to organize a prospective controlled clinical trial to compare the effects of magnesium substitution vs. placebo on the outcome of pregnancy in a randomized, double-blind study.

The magnesium preparation was the Magnesium 5 Longoral oral tablet containing 121.5 mg or 5 mmol, or 10 mval magnesium in aspartate form, a product of the Artesan Company, Lüchow, Federal Republic of Germany. The same company also produced the placebo tablets in an identical form and package. The treatment dose was one tablet, three times daily, i.e., 15 mmol. The randomization occurred according to the participating antenatal clinics: in eight of them magnesium tablets were distributed, and in seven of them placebo tablets. The random code was known only to the principal investigator.

The subjects were recruited and admitted to the study at the time of the first antenatal visit, and they were followed up at every visit (at least four weekly). The admission period lasted from June 1984 to October 1985.

Table 1 contains the composition of the study population. The total number of admissions was 997. Twelve subjects were later excluded: in four cases because they were not pregnant, in seven cases multiple pregnancy was diagnosed, and one case involved an anencephalus. The remaining 985 cases were included in the study.

The randomization was successful. The magnesium and placebo groups did not differ in age, in the obstetric history of the subjects (Table 2), or in gestational age at admission (Figure 1). Consequently, the groups were comparable. The data in Figure 1 indicate that most of the subjects began the treatment in the first trimester.

For different reasons, 129 subjects dropped out of the study and thus the outcome of pregnancy in those cases is unknown. We have information on the outcome of pregnancy in 856 cases (Table 3). In order to achieve a realistic evaluation, we classified the subjects as regular and irregular users. Those were regarded as regular users who took the one tablet three times daily for at least 15 weeks. Those who did not fulfil this criterion were included in the irregular group.

In 796 pregnancies, or 92.9% of the cases, the outcome was parturition, whereas in 60 cases (7.1%) abortion was the outcome. The ratio of abortions was the same in the magnesium

**Table 2**
**OBSTETRIC HISTORY OF SUBJECTS**

| | Magnesium | | Placebo | | |
|---|---|---|---|---|---|
| | n | % | n | % | Total |
| First pregnancy | 234 | 48.4 | 24 | 48.0 | 474 |
| Only term delivery | 113 | 23.3 | 119 | 23.8 | 232 |
| Preterm delivery | 15 | 3.1 | 15 | 3.0 | 30 |
| Only artificial abortion | 24 | 4.9 | 32 | 6.4 | 56 |
| Only spontaneous abortion | 34 | 7.0 | 11 | 2.2 | 45 |
| Other | 65 | 13.4 | 83 | 16.6 | 148 |
| Total | 485 | | 500 | | 985 |

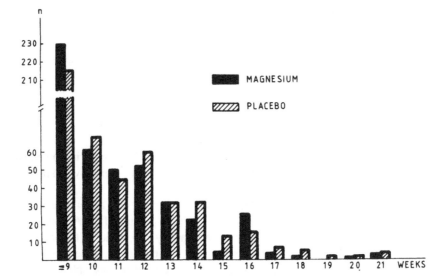

FIGURE 1.   Distribution of subjects in the magnesium and placebo groups according to duration of gestation at admission.

**Table 3**
**OUTCOME OF PREGNANCY**

| | Abortion | | Parturition | | |
|---|---|---|---|---|---|
| | n | % | n | % | Total |
| Magnesium regular | ∅ | 0 | 210 | 100 | 210 |
| Magnesium irregular | 28 | 12.8 | 190 | 87.2 | 218 |
| Placebo regular | ∅ | 0 | 168 | 100 | 168 |
| Placebo irregular | 32 | 12.3 | 228 | 87.7 | 260 |
| Total | 60 | 7.1 | 796 | 92.9 | 856 |

and in the placebo groups. There were no abortions among the regular users. The explanation lies in the definition of regularity: the use for at least 15 weeks. Most of the abortions (41 cases) occurred within the first 4 weeks of treatment.

Figure 2 shows the distribution of the newborns according to birthweight. The ratio of low birthweight infants (<2500 g) is the lowest in the regular magnesium group. Only one-third (36.8%) of the low birthweight infants come from the magnesium group, with two-

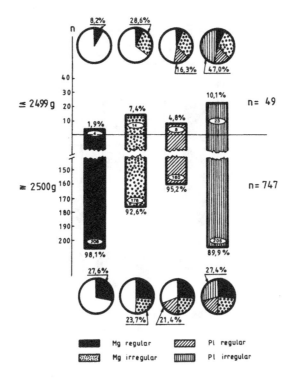

FIGURE 2. Distribution of newborns according to birthweight. Columns indicate the proportions of low and normal birthweight in the treatment groups. Circular diagrams indicate the proportions of the different treatments in the two weight categories.

thirds from the placebo group. Statistical comparison of the results by the $X^2$ test showed a difference of $p < 0.05$.

The comparison of the gestational age at birth (Figure 3) gives the best result in the regular magnesium group. Here the pregnancy ended before the 258th day of gestation in only 7% of the cases, whereas the corresponding figure was 15.6% in the placebo group. The difference in the results is significant at the level $p < 0.05$.

The analysis of the birthweight percentile data is the most important as regards the question of intrauterine growth retardation (Figure 4). The ratio of small-for-date infants (less than 5th percentile) is the lowest in the magnesium group. Most of the newborns in the regular magnesium group are in the 50 to 95th percentile class, whereas the majority in the placebo group are in the 5 to 50th percentile category. These results suggest that the magnesium supplementation supported the intrauterine development of the fetus.

The condition of the newborns at birth is characterized by the Apgar score (Table 4). The regular magnesium group displayed a higher ratio of the eight-ten-score category.

The perinatal mortality was 1.37% of the total population of the study (Table 5). There was no difference between the magnesium and placebo groups. The causes of the five postnatal deaths were as follows: in three cases idiopathic respiratory distress syndrome, in one case intracranial bleeding, and in one case multiple developmental disorders.

Only minor, mainly gastrointestinal side effects were observed (Figure 5). These occurred in almost identical ratios in the magnesium and placebo groups.

The number of discontinuations was high both in the magnesium and in placebo groups (Figure 6). In the magnesium group, 64.9% of the subjects continued the treatment until the end of pregnancy and 35.1% discontinued it; the corresponding figures are similar in the placebo group: 56.4 and 46.3%, respectively. Naturally, the ratio of discontinuation was

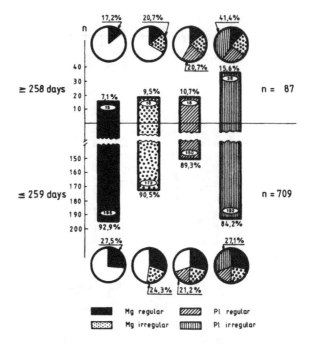

FIGURE 3. Distribution of the cases according to gestational age of birth. Columns indicate the proportions of premature and term deliveries in the treatment groups. Circular diagrams indicate the proportions of the different treatments in the two gestational age categories.

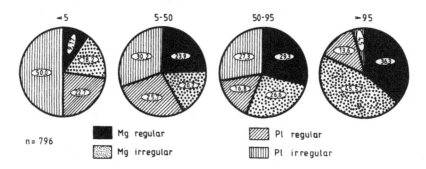

FIGURE 4. Percentage distribution of newborns in the different birthweight percentile categories according to the treatment groups.

### Table 4
### APGAR SCORE (1 MIN) OF THE NEWBORNS

|                     | 0          | 1—5       | 6—7        | 8—10         | Total |
|---------------------|------------|-----------|------------|--------------|-------|
| Magnesium regular   | 2 (0.9%)   | 2 (0.9%)  | 8 (3.8%)   | 198 (94.3%)  | 210   |
| Magnesium irregular | 1 (0.15%)  | 5 (2.6%)  | 10 (5.3%)  | 174 (91.6%)  | 190   |
| Placebo regular     | 1 (0.6%)   | 3 (1.8%)  | 15 (8.9%)  | 149 (88.7%)  | 168   |
| Placebo irregular   | 2 (0.9%)   | 6 (2.6%)  | 15 (6.6%)  | 205 (89.9%)  | 228   |
| Total               | 6 (0.7%)   | 16 (2.1%) | 48 (6.0%)  | 726 (91.1%)  | 796   |

## Table 5
## PERINATAL MORTALITY

| | Antena-tal | Intrapar-tum | Postna-tal | Total |
|---|---|---|---|---|
| Magnesium regular | 2 | 0 | 0 | 2 |
| Magnesium irregular | 1 | 0 | 3 | 4 |
| Placebo regular | 1 | 0 | 0 | 1 |
| Placebo irregular | 2 | 0 | 2 | 4 |
| Total | 6 | 0 | 5 | 11 (1.38%) |

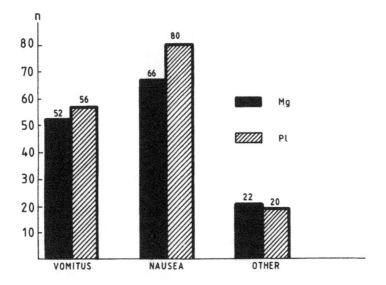

FIGURE 5.   Side effects in the magnesium and placebo treatment groups.

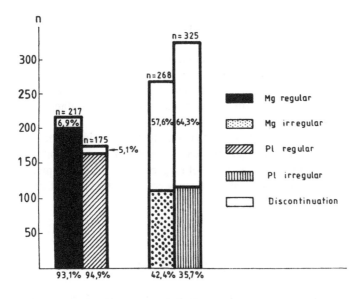

FIGURE 6.   Proportion of discontinuations in the different treatment groups.

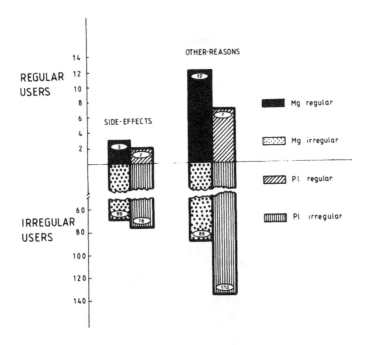

FIGURE 7. Reasons for discontinuations in the different treatment groups.

higher in the irregular groups: most of the subjects were "irregular" because of the discontinuation and consequently the treatment shorter than 15 weeks.

Side effects were the reason for discontinuation in a small proportion of the cases, the major proportion discontinuing for other reasons (Figure 7). Most of them disliked the long-term use of the chewing tablets. This experience suggests that it might be reasonable to test other oral formulations for acceptability, e.g., instant solutions as beverages, because with a more pleasant form of drug administration a better compliance may be achieved.

## V. CONCLUSIONS

In patients receiving magnesium substitution in a daily dose of 15 mmol during pregnancy, the incidence of SFD babies was significantly less than in those patients receiving placebo treatment. Also, in the magnesium-treated group the rate of preterm labor was less, the ratio of low birthweight infants was smaller, and the proportion of infants whose intrauterine growth was retarded was less.

The results seem to lend support to the idea that magnesium supplementation during pregnancy may be justified in antenatal care because of the probability of the frequent occurrence of hypomagnesemia. Addition of magnesium to the diet in pregnancy is a promising treatment for the prevention of intrauterine growth retardation of the fetus.

## REFERENCES

1. **Elliott, J. P.,** Magnesium sulfate as a tocolytic agent, *Am. J. Obstet. Gynecol.,* 147, 277, 1983.
2. **Wilkins, I. A., Goldberg, J. D., Phillips, R. N., Bacal, C. J., and Chervenak, F. A.,** Long-term use of magnesium sulfate as a tocolytic agent, *Obstet. Gynecol.,* Suppl. 67, 38, 1986.
3. **Spätling, L.,** Magnesiumzusatztherapie zur Tokolyse: Klinisch-chemische Überwachungsparameter, *Geburtshilfe Frauenheilkd.,* 44, 19, 1984.

4. **Conradt, A.,** Magnesium sulfate therapy in gestosis (pre-eclampsia), in *Perinatal Care and Gestosis,* Suzuki, M., Ed., Elsevier, Amsterdam, 1985, 55.

5. **Conradt, A., Weidinger, H., and Algayer, H.,** On the role of magnesium in fetal hypotrophy, pregnancy induced hypertension and pre-eclampsia, *Magnesium Bull.,* 6, 68, 1984.

6. **Kuti, V., Balázs, M., Morvay, F., Varenak, Z., Székely, A., and Szücs, M.,** Effect of maternal magnesium supply on spontaneous abortion and premature birth and on intrauterine fetal development: experimental epidemiological study, *Magnesium Bull.,* 3, 73, 1981.

7. **Conradt, A., Weidinger, H., and Algayer, H.,** Reduzierung der Mangelgeburt, sowie der vorzeitigen Amnionruptur und Frühgeburt nach Magnesium-Zusatztherapie bei Betamimetika/Cerclagebehandelten Risiko-Schwangerschaften, *Geburtshilfe Frauenheilkd.* 43, 355, 1983.

8. **Kovács, L., Bódis, L., Szabó, J.,** Magnesium-substitution während der Schwangerschaft "Szegeder Magnesium Studie", in *Magnesium in der Frauenheilkunde,* Weidinger, H., Ed., Münchner Wissenschaftsliche Publikationen, Munich, West Germany, 1985, 110.

9. **Vetter, K. and Spaetling, L.,** Magnesiumsubstitution in der Schwangerschaft. Eine Doppelblindstudie, *Arch. Gynecol.,* 239, 176, 1986.

Chapter 13

# LONG-TERM GLUCOSE INFUSIONS IN THE TREATMENT OF FETAL GROWTH RETARDATION

**V. Šabata and H. Přibylová**

## TABLE OF CONTENTS

## I. FETAL GROWTH RETARDATION

Glucose belongs among the main energy sources of the human fetus.[1] In small-for-date (SFD) fetuses, however, the carbohydrate metabolism is altered. Numerous papers dealing with animal as well as human fetuses bear witness to deviations in their glucose and insulin levels, and in their pancreatic endocrine tissue.

### A. Carbohydrate Metabolism in the SFD Fetus

Lafeber[2] has shown that when growth retardation is caused in the litters of guinea-pigs by means of ligation of the uterine artery, the fetal glucose and insulin levels are decreased. In spontaneously growth-retarded fetuses, hypoglycemia and hypoinsulinemia was even greater (Jones et al.[3]).

In experimentally growth-retarded rat fetuses, hypoglycemia and a decreased content of glycogen in the liver was found (Roux et al.[4]). Also in the amniotic fluid the content of glucose and of insulin was decreased (De Prins et al.[5]). Nitzan and Groffman[6] have shown that the growth-retarded rat litter had considerably lower reserves of glycogen. However, when liver slices were incubatetd in a medium containing labeled glucose, the incorporation of the precursor into glycogen was more than twofold. This suggests that the liver of a growth-retarded rat fetus is enzymatically well equipped for glycogen synthesis, and that the inadequate glucose transport from the mother is the main cause for the poor hepatic glycogen stores.

A series of experimental papers also confirms the importance of glucose for fetal growth. Gruppuso et al.[7] caused chronic hypoglycemia on the 15th to 18th day of the rat pregnancy when administering a constant infusion of insulin. Fetal hypoglycemia, hypoinsulinemia, and growth deceleration took place. The authors conclude that the main cause of the growth deceleration was the limitation of the supply of glucose as a main source of fetal nutrition. This view is also confirmed by other papers. Thus, Oh et al.[8] administered glucose infusions on the last day of pregnancy to rats whose fetuses were SFD due to ligation of uterine artery. The decreased hepatic glycogen content returned to normal level subsequent to the infusion. Dunlop et al.[9] observed a decreased fetal growth in rats who received a dietary supplement of caffeine during pregnancy. If the caffeine was consumed together with sucrose, then growth retardation did not occur. Charlton and Johengen[10] studied pregnant ewes receiving a restricted diet. Intragastric supplementation of aminoacids and of glucose was performed in some of the fetuses. The maternal weight was the same in both groups, but the supplemented fetuses were considerably heavier and exhibited less biochemical evidence of malnutrition.

Similar results and views can be found in papers dealing with human fetuses. Phillips et al.,[11] as well as Garmasheva and Konstantinova,[12] have found hypoglycemia in SFD fetuses. According to Dražančić and Kuvačić[13] the amniotic fluid content of glucose was also decreased.

### B. The Importance of Insulin for Fetal Growth

Picon[15] injected rat fetuses with insulin for 3 d. After the third insulin injection there was a significant increase in fetal weight. Hill[16] found that all fetuses with agenesis of the pancreas had unmeasurable levels of insulin and were severely growth-retarded. Similar results are shown by Sherwood et al.[17] Garmasheva and Konstantinova[12] state that the lack of substrates necessary for the synthesis of new tissues, the stimulator of growth insulin, and of the oxygen necessary for metabolism, represent three basic factors retarding the fetal growth in the course of development. Robinson et al.[18] suppose that the reduction of the supply of nutrients provokes endocrine changes and that these modulate fetal growth. Van Assche and Aerts[14] describe a decreased quantity of endocrine tissue and a smaller number of insulin producing

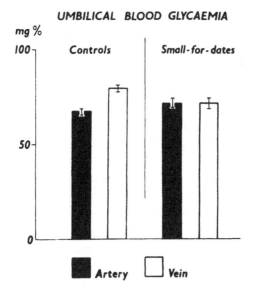

FIGURE 1.   Blood glucose levels in umbilical vessels of healthy and SFD fetuses.

B cells of the Langerhans islets in the pancreas of SFD fetuses. They conclude that insulin is an important growth factor, and that this suggests a new possibility in the treatment of the fetal growth retardation.

To summarize (even with a danger of oversimplification): fetal growth retardation is chiefly connected with an insufficient supply of fetal nutrients and oxygen, and is characterized by hypoglycemia and hypoxia. One consequence is an insufficient stimulation of pancreas and of insulin production. A primary derangement of the development and function of the pancreas, or of target cell receptors, could be also involved. When growth retardation is due to chromosomal and other congenital malformations, the glucose-insulin mechanism is relatively unimportant.

## II. PRELIMINARY STUDIES

### A. Umbilical Cord Blood Values in the SFD Fetuses

Many years ago, when studying carbohydrate and lipid metabolism in human fetuses, the authors found that the values of blood glucose were equal in both umbilical vessels of SFD fetuses. The usual arteriovenous difference which exists under normal conditions was not observed[19] (Figure 1).

A reliable interpretation of these results is rather difficult. Nevertheless, it is probable that the quantity of glucose retained by the SFD fetus is substantially smaller than under normal conditions.

### B. Intrapartal Glucose Infusions

To test whether glucose, administered to the fetus via the mother, could improve the unfavorable metabolic condition of the SFD fetus, we have performed the following studies.

First, we studied the effects of glucose infusions,[20] and glucose with insulin infusions[21] administered during spontaneous deliveries to 20 healthy parturients with healthy fetuses.

Subsequently, 12 parturients with SFD fetuses received a 10% glucose solution at the end of the first stage of labor and during the second stage at an average speed of 1 g glucose per min. The mean duration of infusion was 62 min, the medium weight of the fetuses was 2327 g, and gestational age 39 weeks.[22]

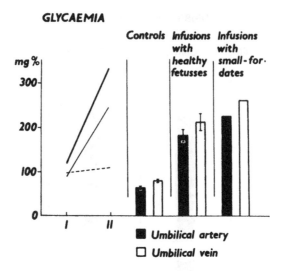

FIGURE 2.   Effect of glucose infusion upon blood glucose levels in the mother and fetus. I: beginning of infusion; II: end of infusion and delivery of the fetus; ($- - -$) levels in uninfluenced parturients; (—) levels in deliveries of healthy fetuses; (■) levels in deliveries of SFD fetuses.

As a control group we used 12 SFD fetuses receiving no prenatal treatment; their average weight was 2177 g and their gestational age 38 weeks.

The increase in blood glucose was practically the same in both groups of parturients with glucose infusions and substantially higher than under normal conditions (Figure 2). Similarly, in the umbilical blood the average glucose level as well as the arteriovenous difference for glucose was, after glucose administration, the same for both the growth-retarded and the healthy fetuses. This shows that, after a glucose load, the response of the maternal organism, the glucose passage across the placental barrier, and the glucose retention by the fetus is equal in healthy and in SFD fetuses. The placenta of the growth-retarded fetus does, consequently, not represent any obstacle to the surplus glucose.

The effect of the infusion upon the metabolism of the newborn in the first few postnatal days was compared with the group of untreated SFD newborns. The blood glucose in the SFD group begins at values significantly higher than in the control group. The value decreases steeply but remains higher than in the untreated group (Figure 3). Free fatty acids are not mobilized to the same extent as in the control group and their level remains low for the first 48 h (Figure 4). It is possible to presume that the surplus glucose provided sufficient carbohydrate to prevent the fetus and newborn from mobilizing its stores of fatty acids. The infusion did not cause a metabolic acidosis of the fetus and newborn. The lactate/pyruvate ratio is actually somewhat lower than in the control group, but the difference is not statistically significant (Figure 5).

These results demonstrate that the SFD fetus and newborn is safely able to retain and metabolize the surplus glucose passing freely through the placental barrier.

What is the practical effect of these results? The favorable influence lasts for a few hours at best, i.e., in the course of labor and for a few days after delivery. An effort to prolong and increase the favorable effect of prenatal glucose administration led us to the next study.

## III. PRENATAL LONG-TERM GLUCOSE INFUSIONS

We started to use long-term glucose infusions many years ago. This has had both advantages and disadvantages. The rather primitive diagnostic and research methods of that time can be considered a sizable disadvantage. Nevertheless, it probably is worth describing the

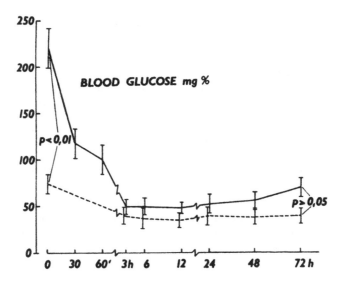

FIGURE 3.   Blood glucose levels in peripheral blood of SFD newborns with (————) and without (− − −) intrapartal glucose infusion.

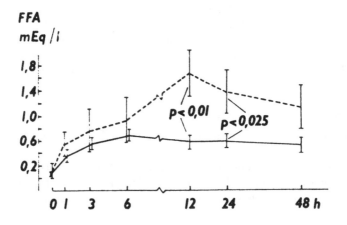

FIGURE 4.   Free fatty acid levels in peripheral blood of SFD newborns with (—) and without (− − −) intrapartal glucose infusion.

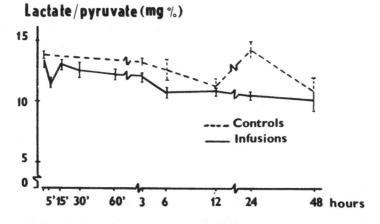

FIGURE 5.   The lactate/pyruvate ratio in peripheral blood of SFD newborns with (—) and without (− − −) intrapartal glucose infusion.

very beginning of our study, if for no other reason than that a 12-year follow-up of the prenatally treated SFD infants might be informative.

## A. Choice of Cases, Methods

Initially, growth retardation was diagnosed by: ultrasound measurement of the biparietal diameter, dehydroepiandrosterone-sulphate test in a modification of Štembera,[23] and some other obsolete tests such as vaginal cytology and step test.

The tests were performed repeatedly, and if the diagnosis of a growth retardation was confirmed, treatment was started. Every day 2 l of a 10% glucose solution were infused intravenously at a speed of 5 ml/min, i.e. 0.5 g glucose per min. This way the infusions lasted for 6 h and 40 min. As a rule, the infusions were performed for 6 d each week. The last day was reserved for repetition of all tests. If the improvement in the course of therapy was very satisfactory, 1 or 2 d in a week were left free without infusions. The total number of infusions varied between 5 and 35, 14.5 on the average. Usually the infusions were performed up to the delivery.

## B. Control Groups

We decided to use as control groups hospitalized women with growth-retarded fetuses who did not receive any glucose infusions.

The first group consisted of 22 pregnant women with growth-retarded fetuses. They were hospitalized for 11 to 114 d (average, 40 d), but did not receive glucose infusions.

The second group involved nine women with SFD fetuses who were hospitalized prior to infusion therapy without receiving any glucose. The hospitalization lasted from 10 to 97 d (average, 47 d). Afterwards glucose infusions were started. In these two groups the urinary estriol levels were assessed.

During hospitalization an insignificant increase in estriol values occurred in both the first group of hospitalized, untreated women, and in the second group before treatment (Figure 6). The increase in estriol levels was significant only after the beginning of prenatal glucose infusions ($t = 2.37$, $p < 0.05$).

The individual pediatric examinations were performed in the course of 12 years. This unusually long spell made it impossible to use a single control group. Therefore, a randomly selected control group of growth-retarded infants of a corresponding age was used for every examination.

## C. Types of Outcome
*1. Pregnancy*

In pregnant women the blood glucose increased in the course of infusions to 150 to 200 mg% (8 to 11 mmol/l). This elevation lasted for approximately 8 h. In sporadic cases a mild, insignificant glycosuria was observed, not influencing the amount of glucose administered. The daily supply of 2 l of liquid did not manifest itself by excessive weight gain or increased blood pressure. Only occasionally was edema seen. The hypertonic solution did not damage the veins. However, usually we used a different vein each day.

The biparietal diameter was measured in the majority of cases several times before the treatment and several times in the course of infusions. The average weekly increase amounted to 0.137 cm (SE 0.02) before treatment, and to 0.225 cm (SE 0.02) in the course of the treatment. This difference is significant ($t = 7.69$, $p < 0.01$). Figure 7 shows several examples of the measurements.

The dehydroepiandrosterone-sulphate test. This assesses the function of the fetoplacental unit. Estriol is measured in six 2-h samples of urine over 12 h. After 4 h, 30 mg of dehydroepiandrosterone-sulphate are administered intravenously. From the resulting estriol levels the value is calculated in points. Values greater than 14 points indicate a healthy

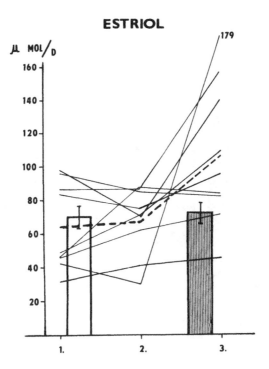

**ESTRIOL**

FIGURE 6. Estriol values in women with a SFD fetus and a long-term hospitalization before the beginning of glucose infusions. 1: beginning of hospitalization; 2: beginning of glucose infusions; 3: shortly before delivery; (− − −) average value. Columns represent estriol values in long-term hospitalized women with a SFD fetus and without glucose infusions.

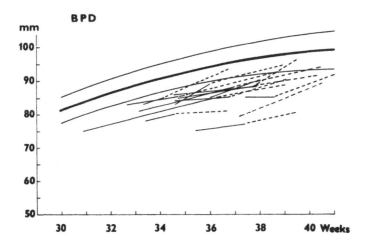

FIGURE 7. Biparietal diameter of the treated SFD fetuses as compared with the average values. (—) Before prenatal therapy, and (− − −) in the course of therapy. (From Šabata, V., *Die Therapie der Intrauterinen Mangelernäh-vung*, Springer-Verlag, Berlin, 1984, 236. With permission.)

fetus. If, however, point values are less than ten, a suspicion of a growth-retarded fetus arises. At the beginning of the pretreatment period, the values in 30 fetuses amounted to 9.6 points (SE 1.26) and decreased shortly before treatment to 6.1 points (SE 0.43). This decrease is significant ($t = 3.04$, $p < 0.01$). In the course of infusions an increase to 12.7 points (SD 0.75) occurred. This elevation is highly significant ($t = 7.69$, $p < 0.01$).

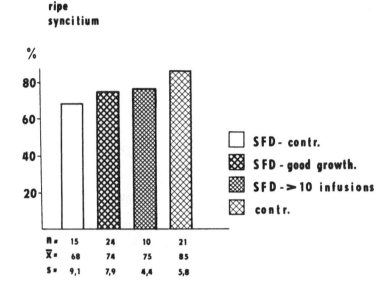

**ripe
syncitium**

FIGURE 8.   The share of ripe syncitium in placentae of SFD fetuses as compared with healthy controls. (From Šabata, V., *Die Therapie der Intrauterinen Mangeler-nährung*, Springer-Verlag, Berlin, 1984, 236. With permission.)

*2. Placenta*

The placentae were studied in cooperation with Leipzig University.[24] The average proportion of ripe, predegenerative, and degenerative syncytium was assessed in enzyme-incubated, toluidine-blue stained semithin sections. In the placenta of healthy fetuses the share of ripe syncytium is significantly greater than in those of SFD fetuses.[25] It is also known that there is a positive correlation between the estriol values, HPL values, and the proportion of ripe syncytium.[26]

Figure 8 shows the effect of long-term glucose infusions. It can be seen that a significant increase in the proportion of ripe syncytium occurred only, when more than ten infusions were administered. The normal values, however, were never attained.

The group of growth-retarded fetuses in whom the glucose infusions caused a considerable acceleration of growth, and who were born with a birthweight >3 kg, exhibit an increased proportion of the ripe syncytium. The values of healthy controls, however, were never attained. Indirectly this can be taken to indicate that these newborns were, indeed, previously growth retarded, and not erroneously treated appropriate for dates (AFD) fetuses.

*3. Newborn*

Due to the growth acceleration, only a few of the treated fetuses were born growth retarded. However, there were also only a few, whose weight was >3000 g. The average weight for the whole group was 2.712 g and all fetuses were born between the 37th and 40th weeks of pregnancy.

Glycogen content of the white subcutaneous adipose tissue was measured in nine prenatally treated SFD newborns, and compared with that of 15 growth-retarded newborns without prenatal treatment, and that of 89 healthy newborns. The subcutaneous adipose tissue from the gluteal region was withdrawn by means of a special needle 16 to 50 h after delivery (27 h on the average).[27] The glycogen content in the wet tissue was assessed by means of diphenylamine.[28] The amount of glycogen was expressed in milligrams of glycogen to 1 g of the wet tissue.

Figure 9 shows that there is practically no difference in the glycogen content of the

## GLYCOGEN RESERVES

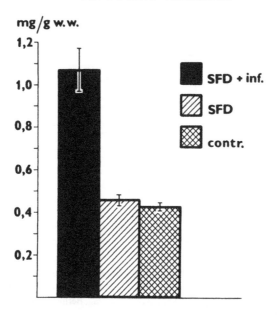

FIGURE 9.  Glycogen content of the white subcutaneous adipose tissue of the treated and untreated SFD newborns, as compared with healthy newborns. (From Šabata, V., *Die Therapie der Intrauterinen Mangelernährung*, Springer-Verlag, Berlin, 1984, 236. With permission.)

subcutaneous adipose tissue between the untreated SFD newborns and the healthy term newborns. However, it is to be taken into account that the total amount of adipose tissue in the SFD newborns is considerably less than in healthy newborns. Consequently, also the absolute content of glycogen is smaller. The prenatal glucose infusions have brought about a significant increase of glycogen reserves.

A glucagon test[29] was performed in the course of the first 12 h of life in nine SFD newborns after prenatal glucose therapy. The results were compared with those from seven untreated SFD fetuses and seven AFD newborns. Glucagon was administered in an amount of 0.3 mg/kg weight. The blood glucose value was measured at the moment of administration, and 5, 15, 30, 60, and 120 min thereafter.

Results are shown in Figure 10. In the SFD newborns without prenatal glucose infusions, the increase of blood glucose is about half of that seen in AFD newborns. In the group of prenatally treated SFD newborns the increase is almost the same as in the AFD newborns. Despite the small number of infants studied, the difference between the treated and untreated SFD infants is significant ($p < 0.02$) 60 min after injection.

These results show that the SFD fetus is able not only to retain, utilize, and store the surplus glucose during intrauterine life, but is also able to use if after delivery.[30] This correlates well with the decreased mobilization of free fatty acids, previously shown in SFD newborns that received a glucose infusion in the course of labor.

### 4. Infant

In cooperation with the pediatric group of our institute, a series of further studies was undertaken upon the infants up to the age of 12 years.

Polygraphic examinations were performed by Paul et al.[31] in three groups of infants: the first one included 11 SFD infants (average birthweight, 2.713 g) who had received prenatal glucose therapy. In the second group were 14 SFD infants without prenatal treatment (average birthweight, 2.440 g). The third group consisted of 22 healthy infants. The average birthweight was 3.411 g.

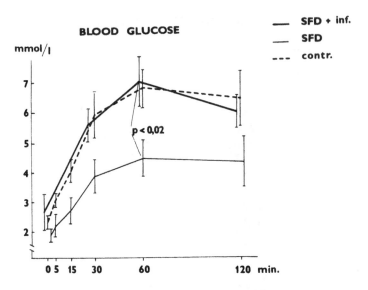

FIGURE 10.    Blood glucose levels in the newborns subsequent to i.v. administration of 0.3 mg Glucagon per kg weight. (From Šabata, V., *Die Therapie der Intrauterinen Mangelernährung*, Springer-Verlag, Berlin, 1984, 236. With permission.)

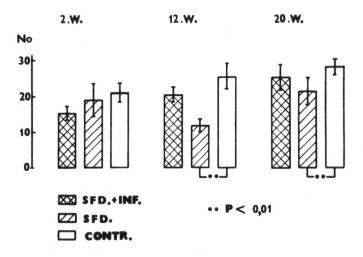

FIGURE 11.    Frequency of rapid eye movements at the age of 2, 12, and 20 weeks. (From Šabata, V., Paul, K., Zezuláková, J., and Dittrichová, J., *Progress in Clinical and Biological Research*, Vol. 163, Alan R. Liss, New York, 1985, 249. With permission.)

The polygraphic examinations were performed in the 2nd, 12th, and 20th weeks, and always lasted 3 h. Two sleep cycles were assessed.

No differences were found between the three groups in the duration and stability of their sleep states.

The frequency of rapid eye movements (REM) represents an important variable of paradoxical sleep. In SFD infants the frequency of REM was significantly decreased, in the 12th and 20th week, when compared with the two other groups. This decrease may express a delay in the development of CNS. In infants who received prenatal glucose infusions the frequency of REM was similar to that observed in control infants (Figure 11).

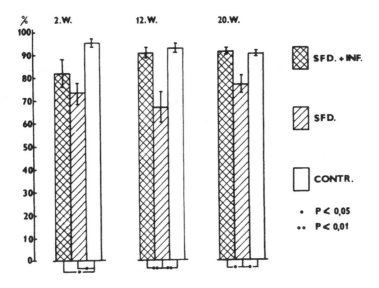

FIGURE 12.  Maturity of electroencephalographic activity at the age of 2, 12, and 20 weeks. (From Šabata, V., Paul, K., Zezuláková, J., and Dittrichová, J., *Progress in Clinical and Biological Research*, Vol. 163, Alan R. Liss, New York, 1985, 249. With permission.)

EEG activity, as shown by Parmelee et al.[32] and Schulte et al.,[33] changes strikingly in the first months after delivery. In the control group of untreated SFD infants, the EEG activity was significantly less mature. In the prenatally treated SFD infants the less mature activity was found only at the age of 2 weeks (Figure 12).

Neurologic development was examined immediately after birth and in the 3rd, 6 to 8th, and 12 to 18th month of life by Zezuláková et al.[34] using the method of Vlach et al.[35] This method involves both developmental and neurologic components.

The study group consists of 10 prenatally treated SFD infants, 76 mature SFD infants, 23 premature SFD infants, and 109 AFD controls.

According to the examination findings, the results were divided into four groups: normal neurologic finding, psychomotor retardation, subtle neurologic deviations, and serious neurologic deviations.

In the group of prenatally treated SFD infants there was no significant difference from the control group of AFD infants (Figure 13). The most favorable results were found at the age of 18 months. At that time, 90% of the treated SFD infants exhibited normal findings. The results were worse in the group of untreated SFD infants and most unfavourable in premature SFD infants.

Psychologic examination. Examinations were performed at the age of 3 years by means of the Terman-Merrill test, fine motor behavior test, and behavior assessment in a strange situation by a modified Kalverboer method.[36] Three groups of infants were studied. The first group consisted of 23 AFD infants, the second of 14 SFD infants without prenatal therapy, and the third of 12 SFD infants receiving prenatal glucose therapy (Dittrichová et al.[37]).

There was no significant difference between the prenatally treated SFD infants and AFD infants. The SFD infants without prenatal glucose therapy had a significantly lower IQ than the other two groups (Figure 14). The Terman-Merrill test gives higher values in our conditions, but this does not influence the differences between the individual groups.

A decreased score in fine motor behavior was found in the group of SFD infants, when compared with both the healthy controls and with the prenatally treated SFD infants (Figure 15). No differences were observed in behavior in a strange situation.

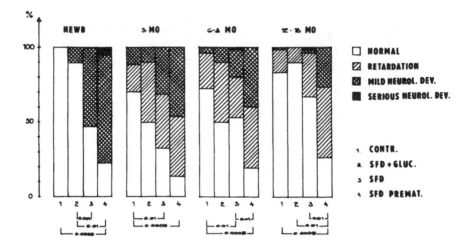

FIGURE 13.   Results of neurologic examinations in the newborns and in infants at the age of 3, 6 to 8, and 12 to 18 months. Beside controls, SFD infants with prenatal glucose infusions, term, and premature SFD infants without prenatal therapy were examined. (From Šabata, V., Paul, K., Zezuláková, J., and Dittrichová, J., *Progress in Clinical and Biological Research*, Vol. 163, Alan R. Liss, New York, 1985, 249. With permission.)

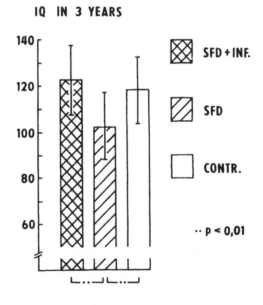

FIGURE 14.   IQ in 3 years. (From Šabata, V., Paul, K., Zezuláková, J., and Dittrichová, J., *Progress in Clinical and Biological Research*, Vol. 163, Alan R. Liss, New York, 1985, 249. With permission.)

Neuropsychic examination was performed in 24 prenatally treated SFD infants and in 29 control SFD infants at the age of 8 to 12 years. Table 1 shows the deviations that were found in the infants studied. Most alarming are the children with minimal brain damage, sensory (eye) defects, and epilepsy confirmed by EEG, who were found among the untreated SFD infants. Other differences were also observed in their fine and gross motor movements and in their attention. The occurrence of acute and chronic diseases and allergies was equal in both groups.

## 5. Clinical Considerations

The relatively long time during which the long-term prenatal glucose infusions were

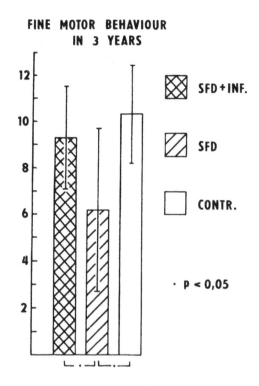

FIGURE 15.   Fine motor behavior in 3 years.

**Table 1**
**RESULTS OF EXAMINATION OF**
**DEVELOPMENTAL HANDICAP IN**
**TREATED AND UNTREATED SFD INFANTS**
**(%) AT THE AGE OF 8 TO 12 YEARS**

|  | Prenatally treated infants | Control infants |
|---|---|---|
| N | 24 | 29 |
| Minimal brain damage | 0 | 13.79 |
| Epilepsy | 0 | 3.45 |
| Febrile seizures | 0 | 6.90 |
| Sensor defects | 0 | 10.34 |
| Fine motor behavior | 12.50 | 20.69 |
| Gross motor behavior | 4.17 | 17.24 |
| Attention deficits | 4.17 | 13.79 |

routinely used in our institute has made it possible to evaluate the effect of the procedure upon the clinical situation.

We have analyzed the frequency of deliveries of SFD fetuses after the 37th week of pregnancy. In the years 1968—1972, i.e., before the introduction of treatment, 2.45% of fetuses delivered after the 37th week were SFD. In the years 1973—1981, only 1.62% of delivered fetuses were SFD. This difference is significant: $t = 4.98$, $p < 0.01$, confirming that prenatal therapy is able to decrease the frequency of deliveries of SFD infants.

The first 60 treated cases were classified into two groups according to the effect of therapy

**Table 2**

**CLINICAL ANALYSIS OF THE RESULTS OF PRENATAL
GLUCOSE ADMINISTRATION IN SFD FETUSES**

| Characteristic | N | % | Therapy | N | % |
|---|---|---|---|---|---|
| Pure FGR | 48 | 80 | Successful | 45 | 75 (94%) |
|  |  |  | Unsuccessful | 3 | 5 (6%) |
| FGR caused by: |  |  |  |  |  |
| Malformations | 9 | 15 |  |  |  |
| Anatomic derangement of | 3 | 5 | Successful | 0 | 0 |
| placenta and umbilical |  |  | Unsuccessful | 12 | 20 |
| cord |  |  |  |  |  |

and the condition of the newborn. In the first group all the SFD fetuses were included in whom growth retardation was the only ascertainable derangement, "pure FGR" (Table 2). There were no perinatal deaths. With the exception of three infants, the effect of glucose infusions can be regarded as favorable. In these three the treatment must be considered unsuccessful because no improvement occurred in the tests. Nevertheless, the fetuses were delivered alive.

The second group includes the infants in whom growth retardation was associated with an anatomical derangement of the fetoplacental unit, predominantly malformations. In this group the treatment did not improve the fetal condition.

## IV. POSSIBLE DANGERS

### A. Hypoxia

A series of papers dealing with nonhypoxic human fetuses has shown that prenatal glucose infusion does not aggravate acidosis.[38-41] Our own earlier studies confirm this.[20,21] Also, in hypoglycemic fetuses, an injection of 50 g of glucose to the mother did not deteriorate the fetal base excess.[42] In hypoxic fetuses, Romney and Gabel[43] found an improvement in the condition of the fetus following glucose administration. Other authors[44-46] did not find any substantial effect upon either the acid-base balance or heart action, but two authors concluded that glucose has a favorable effect upon the fetus.

Consequently, there is little to support the notion of danger from hypoxia in the human fetus, if glucose is administered prenatally. However, in cases of severe intrauterine hypoxia, the fetoplacental circulation may decrease to a third of normal and this substantially worsens the fetal metabolic condition.[47] Secondly if the prenatal glucose load is too great, metabolic acidosis can occur in the human fetus.[48] To discover whether hypoxia or the glucose load we used adversely affected the prenatally treated SFD fetuses, two studies were performed.

The acid-base balance was controlled for the first 24 h of life in 15 SFD newborns after prenatal glucose infusions and in 15 AFD newborns.[49] Table 3 shows that there are no differences in the pH and Base excess values in the two groups. These results, however, relate only to the immediate condition of the newborn. Therefore another study was performed.

Erythropoietic activity in the blood from umbilical vessels of the newborn reflects chronic prenatal hypoxia. Three groups were examined: 11 untreated SFD newborns, 12 SFD newborns whose mothers received long-term prenatal glucose infusions, and 36 healthy newborns. The titre of erythropoietin was measured in mixed umbilical cord blood by means of a biologic titration in polycythaemic mice. Also the reticulocyte count was established. The titre of erythropoietin was expressed as the percentage of $^{59}$Fe incorporation into the erythrocytes.[50]

The titre was significantly greater ($p < 0.01$) in the untreated SFD newborns than in the

## Table 3
### pH AND BASE EXCESS VALUES IN THE UMBILICAL ARTERY AND VEIN
### AND DURING THE FIRST 24 H OF LIFE IN SFD NEWBORNS RECEIVING
### PRENATAL GLUCOSE THERAPY AND IN HEALTHY CONTROL NEWBORNS

|    |           |       | A      | V      | 30 min | 60 min | 3 h    | 6 h    | 12 h   | 24 h   |
|----|-----------|-------|--------|--------|--------|--------|--------|--------|--------|--------|
| pH | Infusions | $\bar{x}$ | 7.28   | 7.35   | 7.29   | 7.34   | 7.37   | 7.38   | 7.38   | 7.40   |
|    | Controls  | $\bar{x}$ | 7.23   | 7.31   | 7.29   | 7.35   | 7.37   | 7.37   | 7.40   | 7.42   |
| BE | Infusions | $\bar{x}$ | −8.02  | −7.19  | −7.27  | −4.86  | −4.57  | −4.26  | −3.0   | −1.8   |
|    | Controls  | $\bar{x}$ | −9.53  | −7.67  | −7.83  | −4.57  | −3.25  | −2.77  | −1.59  | −0.86  |

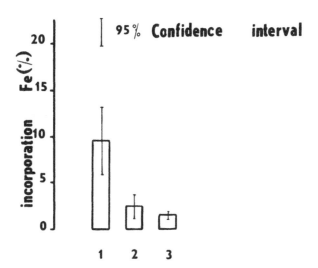

FIGURE 16. Titer of erythropoietine in mixed umbilical cord blood. 1: SFD without prenatal treatment; 2: SFD with prenatal glucose infusions; 3: healthy controls. (From Šabata, V., *Die Therapie der Intrauterinen Mangelernährung*, Springer-Verlag, Berlin, 1984, 236. With permission.)

treated ones (Figure 16) who had practically the same value as the control group. Similar results were found upon analyzing the reticulocyte count. The lower value in the treated SFD newborns can be considered as a sign of compensation of the chronic hypoxia.

These results reveal no adverse effect of the long-term prenatal glucose infusions in the SFD fetus. Nonetheless, the prenatal infusions should not be used in cases with a severe intrauterine hypoxia, and the dose we have used (0.5 g glucose per min) should not be exceeded.

## B. Diabetogenic Effect

According to Freinkel and Metzger,[51] some fetal cells can be considered as terminal structures since they have a limited replicative capability. The brain, fat, and muscle cells, and probably also the B cells of the Langerhans islets belong among them. Their function can be influenced by intrauterine conditions and by nutrients supplied to the fetus via the mother. Consequently, pregnancy provides a unique possibility for nutritional and biochemical engineering. Indeed, no other spell in human development yields a greater potential for promoting long-lasting influences by means of a short metabolic intervention.

Even though there are no other theoretical presumptions of a diabetogenic effect caused by prenatal glucose administration, we felt it necessary to perform in the prenatally treated newborns and infants glucose-tolerance tests.

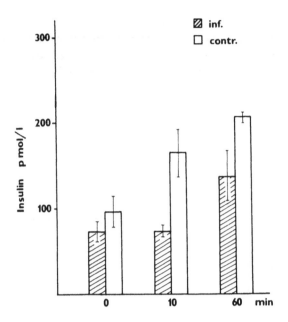

FIGURE 17.    Insulin levels in the course of intravenous glucose-tolerance test in prenatally treated SFD newborns (hatched columns) and in healthy newborns (white columns).

Intravenous glucose-tolerance tests were performed at the age of 6 to 32 h in eight newborns whose mothers received long-term glucose infusions in the course of pregnancy and in ten AFD newbornes (Přibylová and Šabata[52]). A 20% glucose solution was administered into the peripheral vein at a dose of 1 g/kg weight. The administration lasted for 2 to 3 min. Glucose and insulin levels were assessed 10, 20, 30, 40, 50, 60, 90 and 120 min after the injection.

From the glucose values the assimilation coefficient K was calculated. The K values were 1.11 ± 0.09 for the prenatally treated SFD newborns and 1.48 ± 0.11 for the control newborns. A low coefficient can be found in situations when a small quantity of insulin is released. Gentz et al.[53] have found low K values in SFD and premature newborns. In diabetic newborns, on the other hand, the K values are elevated (Thalme and Edström[54]). In an earlier paper (Přibylová et al.[55]) the K values 1.84 ± 0.19 were found for newborns of diabetic mothers.

The insulin levels are increased in newborns of diabetic mothers.[56] However, the levels found in the prenatally treated SFD newborns (Figure 17) were less than in the healthy term newborns.

In summary, the reduced utilization of glucose plus the low insulin levels, indicate the presence of sufficient glycogen stores without hyperplasia of the pancreatic islets. No changes suggesting a diabetogenic influence were found. However, since such an effect could become manifest later on, a test was performed also in the group of oldest infants.

When aged 8 to 12 years, oral glucose-tolerance tests (OGTT) were performed in 24 SFD infants who received prenatal therapy, and in 29 SFD infants without prenatal glucose administration. In order to obtain reliable results, the group of treated infants included only those whose mother received at least eight infusions. A detailed OGTT was used lasting 3 h and assessing five blood glucose values (Přibylová et al.[57]).

In two of the 24 SFD infants receiving prenatal glucose infusions, one value of the test was always in the limits of an impaired glucose tolerance. On repeating the test after 6 weeks in these two infants, the results were normal. In the control group of 29 untreated SFD infants, an impaired glucose tolerance was found in four. On repeating the test after

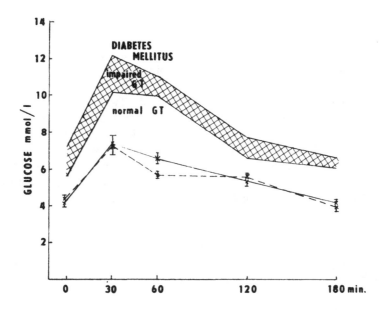

FIGURE 18.   Blood glucose levels in the course of peroral glucose-tolerance tests in prenatally treated SFD infants (—) and in SFD infants without prenatal glucose infusions (− − −). Borderlines of normal glucose tolerance, of impaired glucose tolerance, and of diabetes are shown.

6 weeks, normal values were found in three, and the one remaining child was transferred to the pediatric clinic with suspected diabetes.

The average blood glucose levels of both studied groups were in the normal limits (Figure 18). In the prenatally treated infants, 60 min after glucose administration the glucose level was significantly less than in the untreated SFD infants. This may be interpreted as a better response of the infants' pancreas to a glucose load.

These results do not suggest that prenatal glucose infusions have a diabetogenic effect. However, this type of treatment is not recommended for diabetic pregnant women with a SFD fetus.

## C. EPH Gestosis

It is well known that EPH gestosis is a frequent cause of FGR. When analyzing the cases in this study, in which late gestosis was present, we found that glucose treatment is successful in women without proteinuria. In pregnant women with proteinuria, the treatment continues to have a favorable effect upon the fetus, but the maternal situation deteriorates. In these cases the glucose infusions should therefore be avoided.

## V. PERSPECTIVES

## A. Glucose Infusions

Australian workers have confirmed favorable effect of prenatal glucose or dextrose administration upon the development of the SFD fetus.[58-61] The treatment also received support from other authors.[62-65] It is recommended by Iffy and Kaminetzky,[66] and Moll[67] even feels that glucose is the most appropriate means of prenatal treatment.

Several problems remain, however, to be solved in the future. These include:

1.   Determining the effect of prenatal glucose infusions upon aminoacid levels
2.   A study of the effect of infusions started prior to the 35th week of gestation
3.   To find a possibility to predict the effect of therapy after several days of treatment
4.   To evaluate the treatment in selected cases of imminent premature labor

## B. General Considerations

### 1. Prenatal Therapy — Yes or No?

Van Assche and Robertson edited the proceedings of a symposium held in Leuven in 1980 which focused solely on FGR.[68] In the concluding questionnaire, referring to the latest papers of Beischer et al.,[69,70] it was asked: is there a place for nutrient supplementation after a diagnosis of IUGR? Eight participants answered "yes". Two participants said "yes", but only on special indications (undernourished women). Three participants thought it an interesting idea, but had no personal experience. Six participants answered "no", or had no opinion to offer. Plainly, even a well informed group does not yet hold a unanimous view. However, caution must continue to be exercised because of numerous papers dealing with the unfavorable late sequellae of the adverse intrauterine conditions, e.g., Fitzhardinge and Steven,[71] or Pollak et al.[72] Because of this, treatment does seem advisable in selected patients.

### 2. Prenatal Therapy — When?

After the 33rd week of pregnancy, some obstetricians claim therapy is no longer necessary since it is already possible to terminate the pregnancy. It must not be forgotten, however, that the combination of SFD and prematurity gives the worst results for the infant.

### 3. Prenatal Therapy — Which Method?

The first attempts at some kind of prenatal treatment were made 15 years ago. For the time being any of the successful treatments should be used. At least another 10 years are needed for the decision which of the treatments, or combination of what treatments is most suitable.

# REFERENCES

1. **Šabata, V., Wolf, H., and Lausmann, S.,** The role of free fatty acids, glycerol, ketone bodies and glucose in the energy metabolism of the mother and fetus during delivery, *Biol. Neonate,* 13, 7, 1968.
2. **Lafeber, H. N.,** Experimentelle intrauterine Wachstumsretardierung beim Meerschweinchen, *Ann. Nestlé,* 40, 48, 1982.
3. **Jones, C. T., Lafeber, H. N., Rolph, T. P., and Fellows, F. G.,** The timing of biochemical changes in development and their alteration by the growth rate of the fetus, in *Fetal Medicine,* Salvadori, B. and Merialdi, A., Eds., American Express, Rome, 1981, 86.
4. **Roux, J. F., Tordet, C. C., and Chanez, C.,** Studies of experimental hypotrophy in the rat. I. Chemical composition of the total body and some organs in the rat fetuses, *Biol. Neonate,* 15, 342, 1970.
5. **de Prins, F., van Assche, A., and Milner, D.,** Fetal endocrine factors in intrauterine growth retardation, *Eur. J. Obstet. Gynecol. Reprod. Biol.,* 15, 373, 1983.
6. **Nitzan, M. and Groffman, H.,** Glucose metabolism in experimental intrauterine growth retardation, *Biol. Neonate,* 17, 420, 1971.
7. **Gruppuso, P. A., Migliori, R., Susa, J. B., and Schwartz, B.,** Chronic maternal hyperinsulinaemia and hypoglycaemia. A model for experimental intrauterine growth retardation, *Biol. Neonate,* 40, 113, 1981.
8. **Oh, W., D'Amodio, M. D., Ayp, L. L., and Hohenauer, L.,** Carbohydrate metabolism in experimental intrauterine growth retardation in rats, *Am. J. Obstet. Gynecol.,* 108, 415, 1970.
9. **Dunlop, M., Court, J. M., and Larkins, R. G.,** The effect of maternal carbohydrate (sucrose) supplementation on the growth of offspring of pregnancies with habitual caffeine consumption, *Biol. Neonate,* 40, 196, 1981.
10. **Charlton, V. and Johengen, M.,** Effects of intrauterine nutritional supplementation on fetal growth retardation, *Biol. Neonate,* 48, 125, 1985.
11. **Phillips, L., Lumley, J., Peterson, P., and Wood, C.,** Fetal hypoglycaemia, *Am. J. Obstet. Gynaecol.,* 102, 371, 1968.
12. **Garmasheva, N. L. and Konstantinova, N. N.,** *Pathophysiological Mechanisms of the Protection of Human Intrauterine Development* (in Russian), Medicina, Leningrad, 1985, 157.
13. **Dražančić, A. and Kuvačić, I.,** Amniotic fluid glucose concentration, *Am. J. Obstet. Gynecol.,* 120, 40, 1974.

14. **van Assche, F. A. and Aerts, L.**, The fetal endocrine pancreas, *Contrib. Gynecol. Obstet.*, 5, 44, 1979.
15. **Picon, L.**, Effect of insulin on growth and biochemical composition of the rat fetus, *Endocrinology*, 81, 1419, 1967.
16. **Hill, D. E.**, Fetal endocrine pancreas, *Clin. Obstet. Gynecol.*, 23, 837, 1980.
17. **Sherwood, W. C., Chance, G. W., and Hill, D. E.**, A new syndrome of pancreatic agenesis: the role of insulin and glucagon in somatic and cell growth, *Pediatr. Res.*, 8, 360, 1974.
18. **Robinson, J. S., Falconer, J., and Owens, J. A.**, Intrauterine growth retardation: clinical and experimental, *Acta Paediatr. Scand.*, 319, 135, 1985.
19. **Šabata, V. and Štembera, Z. K.**, Parameters of glucose and lipid metabolism in deliveries of hypotrophic newborns, in *Intra-uterine Dangers to the Fetus*, Horský, J. and Štembera, Z. K., Eds., Excerpta Medica, Amsterdam, 1966, 561.
20. **Šabata, V., Štembera, Z. K., Hodr, J., and Novák, M.**, Die Wirkung von Glukoseinfusionen auf den Lipoid- und Kohlenhydratstoff wechsel der Gebärenden und der Frucht, *Z. Geburtshilfe Gynäekol.*, 162, 253, 1964.
21. **Šabata, V., Štembera, Z. K., Hodr, J., and Novák, M.**, Die Wirkung von Glucose- und Insulininfusionen auf den Lipoid- und Kohlenhydratstoffwechsel der Gebärenden und der Frucht, *Z. Geburtshilfe Gynäekol.*, 164, 152, 1965.
22. **Šabata, V., Znamenáček, K., Přibylová, H., and Melichar, V.**, The effect of glucose in the prenatal treatment of small-for-dates fetuses, *Biol. Neonate*, 22, 78, 1973.
23. **Štembera, Z. K. and Herzmann, J.**, Evaluation of the DHEA-S test as an index of fetoplacental insufficiency, *J. Perinat. Med.*, 1, 192, 1973.
24. **Ruckhäberle, K. E., Šabata, V., Viehweg, B., Scheuner, G., Keller, F., and Gottwald, H. J.**, Characteristics of the trophoblast in placental resorption villi after antepartum glucose infusions: Possibilities for the therapy of chronic placental insufficiency, *J. Perinat. Med.*, 9, 211, 1981.
25. **Ruckhäberle, K. E., Scheunner, C., Franke, J., Viehweg, B., Pickenhain, R., and Gerl, D.**, Quantitative Veränderungen des Zottentrophoblasten bei unter- und normgewichtigen Neugeborenen nach Risikoschwangerschaft und antepartaler Therapie, *Z. Geburtshilfe Perinatol.*, 182, 224, 1978.
26. **Ruckhäberle, K. E., Bilek, K., Scheuner, G., Franke, J., Viehweg, B., Pickenhein, R., Kühndel, K., Schlegel, C., and Rothe, K.**, Beziehungen zwischen HPL-Bestimmung im mütterlichen Serum und Zustand des zugehörigen plazentaren Zottentrophoblasten, *Zentralbl. Gynäekol.*, 100, 1245, 1978.
27. **Novák, M. and Melichar, V.**, Technique for sampling of human adipose tissue, *Physiol. Bohemoslov.*, 12, 84, 1963.
28. **Novák, M. and Monkus, E.**, Metabolism of subcutaneous adipose tissue in the immediate postnatal period of human newborns. I. Developmental changes in lipolysis and glycogen content, *Pediatr. Res.*, 6, 73, 1972.
29. **Melichar, V. and Novák, M.**, Einfluss von Adrenalin und Glucagon auf den Kohlenhydrat- und Fettstoffwechsel bei Neugeborenen, in *Stoffwechsel des Neugeborenen*, Joppich, G. and Wolf, H., Eds., Hippokrates, Stuttgart, 1968, 360.
30. **Melichar, V., Přibylová, H., and Šabata, V.**, Prenatal therapy of fetal growth retardation by long-term glucose infusions. VI. Effect of infusions upon the glycogen reserves of the newborn (in Czech), *Cesk. Gynekol.*, 46, 681, 1981.
31. **Paul, K., Dittrichová, J., and Šabata, V.**, Prenatal therapy of fetal growth retardation by long-term glucose infusions. VIII. The development of sleep polygram of growth-retarded infants in the first months of life (in Czech), *Cesk. Gynekol.*, 47, 730, 1982.
32. **Parmelee, A. H., Schulte, F. J., Akiyama, Y., Wenner, W., Schulz, M., and Stern, E.**, Maturation of EEG activity during sleep in premature infants, *Electroencephalogr. Clin. Neurophysiol.*, 24, 319, 1968.
33. **Schulte, F. J., Hinze, G., and Schrempf, G.**, Maternal toxemia, fetal malnutrition and bioelectric brain activity of the newborn, *Neuropaediatrie*, 2, 439, 1971.
34. **Zezuláková, J., Tautermanová, M., and Šabata, V.**, Prenatal therapy of fetal growth retardation by long-term glucose infusions. IX. Neurologic development of the infants up to the age of 18 months (in Czech), *Cesk. Gynekol.*, 48, 89, 1983.
35. **Vlach, V., Zezuláková, J., and Dolanský, J.**, Neurologic diagnostics, in *High-Risk Pregnancy and Child*, Štembera, Z. K., Poláček, K., and Vlach, V., Eds., Avicenum, Prague, 1979, 250.
36. **Kalverboer, A. P.**, Observation of exploratory behaviour of preschool children alone and in the presence of mother, *Psychiatr. Neurol. Neurochir.*, 74, 47, 1971.
37. **Dittrichová, J., Paul, K., Tautermanová, M., and Šabata, V.**, Prenatal therapy of fetal growth retardation by long-term glucose infusions. X. Neuropsychic development and behaviour of infants at the age of three years (in Czech), *Cesk. Gynekol.*, 48, 327, 1983.
38. **Bossart, H.**, Glucose tolerance tests during labour, in *Perinatal Medicine*, Huntingford, P. J., Hüter, K. A., and Saling, E., Eds., Georg Thieme Verlag, Stuttgart, 1969, 180.
39. **Feige, A., Künzel, W., and Mitzkat, H. J.**, Fetal and maternal blood glucose, insulin and acid base observations following maternal glucose infusion, *J. Perinat. Med.*, 5, 84, 1977.

40. **Gärdmark, S., Gennser, G., Jacobson, K., Rooth, G., and Thorell, J.,** Influence on fetal carbohydrate and fat metabolism and on acid-base balance of glucose administration during labour, *Biol. Neonate,* 26, 129, 1975.

41. **Moretti, M., Zinelli, G., Mansani, F. E., Bevilaqua, G., Ottaviani, A., and Pecorari, D.,** La glicemia del feto e del neonato ed effetti della infusione di glucosio alla madre intra partum, *Monit. Ostet. Ginecol. Endocrinol. Metab.,* 5 (Suppl. 38), 45, 1967.

42. **Phillips, L., Lumley, J., Paterson, P., and Wood, C.,** Fetal hypoglycaemia, *Am. J. Obstet. Gynecol.,* 102, 371, 1968.

43. **Romney, S. L. and Gabel, P. V.,** Maternal glucose loading in the management of fetal distress, *Am. J. Obstet. Gynecol.,* 96, 698, 1966.

44. **Anderson, G. G., Cordero, L., and Hon, E. H.,** Hypertonic glucose infusion during labor. Effect on acid-base status, fetal heart rate and uterine contractions, *Obstet. Gynecol.,* 36, 405, 1970.

45. **Paterson, P., Phillips, L., and Wood, C.,** Relationship between maternal and fetal blood glucose during labor, *Am. J. Obstet. Gynecol.,* 98, 938, 1967.

46. **Zakut, H., Maschiach, S., Plankenstein, J., and Serr, D. M.,** Maternal and fetal response to rapid glucose loading in pregnancy and labor, *Isr. J. Med. Sci.,* 11, 632, 1975.

47. **Štembera, Z. K., Hodr, J., and Janda, J.,** Umbilical blood flow in newborn infants who suffered intrauterine hypoxia, *Am. J. Obstet. Gynecol.,* 101, 546, 1968.

48. **Lawrence, G. F., Brown, V. A., Parsons, R. J., and Cooke, I. D.,** Feto-maternal consequences of high-dose glucose infusion during labour, *Br. J. Obstet. Gynaecol.,* 89, 27, 1982.

49. **Schlegelová, Ch., Šabata, V., and Schulzeová, G.,** Prenatal therapy of fetal growth retardation by long-term glucose infusions. III. Effect of long-term therapy upon the metabolic parameters of the fetus and newborn (in Czech), *Cesk. Gynekol.,* 46, 96, 1981.

50. **Šabata, V.,** Die Therapie der intrauterinen Mangelernährung, *Gynäkologe,* 17, 236, 1984.

51. **Freinkel, N. and Metzger, B. E.,** Pregnancy as a tissue culture experience. The critical implications of maternal metabolism to fetal development, in *Pregnancy Metabolism, Diabetes and the Fetus, Ciba Foundation Symposium 63,* Excerpta Medica, Amsterdam, 1979, 3.

52. **Přibylová, H. and Šabata, V.,** Prenatal treatment of fetal growth retardation by long-term glucose infusions. VII. Glucose-tolerance tests in prenatally treated SFD newborns (in Czech), *Cesk. Gynekol.,* 47, 256, 1982.

53. **Gentz, J., Warrner, R., Persson, B., and Cornblath, M.,** Intravenous glucose tolerance, plasma insulin, free fatty acids and beta-hydroxybutyrate in underweight newborn infants, *Acta Paediatr. Scand.,* 58, 481, 1967.

54. **Thalme, B. and Edström, K.,** Intravenous glucose tolerance test and its relation to a scoring system for the degree of diabetic fetopathy in newborn infants, *J. Perinat. Med.,* 2, 233, 1974.

55. **Přibylová, H., Šternová, H., and Kimlová, I.,** Plasma insulin, carbohydrate and free fatty acid changes in newly born infants of diabetic and non-diabetic mothers after loading with glucose, fructose and galactose, *Physiol. Bohemoslov.,* 28, 113, 1979.

56. **Mølsted-Pedersen, L. and Jørgensen, K. R.,** Aspects of carbohydrate metabolism in newborn infants of diabetic mothers. III. Plasma insulin during intravenous glucose tolerance tests, *Acta Endocrinol., (Copenhagen),* 71, 115, 1972.

57. **Přibylová, H., Šabata, V., Cajthamlová, J., and Chotašová, L.,** The effect of prenatal glucose infusions upon the carbohydrate metabolism of the fetus and infant. II. Glucose-tolerance tests and somatic development of infants after prenatal therapy at the age of 8 to 12 years (in Czech), *Cesk. Gynekol.,* 53, 243, 1988.

58. **Beischer, N. A. and O'Sullivan, E. F.,** The effect of rest and intravenous infusion of hypertonic dextrose on subnormal estriol excretion in pregnancy, *Am. J. Obstet. Gynecol.,* 113, 771, 1972.

59. **Beischer, N. A., Drew, J. N., and Kenny, J. M.,** The effect of rest and intravenous infusion of hypertonic dextrose on subnormal estriol excretion in pregnancy, *Clin. Perinatol.,* 1, 253, 1974.

60. **Abell, D. A. and Beischer, N. A.,** The influence of abnormal glucose tolerance (hyperglycaemia and hypoglycaemia) on pregnancy outcome when estriol excretion in subnormal, *Br. J. Obstet. Gynaecol.,* 82, 936, 1975.

61. **Chang, A., Abell, D., Beischer, N. A., and Wood, C.,** Trial of intravenous therapy in women with low urinary estriol excretion, *Am. J. Obstet. Gynecol.,* 127, 793, 1977.

62. **Murooka, H., Araki, T., and Shigeta, H.,** New trials of treatment for prevention of SFD, Paper presented at the Asia-Oceania Congress of Perinatology, Singapore, November 25 to 28, 1979.

63. **Ruckhäberle, K. E., Petzold, J., Viehweg, B., Ruckhäberle, B., Robel, R., Langanke, D., and Faber, R.,** Therapeutische Bemühungen um präpartale Beeinflussung ausgewählter gestörter fetomaternaler Beziehungen, *Zentralbl. Gynaekol.,* 107, 803, 1985.

64. **Schlegel, L., Weissbach, R., and Beyreiss, K.,** Glukose-infusion bei Verdacht auf chronische Plazentainsuffizienz, *Wiss. Z. Karl Marx Univ. Leipzig, Math. Naturwiss, Reihe,* 25, 137, 1976.

65. **Nikolaev, A. A. and Abramčenko, V. V.,** Application of glucose solution in prevention and treatment of fetal hypoxia (in Russian), *Akush. Ginekol. (Moscow),* 12, 8, 1985.

66. **Iffy, L. and Kaminetzky, H. A.**, *Principles and Practices of Obstetrics and Perinatology*, John Wiley & Sons, New York, 1981.

67. **Moll, W.**, Ist die Therapie mit Glucose, Aminosäuren und Heparin sinnvoll? *Arch. Gynaekol.*, 235, 559, 1983.

68. **van Assche, F. A. and Robertson, V. B., Eds.**, Fetal Growth Retardation, Churchill Livingstone, Edinburgh, 1981.

69. **Beischer, N. A., Abell, D. A., and Drew, J. H.**, Management of fetal growth retardation, *Med. J. Aust.*, 2, 641, 1977.

70. **Beischer, N. A.**, Treatment of fetal growth retardation, *Aust. N. Z. J. Obstet. Gynecol.*, 18, 28, 1978.

71. **Fitzhardinge, P. M. and Steven, E. M.**, The small-for date infant. II. Neurological and intellectual sequellae, *Pediatrics*, 50, 50, 1972.

72. **Pollak, A., Knoll, E., Barsegar, B., Havelec, L., and Uhlig, G.**, Ergebnisse einer Untersuchung von small-for-date Babies. Psychisch-intellektuelle Entwicklung, *Geburtshilfe Perinat.*, 179, 372, 1975.

Chapter 14

# POSTNATAL SEQUELAE OF FETAL GROWTH RETARDATION

## H. Přibylová

## TABLE OF CONTENTS

# I. INTRODUCTION

Antenatal diagnosis of fetal growth retardation is a problem for the obstetrician who must recognize not only the degree of retarded growth, but also, then ensure adequate treatment, and select the correct time and manner of delivery before the onset of intrauterine asphyxia. It has been suggested that fetal malnutrition (lasting through parturition) may significantly alter the potential for postnatal growth, thus accounting for the lack of catch-up growth. It also has been proposed that fetal acute and/or chronic asphyxia, and the stresses that these infants encountered during the neonatal period, may account for their subsequent unfavorable neurologic and developmental outcome.[1,2,3]

Most outcome studies evaluate the small-for-date (SFD) newborn on the basis of birthweight. The most frequently used norms are those published by Lubchenco et al.,[4] Thomson et al.,[5] and Usher and McLean.,[6] which represent the distribution of birthweight between 26 and 43 weeks' gestation. Some alternative definitions have been suggested and used. For example, infants whose birthweight is more than 2 SD below the mean birthweight, or below the third, fifth, or tenth percentiles, respectively, for birthweight at a given gestation.

Since different ethnic groups may vary in both size and body weight, the exact characteristics of the group of infants studied must be formulated, and corresponding charts used. Meredith[7] reported a dispersion of almost 1 Kg above the mean values of body weight at birth in various ethnic groups. Perinatal weight charts have been created by Dunn[8] to serve as an international standard (Chapter 6).

From the pediatrician's viewpoint, growth-retarded fetuses are a high-risk population group, requiring careful follow-up. Their perinatal mortality and morbidity increase, and their long-term prognosis gets worse, as gestational age and weight diminish.

# II. NUTRITIONAL STATUS AT BIRTH

Birthweight for gestational age fails to reflect the nutritional status of many newborns at birth. Some SFD newborns are of normal length but look wasted and, therefore, disproportionally small. Others are proportionally small. Gruenwald[9] introduced the terms "subacute" and "chronic" fetal distress, to describe "disproportionate" and "proportionate" IUGR at birth.

To facilitate the diagnosis of intrauterine malnutrition at birth, it is useful to incorporate body length in the assessment and to calculate Rohrer's Ponderal Index (PI).

$$PI = \frac{\text{weight (g)} \times 100}{(\text{length (cm))}^3}$$

This formula assesses whether an infant is relatively fat or thin.[9,10] Also, it is relatively independent of race, sex, birth rank, and gestational age.

Neonates with a ponderal index below the third percentile tend to be relatively long, rather than symmetrically formed. This group embodies about 50% of all babies born as SFD. Their appearance and their substantially reduced amount of subcutaneous adipose tissue, their dry skin and wizened, old, worried appearance, suggests Clifford's syndrome.[11] The perinatal mortality rate of these disproportionately long newborns is much greater than that of infants of the same birthweight but who are of appropriate length.[12-14]

As a tool for predicting neonatal problems, the PI is equal to, or even surpasses birthweight for gestational age especially in those infants whose birthweight falls below the fifth percentile. Infants with a ponderal index below the third percentile are more frequently affected by asphyxia, hypoglycemia, and hypothermia, and therefore constitute a high-risk group among SFD infants.[11,15,16] In this connection Járai et al.[17] directed attention to the significance of soft tissue wasting, rather than low birthweight itself, in the development of neonatal hypoglycemia. Asymmetrical growth retardation is chiefly a problem in well-nourished mothers.[18] By contrast in undernourished mothers in a South African population, the majority of SFD infants were found to be proportionally grown.[19]

## III. INTRAUTERINE DEVELOPMENT

Many factors determine both normal growth and the accelerated velocity required for eventual catchup growth. During the last trimester of fetal life a rapid growth of brain cells takes place in the forebrain, cerebellum, and brain stem.[20] Thus, general growth retardation, which first becomes manifest in the bodily proportions and individual large organs, may also be expected to affect the brain, not only rapid cell division, but also the developmental organization of the brain cells, including cell migration, differentiation, and myelination.

In growth-retarded babies, Winick and Rosso[21] have observed a decrease in the number of brain cells, and other authors[22] have found a reduced brain weight. These results were obtained from autopsy material in newborns, and a better understanding of these findings may be obtained experimentally using malnourished animals.

The potential for catch-up growth depends on the timing, duration, and severity of growth failure. Catch-up growth does not occur when undernutrition is induced during the brain growth spurt. If it occurs during the subsequent body growth spurt, rapid catch-up growth is possible.[23] Winick[24] has shown in animal studies, and in pathological studies of infants dying in the first 6 months of life, that the critical phase of brain growth takes place before birth, and that all growth involving DNA synthesis and cell division is completed within the first few months of life. He showed that interference with growth during the phase of active cell division usually resulted in permanent stunting, but that similar interference during the later phase of individual cell enlargement resulted in a reversible growth impairment.[25]

Sarma and Rao[26] described a notable reduction in the absolute value of total gangliosides in SFD newborns. The distribution pattern in individual gangliosides indicated a significant reduction in the concentration of trisialogangliosides in the cerebrum and cerebellum, as compared to appropriate-for-date (AFD) infants. These alterations in ganglioside profiles might reflect the functional maturity of the developing brain.[27,28]

## IV. PERINATAL COMPLICATIONS

Several studies have examined the relationship between complications arising in pregnancy and labor, perinatal complications, and developmental outcome. It is often difficult to decide which of the factors are most important in long-term prognosis. SFD infants have a greater incidence of perinatal problems. Perinatal complications occurred more than twice as often in SFD newborns as compared to AFD newborns.[29] Pasamanick et al.[30] reported an association between the course of pregnancy, perinatal complications, and a wide range of intellectual, neurological, behavioral, and medical conditions in children. Similar outcomes were reported by Werner et al.[31]

Barker and Edwards[32] using the Birmingham data on 50,000 children, achieved more precise results when they related verbal reasoning scores, at 11 years of age, to specified pregnancy and perinatal events. They described five obstetric complications which seemed to be associated with impaired developmental outcome. These were a short gestation period, a prolonged gestation period, toxemia of pregnancy, occipito-posterior presentation, and delivery in an ambulance. Neligan et al.[33] noted a possible association with antepartum hemorrhage, breech delivery, and fetal distress in labor.

Temporary hypoglycemia constitutes a separate problem during the neonatal period of SFD infants. Based on the reports of SFD infants who suffered hypoglycemia, and who have been followed for a relatively brief period of time, approximately 33% with symptomatic hypoglycemia, and about 20% with asymptomatic hypoglycemia, have some sequelae in later life.[34] However, in contrast to the relatively poor prognosis for SFD infants who have had hypoglycemia due to reduced glycogen and fat stores, it seems that hypoglycemic infants of diabetic mothers have a relatively good prognosis, independently of the presence of symptoms.[35] The outcome of asymptomatic hypoglycemic infants, as reported by Koivisto et al.[36] indicates that the children who have been followed are doing well. By contrast, 50% of those who were symptomatic had significant central nervous system damage.

Many symptoms have been ascribed to polycythemia and hyperviscosity in SFD infants. A central nervous system manifestation in 72% of polycythemic neonates was described by Gross et al.[37] Of 14 symptomatic polycythemic newborns, 29% had motor and/or mental retardation. In a further study of 78 infants, with neonatal hyperviscosity syndrome, and followed for 1 to 3 years, 30% had gross motor delays, and neurologic abnormalities were present in 25%.[38]

Antenatal fetal monitoring — biochemical testing of fetoplacental function and cardiotocography — has emerged as the most effective means of reducing the number of stillbirths and improving the quality of survival of infants who were born alive. Clinical acumen, combined with biochemical and ultrasonographic testing, will identify about 70% of IUGR fetuses.

With present methods of antenatal diagnosis, treatment, timing the delivery, and intensive postnatal care, the physical and intellectual prognosis of SFD infants is reasonably satisfactory. New follow-up studies have shown that only about 2% of such infants are severely handicapped.[39] In another study, comparing 33 SFD and 33 matched control newborns, the results of neurologic and cognitive testing show that full-term, nonasphyxiated SFD infants have an impaired potential for physical growth. However, their prognosis for neurologic and cognitive development is good.[40]

## V. PHYSICAL DEVELOPMENT

Physical growth and body size are influenced by genetic potential. Also, they are indicators of the effect of the early environment on the developing organism.

At birth the normal infant grows at a rate greater than in any other time of its postnatal life. It appears that a normal child is destined to set its growth curve within the first few years of life, and thereafter is rarely deflected away from this curve. Although the general growth pattern of SFD infants and children is similar to infants with average body weight, i.e., the greatest velocity of growth occurs in the first 6 months, growth retardation has been noted by many authors in all types of longitudinal observations.[16,41-46] By contrast, in 28 preterm SFD infants and 110 AFD infants, whose birthweight was 1195 ± 190 g, Vohr et al.[47] found that the weight, length, and head circumference of the SFD infants attained the tenth percentile by 6 to 8 months, and were similar to the AFD group. Ounsted et al.,[48,49] in studies of growth in both SFD and LFD (large-for-date) babies, from birth up to 4 years, showed that there is a general tendency for somatic measurements at both extremes to revert towards the mean after birth. Thus, SFD children were significantly smaller, and LFD children significantly larger, than AFD children. Also, within each extreme group there was a great diversity in postnatal growth patterns. At 4 years, about half the SFD children were within ± 1 SD of the mean for weight, 59% within 1 SD of the mean of height and 47% within 1 SD of the mean of head circumference. About 10% were still very small for all three measures.

After birth SFD infants grow quickly. Their mean weight loss in the first few days is minimal, and they attain a faster weight gain.[44,47] In the study of Hack et al.,[50] somatic development at the third year of life in 46% of very low birthweight infants remained subnormal. These authors showed that the potential for the catch-up growth in SFD population seemed limited to infancy. Kitchen et al.[51] described some catch-up growth, between 2 and 8 years of age, in both SFD and AFD infants weighing 1 to 1.5 kg at birth. However, in a prospective study of 96 SFD infants, it was shown that the later growth cannot be predicted by the degree of weight retardation, though it does bear a relationship to the rate of growth in the first 6 months.[43]

At the age of 6-12 years one-third of 58 SFD babies who were followed up still had deficits in body weight and height.[52] Rantakallio[53] reported, from a birth cohort of 12,000 children, that at 14 years of age, the mean height of healthy boys, whose birthweight was less than 2 SD below the mean was greater than the 25th percentile. The corresponding height for girls was below the 25th percentile. The preterm children were significantly shorter at the age of 14 than the term infants. This is not, however, necessarily true for the individual final height, because children at 10 to 14 years of age show great variations in height anyway, and this widens the percentile limits.

The sex differences for weight and length may be found by Ounsted et al.:[54] weight gain is greater for boys than for girls, so that by 1 year there is a highly significant difference between the two sexes.

The etiological factors responsible for the differences in height, between children in different weight percentiles at birth, are partly genetic and partly social. The findings of poor catch-up growth, in SFD infants who suffered from early, prolonged, and severe intrauterine growth failure, supports the concept that the timing, duration, and severity of growth failure affects later catch-up growth.[50]

According to Lubchenco,[55] later physical development is frequently similar to primary development. Thus, infants with body weight at the tenth percentiles at birth continue to show similar level of development at the age of 9 to 10 years, i.e., about the tenth percentile. The physical growth outcome in premature SFD infants is dependent on the gestational age at birth. Thus, whereas after 1 year, only 8% AFD infants of very low birthweight (1250 g or less) had a weight under the third percentile,[56] the corresponding figure in SFD infants was 46%.

## VI. PSYCHOMOTOR DEVELOPMENT

The problem of mental development in newborns weighing 2500 g or less has been a matter of concern for many years, but only relatively recently have SFD infants been differentiated within this group.

Many studies point out the relationship between the circumference of the head and the neurological development of the child, and especially, of its intellect.[57-59] Long-term follow-up of these children may detect neurological alterations which appear at various ages. For example, infants whose intrauterine head growth was retarded before 26 weeks' gestation, performed less well at school than those who had normal head growth.[60] Brandt[61] studied the postnatal growth and development of 43 preterm SFD babies, of whom 21 showed catchup growth in head circumference with favorable development, whereas 22, without catchup growth, had less favorable development. Growth differences were not attributable to differences in mean head circumference at birth, nor to genetic influences.

Following studies which centered chiefly upon the measurements of head circumference,[62,63] there appeared a series of prospective works which related psychomotor development to head and general body development. It is now clear that there is a generally increased risk of later disability among infants who show neurological abnormality in the newborn period, especially those with a certain constellation of neurological signs.[58,64-66] However, the prognostic value of various neurological deviations remains variable for each individual. Thus, although a normal neurological finding in a newborn usually offers a good prognosis, an abnormal finding has to be followed up meticulously.[64,67]

The EEG provides a noninvasive method of studying brain development, which may unveil some hidden brain alterations. In an extensive study, comprising the follow-up of 96 term SFD infants, Fitzhardinge and Steven[68] observed that EEG abnormalities were more than twice as common in SFD infants as in the controls. Schulte et al.[69] reported that, in the SFD infant, EEG maturation is retarded.

Anomalies of the duration and stability of the stages of sleep may represent manifestations of altered homeostatic and coordinatory functions of the brain stem.[70] Fitzhardinge et al.[68,71] showed that, aside from the EEG tracing alterations, there was a minimal brain damage in 25% of SFD infants, and speech defects were five times more frequent than in normal children.

It seems that growth and development is less favorable, the earlier that growth failure occurs. It is not only the severity of the insult to the fetus which matters, but also the duration and timing of the insult. Thus maternal complications that occur before the third trimester and continue until pregnancy is terminated probably have the most devastating effect.[72] Children whose head growth slows before 26 weeks' gestation, have significantly lower scores on the general cognitive index, than control children. This does not occur in children whose head growth slows later in gestation. Prolonged slow growth *in utero* affects a child's later development and abilities, in particular, perceptual performance and motor ability.[73]

The duration of gestation is also very important with regard the newborn's further development. There are neurological and developmental differences between full-term and premature SFD infants. A series of studies has shown that the term SFD infants have no major handicap.[70,74-76] For example, Neligan et al.,[33] observed in 333 SFD infants who were followed up for 7 years, that severe damage occurred in only 0.6% but there were IQ alterations, changes in verbal expression, in visuo-motor errors, in activity, and neurological abnormalities.

Studies comprising large groups show that cerebral palsy is not more frequent in term SFD infants than in term AFD ones. However, the former exhibit spastic diplegia more frequently.[58,77,78]

In the course of IQ testing of preschool, and school-age children, certain authors have reported differences. Only Neligan et al.[33] and Hill et al.[79] have demonstrated a statistically significant difference. Westwood et al.[40] reported a lowered IQ, with 0.05 significance, at the ages of 13 to 19 years. Low et al. did not record any IQ differences in five year old children. Similar results in 7-year-olds were observed by Rubin et al.[80]

In term SFD infants most studies have not revealed any major handicap. Term SFD infants tend to follow postnatal development patterns that are associated with their physical characteristics at birth.[81] However, in some of the groups studied a minimal cerebral dysfunction was seen which manifested itself mostly by speech defects and language problems,[68] At school age, problems related to attentiveness appear, so that children may have lower grades in school, even though their IQ is not altered.

Studies in premature SFD infants are difficult to interpret. Smaller groups are being compared and these are heterogenous. It is often impossible to differentiate the effects of prematurity from the neonatal complications due to growth retardation.

In the younger SFD infants most studies show worse results when compared to preterm AFD infants.[47,82,83] IQ differences appear in some studies,[68,84,85] whereas other authors record no significant IQ differences.[47,82,83] Drillien[42] suggests that in the middle socioeconomic classes, the IQ of both preterm SFD and preterm AFD, correspond to 95.8 while in infants born to parents of a low socioeconomic status, the IQ of preterm SFD infants was only 88.5, against that of 95.8 in term SFD infants.

The additional environmental effects of low social class and multiple birth probably further impaired catch-up growth and development in the SFD population.[50,86]

Lower absolute birthweight, shorter gestational age, and smaller head circumference at birth, correlate with poorer outcome.[87]

Certain of the more severe complications in SFD babies, such as hydrocephalus, congenital inborn developmental errors, and many others, may be related to the primary cause of growth retardation, i.e., genetic causes, congenital infections, maternal diseases or ingestions, and placental insufficiency. Other major handicaps, such as retrolental fibroplasia, can result from protracted oxygen therapy in severe primary hypoxia. Artificial ventilation in extremely immature LBW infants contributes to the increase of survivors with later handicaps.[88]

## REFERENCES

1. **Lubchenco, L. O., Delivoria-Papandopoulos, M., and Searls, D.,** Long-term follow-up studies of prematurely born infants. II. Influence of birth weight and gestational age on sequelae, *J. Pediatr.,* 80, 509, 1972.
2. **Allen, M. C.,** Developmental outcome and follow-up of the small for gestational age infant, *Semin. Perinatol.,* 3, 123, 1984.
3. **Taylor, D. S.,** Low birthweight and neurodevelopmental handicap, *Clin. Obstet. Gynaecol.,* 11, 525, 1984.
4. **Lubchenco, L. O., Hansman, C., and Boyd, E.,** Intrauterine growth in length and head circumference as estimated from live births at gestational ages from 26-42 weeks, *Pediatrics,* 37, 403, 1966.
5. **Thomson, A. M., Billewicz, N., and Hytten, F. E.,** The assessment of fetal growth, *J. Obstet. Gynaecol. Br. Commonw.,* 75, 903, 1968.
6. **Usher, R. H. and McLean, F. H.,** Normal fetal growth and the significance of fetal growth retardation, in *Scientific Foundations of Paediatrics,* Davis, J. A. and Dobbing, J., Eds., William Heinemann, London, 1974, chap. 6.
7. **Meredith, H. V.,** Body weight at birth of viable human infants. A worldwide comparative treatise, *Hum. Biol.,* 42, 217, 1970.
8. **Dunn, P.,** A perinatal growth chart for international reference, *Acta Paediatr. Scand. Suppl.,* 319, 180, 1985.
9. **Gruenwald, P.,** Pathology of the deprived fetus and its supply line, in *Size at Birth, Ciba Foundation Symp. 27,* Elliott, K. and Knith, S., Eds., Elsevier, Amsterdam, 1974, 3.
10. **Battaglia, F. C. and Lubchenco, L. O.,** A practical classification of newborn infants by weight and gestational age, *J. Pediatr.,* 71, 159, 1967.
11. **Clifford, S.,** Postmaturity with placental dysfunction, Clinikal syndrome and pathologic findings, *J. Pediatr.,* 41, 1, 1954.
12. **Walther, F. J. and Remaekers, L. H. J.,** Neonatal morbidity of SGA infants in relation to their nutritional status at birth, *Acta Paediatr. Scand.,* 71, 437, 1982.
13. **Ounsted, M. and Ounsted, C.,** On fetal growth rate: its variations and their consequences, in *Clinics in Developmental Medicine No. 46, Spastic International Medical Publications,* Heinemann, London, 1973.
14. **Walther, J. F. and Ramaekers, L. J. H.,** The ponderal index as a measure of the nutritional status at birth and its relation to some aspects of neonatal morbidity, *J. Perinat. Med.,* 10, 42, 1982.
15. **Miller, H. C. and Hassanein, K.,** Diagnosis of impaired fetal growth in newborn infants, *Pediatrics,* 48, 511, 1971.
16. **Litschgi, M., Beuz, J. J., and Glatthaar, E.,** Aktuelle und prognostische Bedeutung des arteriellen Nabelschnur-p-H für die postpartale Zustandsdiagnostik, *Z. Geburtshilfe Perinatol.,* 178, 23, 1974.
17. **Járai, I., Mestyán, J., Schultz, K., Lazar, A., Halász, M., and Kraussy, I.,** Body size and neonatal hypoglycemia in intrauterine growth retardation, *Early Hum. Dev.,* 1, 25, 1977.
18. **Davies, D. P., Platts, P., Pritchard, J. M., and Wilkinson, P. W.,** Nutritional status of light-for-date infants at birth and its influence on early postnatal growth, *Arch. Dis. Child.,* 54, 703, 1979.
19. **Woods, D. L., Malan, A. F., and deVheese, H.,** Patterns of retarded fetal growth, *Early Hum. Dev.,* 3, 257, 1973.
20. **Dobbing, J. and Sands, J.,** Quantitative growth and development of human brain, *Arch. Dis. Child.,* 48, 757, 1973.
21. **Winick, M. and Rosso, P.,** The effect of severe early malnutrition on cellular growth of human brain, *Pediatr. Res.,* 3, 181, 1969.

22. **Larroche, J. C. and Korn, G.**, Brain damage in intrauterine growth retardation, in *Intrauterine Asphyxia and the Developing Fetal Brain*, Gluck, L., Ed., Year Book Medical Publishers, Chicago, 1977, 25.

23. **McCance, R. A. and Widdowson, E. M.**, Nutrition and growth, *Proc. R. Soc. London Ser. B*, 156, 326, 1962.

24. **Winick, M.**, Changes in nucleic acid and protein content of the human brain during growth, *Pediatr. Res.*, 2, 352, 1968.

25. **Winick, M.**, Cellular growth of the human placenta. III. Intrauterine growth failure, *J. Pediatr.*, 71, 390, 1967.

26. **Sarma, M. K. J. and Rao, P. S.**, Gangliosides in different regions of brains of small-for-dates infants, *Indian J. Med. Res.*, 75/6, 816, 1982.

27. **Wagen, A., Okken, A., Zweens, J., and Zijlstra, W. G.**, Composition of postnatal weight loss and subsequent weight gain in small-for-dates newborn infants, *Acta Paediatr. Scand.*, 74, 57, 1985.

28. **Brinkman, G. L., Bowie, M. D., Friis-Hansen, B., and Hansen, J. D. L.**, Body water composition before and after loss of edema, *Pediatrics*, 36, 94, 1965.

29. **Ounsted, M., Moar, V., and Scott, W. A.**, Perinatal morbidity and mortality in small-for-dates babies: The relative importance of some maternal factors, *Early Hum. Dev.*, 5, 367, 1981.

30. **Pasamanick, B., Knobloch, H., and Lilienfeld, A. M.**, Socioeconomic status and some precursors of neuropsychiatric disorder., *Am. J. Orthopsychiatry*, 26, 594, 1956.

31. **Werner, E., Simonian, K., Bierman, J. M., and French, F. E.**, Cumulative effect of perinatal complications and deprived environmental on physical, intellectual and social development of pre-school children, *Pediatrics*, 39, 490, 1967.

32. **Barker, D. J. P. and Edwards, J. H.**, Obstetric complications and school performance, *Br. Med. J.*, 3, 695, 1967.

33. **Neligan, G. A., Kolvin, I., Scott, D., and Garside, R. F.**, Born too soon or born too small. A follow-up study to seven years of age, in *Spastic International Medical Publications*, Lippincott, Philadelphia, 1967, 66.

34. **Beard, A., Cornblath, M., Gentz, J., Kellum, M., Persson, B., Zetterström, R., and Haworth, J. C.**, Neonatal hypoglycemia: a discussion, *J. Pediatr.*, 79, 314, 1971.

35. **Přibylová, H.**, The infant of diabetic mother (in Czech.), Avicenum, Prague, 1982, 46.

36. **Koivisto, M. M., Blanco-Sequeiros, M., and Krause, U.**, Neonatal symptomatic and asymptomatic hypoglycemia: a follow-up study of 151 children, *Dev. Med. Child Neurol.*, 14, 603, 1972.

37. **Gross, G. P., Hathaway, W. E., and McGaughey, H. R.**, Hyperviscosity in the neonate, *J. Pediatr.*, 82, 1004, 1973.

38. **Black, V. D., Lubchenco, L. O., Luckey, D. W. et al.**, Developmental and neurologic sequelae of neonatal hyperviscosity syndrome, *Pediatrics*, 69, 426, 1982.

39. **Beisher, N. A., Abel, D. A., and Drew, J. H.**, Intrauterine growth retardation, *Aust. N. Z. J. Obstet. Gynaekol.*, 23, 191, 1983.

40. **Westwood, M., Kramer, M. S., Munz, D. et al.**, Growth and development of full-term nonasphyxiated small-for-gestational-age newborns: follow-up through adolescence, *Pediatrics*, 71, 376, 1983.

41. **Sinclair, J. C. and Coldiron, J. S.**, Low birth weight and postnatal physical development, *Dev. Med. Child Neurol.*, 11, 314, 1969.

42. **Drillien, C. M.**, The small for date infant: etiology and prognosis, *Pediatr. Clin. North. Am.*, 17, 9, 1970.

43. **Fitzhardinge, P. M. and Steven, E. M.**, The small-for-date infant. I. Later growth patterns, *Pediatrics*, 49, 671, 1972.

44. **Lubchenco, L. O.**, The high risk infant, in *Major Problems in Clinical Pediatrics*, Vol. 14, W. B. Saunders, Philadelphia, 1976.

45. **Poláček, K. and Syrovátka, G.**, Wachstums der Kinder mit niedrigen Geburts-gewicht im Alter von 10 jahren, *Monatsschr. Kinderheilkd.*, 124, 151, 1976.

46. **Szotowa, W.**, *Growth and Nutrition of Small-for-Date Infants*, Polish Medical Publications, Warsaw, 1977, 143.

47. **Vohr, B. R., Oh, W., Rosenfiels, A. G., and Cowett, R. M.**, The preterm small-for-gestational age infant: a two-year follow-up study, *Am. J. Obstet. Gynecol.*, 133, 425, 1979.

48. **Ounsted, M., Moar, V., and Scott, A.**, Growth in the first four years. II. Diversity within groups of small-for-dates and large-for-dates babies, *Early Hum. Dev.*, 7, 29, 1982.

49. **Ounsted, M., Moar, V., and Scott, A.**, Growth in the first four years. III. The effects of maternal factors associated with small-for-dates and large-for-dates pregnancies, *Early Hum. Dev.*, 7, 347, 1982.

50. **Hack, M., Merkatz, I. R., McGarth, S. K., Jones, P. K., and Fanaroff, A. A.**, Catch-up growth in very-low-birth-weight infants, *Am. J. Dis. Child.*, 138, 370, 1984.

51. **Kitchen, W. H., McDougall, A. B., and Naylor, F. D.**, A longitudinal study of very low-birthweight infants. III. Distance growth at 8 years of age, *Dev. Med. Child Neurol.*, 22, 163, 1980.

52. **Schlauseil-Zipf, U., Hamm, W., Mandl-Kramer, S., Glatke, E., and Bolte, A.,** Nachuntersuchungsergebnisse ehemaliger prenatal dystropher Neugeborener im Alter von 6-12 Jahren, *Monatsschr. Kinderheilkd.,* 133, 93, 1985.

53. **Rantakallio, P.,** A 14-year follow-up of children with normal and abnormal birth weight for their gestational age. A population study, *Acta Paediatr. Scand.,* 74, 62, 1985.

54. **Ounsted, M., Moar, V., and Soctt, A.,** Growth in the first year of life: Effects of sex and weight for gestational age at birth, *Dev. Med. Child Neurol.,* 24, 356, 1982.

55. **Lubchenco, L. O.,** Assessment of gestational age and development at birth, *Pediatr. Clin. North Am.,* 17, 125, 1970.

56. **Kumar, S. P., Anday, E. K., Sacks, L. M., Ting, R. Y., and Delivoria-Papandopoulos, M.,** Follow-up studies of very low birth weight infants (1,250 grams or less) born and treated within a perinatal center, *Pediatrics,* 66, 438, 1980.

57. **Davies, H. and Kirman, S. W.,** Microcephaly, *Arch. Dis. Child.,* 37, 623, 1962.

58. **Nelson, K. B. and Ellenberg, J. H.,** Neonatal signs as a predictor of cerebral palsy, *Pediatrics,* 64, 225, 1979.

59. **Allen, N.,** Developmental and degenerating diseases of the brain, in *Pediatric Neurology,* Farmer, T. W., Ed., Harper & Row, New York, 1964, 176.

60. **Parkinson, C. E., Walis, S. H., and Harvey, D.,** School achievement and behaviour of children who were small-for-dates at birth, *Dev. Med. Child Neurol.,* 23, 41, 1981.

61. **Brandt, I.,** Growth dynamics of low birthweight infants with emphasis on the perinatal period, in *Human Growth,* Vol. 2, Falkner, F. and Tanner, J. M., Eds., Plenum Press, London, 1978, 557.

62. **Weinberg, W. A., Dietz, S. G., Penick, E. C., and McAlister, W. H.,** Intelligence, reading, achievement, physical size and social class, *J. Pediatr.,* 85, 482, 1974.

63. **Ounsted, M., Moar, V. A., and Scott, A.,** Children of deviant birth weight at the age of seven years: health, handicap, size and developmental status, *Early Hum. Dev.,* 9, 323, 1984.

64. **Prechtl, H. F. R.,** The neurological examination of the full-term newborn infant, in *Clinics in Developmental Medicine No. 63,* 2nd ed., William Heinemann, London, 1977.

65. **Volpe, J. J.,** Value of the neonatal neurologic examination, *Pediatrics,* 64, 547, 1979.

66. **Illsley, R. and Mitchell, R. C.,** Low birth weight. A medical, psychological and social study, John Wiley & Sons, Chichester, 1984.

67. **Dennis, J.,** Neonatal convulsions: aetiology, late neonatal status and long-term outcome, *Dev. Med. Child Neurol.,* 20, 143, 1978.

68. **Fitzhardinge, P. M. and Steven, E. M.,** The small for date infant. II. Neurological and intellectual sequelae, *Pediatrics,* 50, 50, 1972.

69. **Shulte, F. L., Schempf, G., and Hinze, G.,** Maternal toxemia, fetal malnutrition, and motor behavior of the newborn, *Pediatrics,* 48, 871, 1971.

70. **Prechtl, H. F. R., Theorel, K., and Blair, A. W.,** Behavioural state cycles in abnormal infants, *Dev. Med. Child Neurol.,* 15, 606, 1973.

71. **Fitzhardinge, P. M., Kalman, E., Ashby, S., and Pape, K.,** Present status of the infant of very low birth weight treated in a referral neonatal intensive care unit in 1974, in *Major Mental Handicap: Methods and Costs of Prevention,* Elsevier/North-Holland, Amsterdam, 1978, 139.

72. **Beargie, R. A., Vernon, L. J., and Greene, J. W.,** Growth and development of small-for-date newborns, *Pediatr. Clin. North Am.,* 17, 159, 1970.

73. **Harvey, D., Prince, J., Bunton, J. et al.,** Abilities of children who were small-for-gestational-age babies, *Pediatrics,* 69, 296, 1982.

74. **Babson, S. G. and Henderson, N. B.,** Fetal undergrowth: relation of head growth to later intellectual performance, *Pediatrics,* 53, 890, 1974.

75. **Walther, F. J. and Ramaekers, L. H. J.,** Developmental aspects of subacute fetal distress: behaviour problems and neurological dysfunction, *Early Hum. Dev.,* 6, 1, 1982.

76. **Low, J. A., Galbraith, R. S., Muir, D. et al.,** Intrauterine growth retardation: A study of long-term morbidity, *Am. J. Obstet. Gynecol.,* 142, 670, 1982.

77. **Nelson, K. B. and Deutschberger, J.,** Head size at one year as a predictor of four year IQ, *Dev. Med. Child Neurol.,* 12, 487, 1970.

78. **Nelson, K. and Broman, S.,** Perinatal risk factors in children with serious motor and mental handicaps, *Ann. Neurol.,* 2, 374, 1977.

79. **Hill, R. M., Verdinaud, W. M., Deter, R. L. et al.,** The effect of intrauterine malnutrition on the term infant. A 14-year progressive study, *Acta Paediatr. Scand.,* 73, 482, 1984.

80. **Rubin, R. A., Rosenblatt, C., and Balow, B.,** Psychological and educational sequelae of prematurity, *Pediatrics,* 52, 352, 1973.

81. **Villar, J., Smeriglio, V., Martorell, R. et al.,** Heterogenous growth and mental development of intrauterine growth-retarded infants during first 3 years of life, *Pediatrics,* 74, 783, 1984.

82. **Eaves, L. C., Nuttal, J. C., Klonoff, H. et al.,** Development and psychological test scores in children of low birth weight, *Pediatrics,* 45, 9, 1970.

83. **Calame, A., Ducret, S., Jaunin, L., and Plancherel, B.,** High risk appropriate for gestational age (AGA) and small for gestational age (SGA) preterm infants. Neurological handicap and developmental abnormalities at five years of age, *Helv. Paediatr. Acta,* 38, 39, 1983.

84. **Commey, J. O. and Fitzhardinge, P. M.,** Handicap in the preterm small-for-gestational age infants, *J. Pediatr.,* 94, 779, 1979.

85. **Silva, P. A., McGee, R., and Williamd, S.,** A seven year follow-up study of the cognitive development of children who experienced common perinatal problems, *Aust. Paediatr. J.,* 20, 23, 1984.

86. **Patterson, R. M., Gibbs, C. E., and Wood, R. C.,** Birth weight percentile and perinatal outcome: recurrence of intrauterine growth retardation, *Obstet. Gynecol.,* 68, 464, 1986.

87. **Lipper, E., Lee, K., Gartner, L. M., and Grellong, B.,** Determinants of neurobehavior outcome in low-birth-weights infants, *Pediatrics,* 67, 502, 1981.

88. **DeLeew, R. and Wolf, H.,** Follow-up of extremely immature infants, in *10th European Congr. Perinatal Medicine,* Leipzig, August 12 to 16, 1986, Jährig, K., Ed., Halle, 1986, 267.

# INDEX

Printed and bound by CPI Group (UK) Ltd, Croydon, CR0 4YY

23/10/2024

01778245-0006